THE STORY OF MEDICINE

THE STORY OF
MEDICINE

VICTOR ROBINSON, M.D.

PROFESSOR OF HISTORY OF MEDICINE
TEMPLE UNIVERSITY SCHOOL OF MEDICINE
PHILADELPHIA

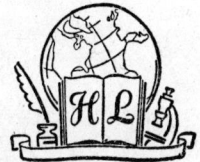

THE NEW HOME LIBRARY
NEW YORK

The New Home Library Edition Published August, 1943

COPYRIGHT, 1931, BY ALBERT & CHARLES BONI
COPYRIGHT, 1943, BY FROBEN PRESS

The New Home Library, 14 West Forty-ninth Street
New York, N. Y.

CL

PRINTED IN THE UNITED STATES OF AMERICA

To
Sir Ronald Ross

Sanitation is not a modern science. The aqueducts built by Agrippa, the writings of the architect Vitruvius on hygiene and plumbing, and the works of Frontius on the water-supply of Rome, testify to the competence of the sanitary engineers of the Caesars. But sophisticated Rome once laughed in the wrong place: the wittiest of Romans, Horace and Juvenal, mocked the mosquito-net—and the mosquito that strikes by twilight, chanted its triumphant hymn amid the ruins of man's greatest empire. It is remarkable how frequently that laughter has echoed down the ages. In the city of Washington, in the latter years of the nineteenth century, it greeted Albert Freeman Africanus King, when he suggested a wire-woven screen to keep out mosquitoes. Advocating the ideas of John Crawford of Maryland, Josiah Clark Nott of Alabama, and Carlos Juan Finlay of Cuba, King advanced nineteen compelling reasons for his belief in the mosquital origin of certain diseases. These men were guessing: they guessed right, but they had little evidence to offer. They received no more credence among the Americans than had Varro among the Ancients.

Sanitarians have realized that the malaria-fighter "must learn to think like a mosquito and act like a larva." The most effective of all mosquito-hunters, the man who emerged from the swamps with the truth beneath the cracked eye-piece of his microscope, is Ronald Ross. Obstructed by officials, sick from heat and work and worry, his painful eyes finally looked at the cause of malaria. Mosquito Day—August 20, 1897—must be regarded as the birthday of a new era in public health. The spirit of Ross sent Walter Reed on his Cuban adventure, from which he returned with proof that in the bite of the mosquito lies the mystery of yellow fever. The work of Ross was the inspiration of Gorgas in the uncertain years on the fatal Isthmus. After ships began to sail through the interoceanic waterway, Gorgas never hesitated to state that the preventive discovery of Ross enabled the building of the Panama Canal.

In this Machine Age, swollen with endless wealth, one of the greatest benefactors in human history is passing his wintry years in poverty. Sir Ronald Ross, Nobel prizeman in medicine a generation ago, scientist, poet, painter, novelist, musician and mathematician, amid his astonishing versatility lacks the money-making gift. He who saved the tropical world, and created untold fortunes for others, has not known how to line his own pocketbook. Had he devoted himself to ledgers instead of laboratory notebooks, had he camped on fashionable Harley Street instead of the sun-scorched rocks of Secunderabad, he might be enjoying a comfortable income today. However, he is certain to receive monuments after his death, and thus he will carry on an ancient tradition.

The author is gratified that Ronald Ross, one of the most romantic and important figures in the history of public health, has accepted the dedication of this Story of Medicine.

CONTENTS

CHAPTER	PAGE
I. MEDICINE IN THE STONE AGE	1
II. MEDICINE IN ANCIENT EGYPT	11
III. MEDICINE IN ANCIENT GREECE	28
IV. GREEK MEDICINE IN ALEXANDRIA	61
V. GREEK MEDICINE IN ROME	83
VI. ARABIAN MEDICINE IN THE MIDDLE AGES	134
VII. EUROPEAN MEDICINE IN THE MIDDLE AGES	193
VIII. MEDICINE IN THE RENAISSANCE	238
IX. MEDICINE IN THE SEVENTEENTH CENTURY	280
X. MEDICINE IN THE EIGHTEENTH CENTURY	327
XI. MODERNIZATION OF MEDICINE	371
XII. MEDICINE IN AMERICA	443
XIII. SOCIOLOGY IN AMERICA	486
BIBLIOGRAPHICAL NOTES	521
INDEX OF INDIVIDUALS AND SUBJECTS	543

THE STORY OF MEDICINE

THE STORY OF MEDICINE

I

MEDICINE IN THE STONE AGE

THE first cry of pain through the primitive jungle was the first call for a physician.

Early man moistened his bruises with saliva, he extracted the thorns which lodged in his flesh, he used a pointed stick to dig sandfleas from his skin, he put leaves or mud or clay on his wounds, he tasted herbs and some he spat out and some he swallowed, he was rubbed or stroked when in pain, his broken bones were splinted with branches, and when bitten by a venomous animal he sucked the poison from his body or his fellows did it for him. Medicine is a natural art, conceived in sympathy and born of necessity; from these instinctive procedures developed the specialized science that is practised today.

Earth is her own historian, and in every age writes her story in forests and deserts, on rocks and in river-beds. Ancient man knew nothing of this language, and modern man understands only fragments of its alphabet. From time to time we discover a fossil that has kept its secret for a million years, but nearly all of nature's infancy is veiled from human eyes. Of the life of ape-man we know little, and it is not until our progenitors are well within the Stone Age that we are able to follow their vanishing footsteps.

What sort of creature was man in his eolithic, paleolithic and neolithic condition? To what extent are we interested in this low-browed, heavy-jawed, hairy-chested ancestor? How important culturally is this cave-man who killed his food with stone-hammer and flint weapons, who raped his women and did not know his own children? He is the origin of archeology and anthropology: every scratch he made on a cavern-wall is discussed by the learned moderns of all nations, every finding of one of his broken bones excites international scholarship. Beneath stalagmite floors, in river-gravel and in glacial mud lie centuries of our racial history, and the most valuable historians of today are the cave-hunters who reveal the past with pick-axe and spade.

Primitive man, wondering and blundering, passed his days in fear and bewilderment. The rains fell on his naked body, the winds swept over him, and while he watched the cloud-covered stars the angry lightning jumped at him. Gliding up from the ground, springing down from the trees, wild beasts attacked him. But his lusts and appetites were strong, and he forgot his troubles when he summoned his clan to a meat-kill, or captured a woman from another tribe: man is the only animal that makes love in all the seasons, and then he felt the joy of life within him. It was good to leap and swim, to eat and mate, to shout and fight.

Health and strength were desirable above all things, but primitive man had enemies who took these gifts from him. What were these sudden pains? What were these spasmodic seizures? Why did he faint and fall? What was gnawing at his vitals? What was hammering within his head? What suffocated him so he could not breathe? Why did he awake at night sweating and screaming? What were those cramps, stronger and tighter? What was growing on his flesh that pricked and burned? What was swelling up within him? What held him, so he could no longer hunt the bison? What blinded him, so he could no longer see the mammoth that passed before his very eyes? Why had he become as helpless as a wounded goose?

Aboriginal man could not grasp the conception of natural death. Disturbance or stoppage of physical life was due to supernatural causes—to the wrath of the dead, the uncanny powers of human enemies, the revenge of offended spirits. Terrifying as were the crocodile and hyena, he could see them and understand them and cope with them, but against witchcraft he had no weapon. Disease-demons were more numerous than the leaves of the forest, and they pursued him every moment of the day and night. He could escape the long serpent that awaited him, but not the ghosts and their magic. Though he climbed the tallest trees or dived in the deepest water, though he hid in the darkest caves or ran till he could run no more, the ghosts never left him—they were in the food he ate, in the water he drank, in the air he breathed. He must be infinitely careful, for without intention he might arouse the wrath of the swarming disease-demons. It was too much for him, he could not fight the ghosts alone, he must have protection. He realized his most important duty was to guard himself against witchcraft, to oppose the magic of his enemies with the superior magic of his friends. Out of primitive man's need, thus arose the first professional class—antedating even prostitution and older than any religion—the profession of the magician or mystery-man, the Medicine-Man.

It is characteristic of the primitive mind that it does not change, but remains stationary. There are various primitive races today who know neither metals nor agriculture nor pottery nor domesticated animals—races truly living in their Stone Age, and they enable us to study the origin of the medicine-man.

The medicine-man was chosen on account of some peculiarity: unusual strength or wisdom, or because of his deformities or epileptic fits, or because he went into a trance, or was bitten by a rattlesnake without being poisoned, or because the elders dreamed of him, or because he was not skilful with weapons of war, or because he was a ventriloquist, or because it was observed that he was addicted to solitary wanderings and musings in the forest. At times a youth with natural aptitude or inclination for the art, preferring healing to hunting, would enroll himself as a pupil of a medicine-man renowned for his cures; the course of study was long, arduous and expensive. There were many herbs, many tricks, infinite details of ritual, and a precise bedside manner to be learned. The medicine-man could not be as other men, he must be a man apart. His dress, his food, his habits, his thoughts, must be different. He must not be seen in the routine life of his fellows—he must ever remain the man of mystery. As the ceremonies grew more complicated and sacred with tradition, the medicine-man became the prophet and priest of his people. He knew how to impress his audience with ostentatious fasting and celibacy, and when this was followed by debauchery he had already reached a position where he could explain matters. The novice found the primitive professor a competent teacher.

Primitive man was close to nature, but the fundamental fallacy of his medicine was its interference with nature. He regarded health and disease as a constant conflict between good spirits and bad spirits, each battling for victory. He was human enough to neglect the good spirits, for they wished him well and would do him no harm, but he was much concerned with the others. The sick person was possessed by devils, and at all hazards these devils must be driven from him.

The sick person was thus denied rest and quiet, for the disease-demons must be allowed no peace: they must be frightened away by terrifying masks and grimaces; by strange howls, noises, dances; they must be made uncomfortable by beating, biting, pinching, kicking, strangling their host; they must be smoked out by unbearable smells and fumigations; they must be alarmed by amulets, fetiches and incantations. If they were strong enough to endure all this, then by sorcery they must be lured elsewhere, to take their abode in some scapegoat—an animal, or the patient's enemy, or an inanimate object. If they were too clever to be fooled, then they must be appeased with sacrifices and precious gifts. The medicine-man's treatment was so heroic that often he looked as ill and gaunt as his patient, but he never gave up. Even when the struggles of the patient ceased and the soul left his body, the medicine-man would try to blow it back through the various orifices—the mouth, the ear, the anus. Many patients died in their prime, but this merely meant that the demons had conquered—perhaps the deceased had been disrespectful. On the other hand, the medicine-man had many remarkable cures to his credit, and if he kept testimonials, his medicine-bag must have been full of them. In primitive medicine, as in modern, the patient's faith and the physician's personality are important factors in the cure, and often both are the victims of ignorance and suggestion.

The original practitioners of medicine have disappeared without eponyms or memorials. Who first watched the breath, or accidentally touched the pulse? Who first speculated on blood, mucus, pus, ichor, saliva, and the bodily excretions? The savage who first found he could control hemorrhage by stroking, pressure and tying at a distant spot, deserved the world's first monument of stone, but he is as nameless as the daring founder of experimental pharmacology who first tasted a poisonous plant and searched for the antidote, or his jungle colleague who sutured wounds by having the edges pinched by the keen nippers of ants, while he rapidly severed their bodies. The origin of many medical procedures is forever lost in the early chapters of the book of time.

Looking backward, the life of primitive man appears simple to us, but he was probably sufficiently occupied in keeping himself alive. At any rate, he was either not fastidious, or his women had not learned the art of housekeeping, for the floors of his caves were never swept. With the passing generations, layers of débris were covered by accumulating layers, but what was rubbish then is archeology now. Primitive man lived on the top of prehistory more primitive than himself. When we enter a paleolithic cave and clear away the Azilian floor, we strike the Madelenian period with its wealth of bone and ivory weapons, and as we dig down through the centuries we reach the Solutrean, beneath which lies the Aurignacian—so old that the cave-bear disputed man's dominion—but underneath this dateless stratum is buried the older Mousterian, and then our spade and speculation halt in the lower paleolithic, in those timeless Acheulean and Chellian epochs when man was not fully man, but was Neanderthal.

Rock-shelters and caves were plentiful in those days, and early man had two kinds: one for feeding, propagating, sleeping and dying; and one for his important ceremonies. In the dark recesses of these caverns—some of which now can be reached only by swimming subterranean rivers—he has left many specimens of his handiwork. The wood he used has rotted, the gorgeous feathers are gone, his skins and leather-work are dust, but stone and bone remain. The limestone statuette of a paleolithic woman, dating back about 22,000 B.C., found in the loess of the Aurignacian period, and known as the Venus of Willendorf, should be compared with the living Hottentot Venus of today, since both illustrate the primitive man's penchant for fleshiness in his females. Primitive man himself is depicted as straight and slender, but he liked his women round, and thus the pendulous breasts and overdevelopment of the buttocks were due not only to too much cave-life and too much meat, but to selection. The primitive woman holding the bison-horn, known as the Venus of Laussel, found in a rock-shelter in the Dorgogne, shows the invariable fat-buttocked condition (*steatopygia*). In the Cogul cave is a group of women surrounding a man: the man is naked, but all the women are carefully dressed. In one of the Capsian paintings, a man is seen climbing a tree to collect wild honey; he clings to the tree with his right hand, and in his left holds a bag, probably of leather, while the disturbed bees swarm around him, seemingly in anger. In the Morella la Vella paintings, bowmen are shooting arrows at each other. At the end of the long cave of Trois Frères is a man in a crouching position disguised as a stag, with tail and antlers, and this mystery-man may be the first picture ever drawn of a physician.

On the whole, the human figure occurs seldom in primitive

art, and as a rule the execution is crude. It is when paleolithic man deals with animals that our admiration begins, and the more we study the subject the deeper is our amazement. On horns, bones, shells, clay, stones, on teeth of mammoths and on reindeer antlers, primitive man produced masterpieces. There were times in the various phases of the long Stone Age when the craftsmen seemed to grow weary, and impressionism was substituted for honest labor, but primitive art at its best has never been surpassed. In the morning of mankind, in the world's first art galleries, lit up only by fat-filled stone lamps, nameless artists drew, etched, engraved and sculptured. No amount of praise, no glowing verbal descriptions can give an adequate conception of the skill, vigor, color and beauty of these works. To be understood, these silhouettes, etchings, reliefs, polychrome paintings and sculptures must be seen on the original rocks or in adequate reproduction. Flat stones were their palettes, hollow bones their paint-boxes, and no living man can do with red and yellow ochre what the Madelenians accomplished. The ingenuity with which they took advantage of the concavity or natural bulging of a rock, the skill with which they could depict motion, the neighing horse's head carved on a reindeer antler at Mas d'Azil, the lowing bison, the running boar, the eager wolf, the engraved dissection of a horse's head, the vivid panorama of animals at Altamira over forty-five feet in length, the frightened red deer crossing a stream—the large stag looking behind and sniffing the air, the female in the middle with outstretched neck, and the calf in front playfully leaping as if counting on its parents' protection—all these show positive genius.

Aside from their remarkable artistic quality, these illustrations are of intense interest because they prove the foundation of nature observation, biological knowledge, and dissection of animals in the prehistoric period. The Pindal elephant showing the position of the heart, and the Niaux bisons with arrows embedded in the heart, demonstrate that man early recognized the importance of this organ. The human vertebrae with flint arrows embedded in them show that primitive man knew where to aim. Even pathological scenes are depicted. On a broken reindeer bone is carved a woman in the last stages of pregnancy, but complicated with uterine inertia; in accordance with a superstition of the time, a large deer is seen stepping over her distended abdomen, to hasten delivery.

Men who were so clever with their hands that with the crudest tools they could create marvels in ivory, could not be backward in surgery, and we know how adept some aborigines are in performing infibulation, caesarean section and ovariotomy with a sharp-pointed flint; scarification and blood-letting are practised with ease in a variety of ways. Stone Age man made splints of wood and kept fractures immobilized with clay. He was not dependent upon spontaneous healing, for the evidence shows that a large percentage of prehistoric fractures were restored. We do not know all the diseases to which the flesh of primitive man was heir, but his surviving bones tell us that he suffered much from cave-gout—the caves were often damp—arthritic lesions, rickets, fixation of the segments of the spinal column, dental caries, pyorrhea alveolaris; the dominant disease was inflammation of the bones involving a joint and producing deformity.

By far the most important phase of prehistoric surgery was the operation known as trepanation—the removal of part of the skull vault. Trepanned skulls have been found in considerable numbers, and modern surgeons who have attempted to repeat the procedure with a flint knife or shark's tooth have not entirely succeeded. Some of these primitive skulls show scratches around the circular or oval hole, indicating an inexperienced operator, but many of the trephinations have been performed with consummate skill. Evidence of cicatrization or healing is frequently apparent, and many of these skulls have been perforated several times, demonstrating not only that patients survived this ordeal —which must have lasted at least an hour—but submitted to it again. There is much about trepanation which we do not yet know: whether the operation was performed by boring, sawing, scraping, cutting or chiseling, or by a combination of these methods; why the larger openings are frequently accompanied by smaller ones nearby; and why the female skulls are marked by intersecting depressions or grooves (*sincipital-T*). The disks of bone removed by trepanation were valued as amulets (*rondelles*), and were often polished into various shapes and worn as a protection against disease—one of the earliest forms of prophylaxis.

Charms from those who survived trepanation were especially in demand, and after the death of these individuals their skulls were chipped into rondelles; if the demand was greater than the supply, amulets were slyly forged from other skulls or from the antlers of stags—primitive man was not too primitive to show his human nature. The chief indications for trepanation were infantile convulsions, relief of cerebral tension, cranial injuries, headaches, epilepsy and blindness. The object of the perforation was to give the confined demon an opportunity to escape.

Let us not regard paleolithic man with contempt. We are heirs to centuries of science, and as we think of modern man's absorption in war, of the grade of intelligence exhibited in political campaigns, of the various religious cults which sprang up within recent years, of the quality of periodicals with the largest circulations, of the seances of spiritualists in all countries, of the numerous individuals who earn a livelihood by reading palms and casting horoscopes, we realize that we have little reason to be boastful.

Shall we laugh because the medicine-man, in order to increase his dignity, smeared his body with red paint? Let us rather recall that in the civilized centuries the mark of the physician was a red cloak. Shall we mock his magic stick, the mere sight of which made his people feel better? Not as long as we remember the vogue of its successor, the gold-headed cane. Shall we condemn him because he sought to mystify his patients with wonder-tricks and words they could not understand? Let us reflect on more modern practitioners who give detailed instructions about taking a cathartic pill. In all ages, the invalid quite as much as the attendant, has insisted on a certain amount of hocus-pocus with the treatment.

The recent decompression operation, now so popular for the relief of intracranial pressure, is really the old trepanation, though drill and burr have replaced the scrapers of stone. Primitive man visualized universal disease-demons in the air, but he could not see them: modern man has captured these little demons, stained them red and violet and brown and blue, and upon them has built the structure of scientific medicine: demonology has been transformed into bacteriology. Thus one of the oldest surgical procedures has been modified into one of the most recent, and the first concept of the causation of disease is linked with the latest. Let us study our primitive ancestor and not scorn him, for even in the gross superstitions that held him in thrall, we find the germ of truth. Intellectually, we are but a stone's throw from the Stone Age; and emotionally, we are still living there.

II

MEDICINE IN ANCIENT EGYPT

No excavated quarries, no deciphered hieroglyphics, no obelisks or stelae will ever reveal to us the origin of civilization. How the predynastic Egyptians began to speak and write; how they took moist earth from their river and dried it in the sun to make bricks; how they fashioned pottery, and learned to bake bread and brew beer; how they made glass and prepared leather; how these dark-skinned, thin-limbed people observed the heavens until they realized the solar year consists of 365 days; how they instituted a priesthood and organized prostitution; how they domesticated plants and animals, and established human slavery; how these dwellers in the valley became a great agricultural nation—are all matters that can be discussed only with gaps and question-marks.

Herodotus is the father of history, but when that inquisitive man explored the long African river, the Nile had already carried the secrets of centuries to the sea. Time, the mud of the Delta, and the hunger of white ants have effaced the early records of Egyptian civilization. Copper is native in Egypt, and when this metal is alloyed with tin, either by accident or design, the result is bronze. Much may be done with this amalgam that is impossible with flint and limestone, and the Age of Stone gave way to the Age of Bronze—the cradle of civilization was built of stone, but embellished with bronze.

By the time the Egyptians began to write about medicine, the art was so old that they either forgot or ignored its crude beginnings, and preferred to attribute its origin to the gods. The effort of medicine to extricate itself from magic, runs through our entire story from its dawn to the present day. In Egypt this separation was impossible, for all the physicians were priests, and the gods were ever present. The race which produced such engineers that we modern men do not know how they reared their pyramids, believed that a crocodile which a sorcerer molded from wax, actually ate up an adulterer—in all ages technical skill may be combined with gross credulity.

The most learned Egyptians of the time, versed in mathematics and astronomy, worshiped the sacred bull who lived in the temple at Memphis and was believed to be the reincarnation of Osiris. The date of his birth, the name of his cow-mother, and the time of his enthronement were more carefully recorded than mundane affairs. As this bull was led through the streets in religious procession, scribes and scholars bowed to the earth in reverence. An army of human beings served this bull, bringing him the choicest food—what he really wanted was some good hay—keeping him spotless, making up his chamber and building a costly harem for his cows. When the bull died, though there was famine in the land, he was surrounded by the rarest jewels and embalmed in a sarcophagus hewn from a single block of polished granite of seventy tons. Men starved in Egypt, while a million dollars were spent on a dead bull. Then his successor was chosen, and in Egypt's capital have been found sixty of these sacred bulls. With slight modifications, this is the thing that man has done in all lands and in all ages.

The Egyptians could not eliminate magic from their medicine, or divorce their sacred and secular knowledge. The ibis-headed Thoth, the hawk-headed Horus, the lion-headed Sekhmet, the cat-headed Pacht, the asp-headed Rannu, overwhelmed the laws of science. Never were demons more prolific than on the Nile, and they attacked not only mortals but the healing divinities: Isis, most benevolent and popular of goddesses, was afflicted with an abscess of the breast; her son Hor suffered from dysentery and anal trouble; and even Rē, the sun-god himself would be smitten suddenly with diseases of the eye. More potent than the venerated gods were the all-powerful magicians who by incantations commanded and changed nature. Pyramid texts and papyrus scrolls tell us of priests who raised the dead, opened the earth, stopped the sun, and parted the waters to find the lost jewel of a princess. The Egyptians who saw the workings of nature in the annual inundation of the river which created their nation, cast out nature with occult formulas.

The Egyptians were always inconsistent, and their belief in divine healing did not prevent them from searching for earthly remedies. Their explanation was that every medicine would be more effective if taken with an incantation. "Welcome, remedy, welcome, which destroyest the trouble in this my heart and in these my limbs. The magic of Horus is victorious in the remedy," is an incantation from their best-known papyrus. The invocation from another papyrus—"O Horus, O Rē, O Shu, O Qêb, O Osiris, O Hekaw, O Nut, praise be unto you, ye great gods,"—is suggestive of recent brochures on astrology.

Their drugs of animal origin sound like a witch's materia medica: the Egyptians prescribed flesh of lizards, blood of bat, womb of cat, dung of the crocodile, semen and testicles of asses, vulva of dog, milk of a lying-in-woman. These medicines became so popular that in time the race of man prepared seventy-nine remedies from the hyena. King Zoser's vizier-architect and physician-magician, Imhotep, who was later deified as the Egyptian god of medicine, is depicted as bald, but the Egyptians did not like baldness and treated the condition vigorously. One prescription consisted of writing ink and cerebrospinal fluid; another was composed of toes of dog, ripe dates and asses' hoof; and the following ointment, for partial baldness, required a brave and enterprising apothecary: the fat of lion, hippopotamus, crocodile, goose, snake and Nubian ibex.

If we are surprised that the hygienic Egyptians, who bathed frequently, gave daily attention to their bowels, wore white linen and sandals, and practised circumcision for cleanliness' sake, should be willing to pay high prices for such medicaments, let us open the London Pharmacopeias of the seventeenth century A.D., and we will find that blood of bat and badger still persisted, and that excrements of many animals—our forefathers wrote volumes on the therapeutic virtues of dung—the skulls of malefactors hanged in the moonlight, bee glue, eel grease, wine of he-goat, vipers' flesh, woodlice, wolf's intestines, omentum of the ram, saliva of a fasting man and secundines of a woman, were officially recommended; let us read the most popular French dictionary of drugs of the eighteenth century, and we will note that man himself is being used as a medicine:

"All parts of man, his excrescences and excrements, contain oil and sal volatile, combined with phlegm and earth. Skull, brain, and calculus are employed in medicine, and are referred to in their proper places. Burning hair, smelt by patients, will counteract the vapors. Moss of the human skull, human blood, and human urine all have their uses in medicine. The saliva of a robust young man, taken fasting, is an antidote against the bites of serpents and mad dogs. Wax from the ears is good against whitlows. Nails from the fingers and toes, given internally either in substance or infused in wine, make a good emetic. Women's milk is pectoral, good in phthisis, and useful to apply to inflamed eyes. Fresh urine, two or three glasses drunk in the morning fasting, is good against gout, hysterical vapors, and obstructions. It may also be applied externally in gout and in skin complaints. Excrement of man can be applied to anthrax, plague bubos, and quinsies. Dried and powdered, it is recommended in epilepsy and intermittent fevers. Dose, one scruple to one drachm."

We must not blame the Egyptians for a credulity which is universal. Whoever should undertake to compile a list of all the drugs that have passed through the alimentary canal of man, would in reality be writing a treatise on human folly. Every country has its pharmacologic graveyards, where the panaceas of the past lie buried. Moreover the Egyptians, by their extensive use of animal remedies, became the forerunners of organotherapy: much more testicular, ovarian, hepatic, adrenal and thyroid extract are consumed in the world today than when the Pharaohs were in power.

If Neolithic man surprises us with trepanation which we cannot imitate, the Egyptians astonish us with the lost art of mummification. Not only human beings, but countless cats, snakes, owls, cuckoos, and insects—including of course the sacred dung-beetle or scarab—have been embalmed forever. The Egyptians must have originated embalming in their stone age, for long after they were acquainted with the metal knife, the original incision was performed with an Ethiopic stone: the cutter who thus offended the dead was a man of lowest caste, who ran from the scene as fast as possible, pursued by stones and curses. The respected guild of embalmers—holy men who had access to the temple—then began their work: with an iron hook they extracted the brain through the nostrils, and after opening the abdominal cavity they cleansed it, rinsing it with palm wine and scouring it with spices. The putrescible viscera were removed, and after being returned to the corpse were packed tight with sawdust, linen, mud, aromatic wood or flowers. The salters then immersed the body in a bath of brine for seventy days, after which it was wrapped in bandages and smeared with gum. This method was as costly as a modern funeral, and there was another mode which consisted essentially of injecting quantities of cedar oil through the rectum; the aperture was then closed to hinder the injection from flowing backwards, the body lay in brine for seventy days, and when the cedar oil was drawn out, such was its strength that the dissolved internal organs came with it.

Herodotus, in his second book, concludes his comments on mummification with these paragraphs:

When they use the third manner of embalming, which is the preparation of the poorer dead, they cleanse the belly with a purge, embalm the body for the seventy days and then give it back to be taken away.

Wives of notable men, and women of great beauty and reputation, are not at once given over to the embalmers, but only after they have been dead for three or four days; this is done, that the embalmers may not have carnal intercourse with them. For it is said that one was found having intercourse with a woman newly dead, and was denounced by his fellow-workman.

When anyone, be he Egyptian or stranger, is known to have been carried off by a crocodile or drowned by the river itself, such an one must by all means be embalmed and tended as fairly as may be and buried in a sacred coffin by the townsmen of the place where he is cast up; nor may any of his kinsfolk or his friends touch him, but his body is deemed something more than human, and is handled and buried by the priests of the Nile themselves.

Diodorus Siculus, in his vivid description of embalming, declares: ". . . the beauty and shape of the face seems just as it was before, and may be known, even the hairs of the eyelids and eye-brows remaining as they were at first. By this means many of the Egyptians, keeping the dead bodies of their ancestors in magnificent houses, so perfectly see the true visage and countenance of those that died many ages before they themselves were born, that in viewing the proportions of every one of them, and the lineaments of their faces, they take as much delight as if they were still living among them."

Siculus did not exaggerate; so well preserved are these mummies, that when the bandages were recently unwrapped from Rameses II and Rameses III, their features were recognizable and could be compared with their statues. It is not easy to examine a mummy: hardened cloth and resin must be scraped away, ancient mud and sand must be picked out, and prehistoric dust is irritating to modern lungs.

These long-silent mummies, after sleeping for thousands of years, now tell their story. This one had multiple abscesses in his kidney, and the bacilli can still be stained; this one had gall-stones, and another urinary calculi; this one had appendicitis, and the adhesions are still visible; by the solidification of that lung, it is seen that this one had pneumonia; here is an arch of the aorta hacked away by the embalmer; these lungs are strangely sooty, showing that the mummy, when alive, worked in smoke-laden air; here the embalmers have been careful, there they were in a hurry; this one suffered from constipation, for his intestines are obstructed; the lumen of this subclavian artery is nearly blocked by a clot—he had a narrow escape; arterial lesions were as prevalent then as now—the problems of high blood-pressure are not new. The humpbacked priest of Ammon, with characteristic spinal protrusion and psoas abscess, shows that tuberculosis existed among the Egyptians.

The Egyptians evidently escaped venereal disease. There were laws against contraception, abortion and immorality, but every nation violates these laws. The pharaoh himself, with his hundred wives clad in jewels and veils, many of them being barbaric princesses from distant lands who could not speak a word of Egyptian, set the standard. Sly cartoonists drew the royal harem, picturing the king as a roaring lion surrounded by pretty gazelles. The people were given to voluptuousness, the Horus-Set myth is pederastic, at least one papyrus is frankly pornographic, beautiful slaves were utilized for sexual purposes, religious ceremonies often ended in orgies—dancing girls are still known in every circus as Little Egypt—and it is related that an Egyptian ruler who sought a prescription for sore eyes, which remedy consisted of the urine of a woman faithful to her husband, was compelled to search for ten years. Yet the Egyptians described no disease corresponding to gonorrhea, and not a single ancient bone has been found that is syphilitic.

One of the most splendid of Egyptian sculptures is the seated scribe—black of hair, brown of flesh, with eager alabaster eyes —holding a white papyrus roll in his hands. The scribe figured prominently in Egyptian life, and he who knew the three forms of writing—the pictographic hieroglyphic, the cursive hieratic, and the simplified demotic—was considered a learned man. The practical advice of the old Egyptian, "My son, apply thyself to learning, that thou mayest be a scribe. The people are heavily laden asses, but the scribe is the driver. The scribe is never hungry; he sits at Pharaoh's table, and his belly is filled by reason of his wisdom," may be compared with the scorn for the frivolous student: "Thou forsakest thy books, thou givest thyself up to pleasure, thou goest from tavern to tavern; the smell of beer makes man shun thee; thou drinkest until it dulls thy wits, and art like a broken oar on the deck of a ship." Egypt, in its senescence, wrote copiously. The papyrus plant grew in the Delta: its pith they used for food, from its head they fashioned garlands for the gods, and from its stem they made cord for their artisans, boats for their sailors, and paper for their scribes—paper that has lasted for thousands of years.

A few medical papyri have been preserved by being lost for ages, thus escaping man's vandalism. They have recently been found between the legs of mummies, in piles of rubbish and in potsherds. Much of what we know of Egyptian medicine comes from these plants which once grew carelessly in the Nile, unmindful that their pages would transmit the record of Egyptian medicine to modernity.

The *Veterinary and Gynecological Papyri from Kahun* are the oldest yet discovered, dating back 2160-1788 B.C. The gynecologic portion, written in clear hieratic, is in a fragmentary condition, and though it has been translated, it remains largely unintelligible. The travail of a thousand scholars has not sufficed to find equivalents for many Egyptian technical words. Here are characteristic passages from the third or last column:

To prevent conception (?). Dung of a crocodile, cut up on "hesaauit" soaked ...
Another medicine: 1 "henu" of honey, "kap" on her vulva: do this upon "sehem" (?) (liquid) of natron.
Another ... upon glue "auit," pour upon her vulva.
To cure itching (biting) of womb. Stalks (?) of dates on ... beat it fine on sweet beer (let her) sit upon it, opening her thighs. Knowledge of woman geated ... are her eyes bleared (?) ... upon the left hand of a (person) born in the Fayoum. Pour ... four mornings; cause her to sit upon the water of ... of the lake cause.
To distinguish her who shall conceive from her who will not con-

ceive. Put thou fresh oil upon . . . examine her; if thou findest the muscles of her breast "khasha" (? soft) say thou with regard to it, it is a birth. If thou findest them "kenken" say thou with regard to it she will bear late; but if thou findest them like the color (?) . . . (say thou with regard to it she will never give birth).

The *Papyrus of Mother and Child*, while not devoid of medical interest, is predominantly magical. One of its passages reveals the source from which Moses borrowed his fairy-tales:

King Cheops was sad and his court could not cheer his heart. He called for his magician who came and produced a boat with twenty jeweled ebony oars driven by twenty beautiful maidens, draped in fish net, who rowed King Cheops over a beautiful lake on the border of the desert, and then was King Cheops' heart cheered. But in the midst of the lake the maidens suddenly stopped rowing, all because the maiden at the stroke oar had lost, in the midst of the lake, a jewel of new lapis lazuli where the water was twelve cubits deep. King Cheops was disturbed and called for the wizard to bring up by his magic the lost jewel. So the wizard stretched forth his hands over the lake and said some potent words and struck the waters with his wand and the waters turned over the one side on to the other and the magician walked in between the waters on dry land and picked up the jewel, which was lying in the midst of the lake on a piece of broken earthenware, and he gave the jewel to the maiden, and then the waters still stood up as he walked out, a wall twelve cubits high on one side and twenty-four cubits on the other side. And when he stood on the shore again the magician raised up his hands and spoke some more powerful words and the waters came together, the twenty maidens dipped the twenty jeweled ebony oars into the water again and the heart of King Cheops was cheered.

The *Surgical Papyrus* written about 1600 B.C., is over fifteen feet in length when unrolled, and originally was considerably longer. The writing in black ink is beautiful, and the important words and subsections are in red—the first rubrics. In the eleventh column the scribe omitted a phrase, and inserted the missing words in the upper margin, marking the place in the text with a little red cross. In some papyri, this cross was placed not only where the missing words occurred, but by the words themselves—the original asterisk. The front of this Surgical Papyrus describes ten cases of wounds of the head; seven of the nose; ten of the ear, lips and jaw; six of the neck and throat; five of the collar bone and shoulders; nine of the chest and breast; and one incomplete case of spinal ailment—forty-eight cases in all. It is apparent that the papyrus meant to be a complete copy of a Book on Surgery and External Medicine, beginning with injuries of the head and concluding with the feet. It ends, however, abruptly, at the bottom of the seventeenth column in the middle of a line, and the sentence which was left incomplete 3500 years ago, will never be finished.

Each of the cases begins with the name of the ailment, followed by an examination giving the symptoms, diagnosis, verdict and treatment. In knife-cuts, sword-slashes and battle-axe blows of the skull, the surgeon is instructed, "You should probe the wound." The prognosis is favorable in contusion, doubtful in a penetrating gash, and unfavorable in fracture. Feeble pulse and fever are noted among the symptoms of severe cranial injuries; in fracture of the skull under the skin, the practitioner must elevate the depression outward; a cut in the forehead is treated by a linen bandage prepared by the embalmer and known as the "physicians' skin"; nasal secretions are to be cleared away by swabs, and two rolls of linen dipped in ointment are inserted in the nostrils; the projections of the jaw-bone are likened to the claws of a two-toed bird; fracture of the temporal bone produces deafness; in dislocations of the jaw the attendant is instructed how to force the bones in place; temperature develops from a knife-wound of the gullet, and if the patient drinks water it turns aside, issuing from the mouth of the wound; in dislocations of the vertebrae of the neck, there is loss of control of arms, legs and excretory organs, and the physician can do nothing.

This papyrus is not an original work but a copy of a text that had been produced a thousand years earlier; in the intervening period so many expressions had become obsolete that a commentary was required to explain them. The Book on Surgery and External Medicine therefore, while copied 3500 years ago, actually reveals Egyptian medicine as it was practised 4500 years ago. While the scientific knowledge disclosed is not great, we must admire the frankness of the physicians in pronouncing many of the cases hopeless. The text is sober, and we are about to be grateful that at last we have an Egyptian document free from demonology, but when we turn the papyrus over and look on the back, we find a magic formula for casting out the winds that carry the plagues, and the last two columns are devoted to the "Incantation of Transforming an Old Man into a Youth of Twenty."

In various respects, the *Therapeutic Papyrus of Thebes,* written in 1552 B.C.—a calendar on the back of the first page establishes the date—is the most interesting and important of all the Egyptian scrolls. Nearly sixty-five feet long when found, more than a foot wide, with over one hundred pages of hieratic script totaling 2289 lines, its decipherment opened a long-closed door in ancient medicine. The inevitable incantations mar its scientific value, but it seems the Egyptians could not function without magic. Among the conditions treated are diseases of the viscera and the organs of special sense. The sections on tumors and obstructions, and on diseases of the ear and eye —from which the Egyptians suffered much—are given considerable space. One of these chapters shows that even then medicine was international, for it is entitled: "Ophthalmology treated according to the priest apothecaries, as revealed by a Semite of Kepni." From pains in the head to sore toes, the misfortunes of human flesh are discussed, though we must not expect descriptions of clinical merit. It is interesting to note that one chapter is devoted to diseases of children; diseases of women receive due attention, in which respect this scroll differs from the Surgical Papyrus which was limited to male patients. Skin diseases are included, and chapter twenty contains "remedies for burns and suppurating sores, gangrene and wallops from flogging." There are over seventy cosmetic prescriptions: for sunburn, freckles, wrinkles, and other facial blemishes; perfumes for women, so their clothing and breath would be pleasant; and for the men, of course many remedies for baldness—not only to produce hair and to prevent it from turning gray, but directions for making hair grow on the scars of the scalp.

No doubt the most significant passage is the one which compares pulsation to the inundations of the Nile, which come and go. The conception of the pulse is thus developed: "There is in the heart a vessel leading to every member of the body. If the physician places his finger on the head, neck, arms, hands, feet or body, everywhere he will find the heart, for the heart leads to every member, and speaks in the vessels of every member." This remarkable doctrine occurs also in the Surgical Papyrus.

Seven hundred remedies are mentioned in the Therapeutic Papyrus, and some of these drugs are serving mankind today: opium, indisputably the monarch of drugdom; castor oil, which in spite of a hundred rivals, remains the most valuable of cathartics; copper salts, indispensable in ophthalmology; and such familiar drugs as squill, acacia, calamus, coriander, saffron, hyoscyamus, colchicum, gentian, pomegranate and olive oil, and the salts of various metals.

But although the Egyptians used these drugs, as a rule they did not know their specific indications, and they laid just as much stock—perhaps more—in such agents as fly-specks scraped from a wall, and moisture from a pig's ear. Seven hundred remedies are perhaps too copious a materia medica for an early people to employ with discrimination, and the Egyptians seem to have collected drugs somewhat in the spirit that a child collects toys: they took whatever they could lay their hands on, whether they had any special use for it or not. But it was their glory to have stumbled on a few drugs which will last as long as their pyramids.

Pharaoh succeeded Pharaoh, and though we know their chronology, each resembled the other so much that it is difficult to tell them apart. The outstanding exception, Amenophis IV, who later changed his name to Akhnaton, is the most real and human of them all. The other god-kings were idealized in their paintings and sculptures, but Akhnaton insisted on being represented just as he looked. His peculiar physiognomy—the big head, the elongated chin, the ugly acromegalic face—is a familiar landmark in Egyptian history. Diseased and deformed, there is yet something strangely attractive in his physique, while his character is full of interest. He married the dreamy-eyed, sensuous-lipped Nefertiti, whose charm survives in Thothmes' statue in natural colors. Akhnaton loved this alluring woman, and encouraged the artists to portray him with Nefertiti sitting on his knees, or exchanging kisses. Especially familiar are the affectionate scenes in which Akhnaton and Nefertiti embrace their daughters—they had no sons—and hold them up naked for the blessing of the sun-god. The sun-disk is in the center, and each effulgent ray shining from heaven terminates in a beneficent hand as it touches earth. For Akhnaton, youthful and zealous, was the iconoclast of Egypt, breaking with the traditions of his fathers, closing the temples of the old gods, driving Isis and Osiris from their sacred altars, casting out great Ammon, despoiling the worship of the local deities, and proclaiming one supreme god—the sun-god Aton, god not only of all Egypt, but of all other lands. People and priesthood were aghast at the blasphemy, but it was perhaps greater heresy to oppose a Pharaoh, and shrines which had been worn by the feet of pilgrims were now deserted.

The Egyptians, especially at Heliopolis, had worshiped a sun-god ages before Akhnaton, but Ammon-Ra was one of many competing gods. Akhnaton banished him with the others, and established the new religion of one god, Atonism. Before his time, all the gods were represented in animal or human form, but anthropomorphic mythology was abolished by Akhnaton. This first international monotheist could not endure the atmosphere of the old polytheism, and left Thebes to build a new capital for Aton at the edge of the desert. In El-Amarna he raised his temples, not dark and mysterious as in the past, but with open courts flooded with sunshine. Stepping out from the shade of the palm-trees, Akhnaton and his wife kissed their beloved children and extended them for the health-giving beams of the sun-disk. There was deep reverence in the voice of Akhnaton as he spoke:

O sun, thou alone didst create this earth, and all upon it: men, herbs and flocks, the growing trees and the flying birds. Thy dawning is beautiful in the horizon of the heavens, O living sun, beginning of life. Thou givest breath to the chick within the shell, thou givest him strength to break from within, to chirp and to run on his feet. Up-stream and down-stream sail the barques, every highway is open because thou dawnest, the fish in the river leap up before thee, thy rays are in the midst of the great green sea.

In the underworld thou hast placed a Nile for Egypt, and a Nile in the sky to bring the rain to other lands. Thou madest the countries of Syria and Cush, and upper and lower Egypt; the tongues of men are divided in speech, their form and skin are diverse, for thou hast made the people various. Thou hast set each man in his place, and hast made what he needs, and the length of his life is reckoned.

When thou settest in the western horizon of the sky, the earth is in darkness like the dead; all lie down like those who die, their heads are wrapped up, their nostrils closed until the next day thou awakenest in glory on the eastern horizon of heaven.

All mankind lives at sight of thee, O sum; the whole earth assembles at thy rising, their hands salute thy dawning; the singers and musicians lift up their voices with gladness, and in every temple in Akhetaton are good and fat offerings. All mankind, cattle, flying and fluttering things, with all kinds of reptiles which are on the earth, they live when they see thee.

Let me stay here, O sun, until the paddy-bird turns black and the crow turns white, until the sea walks on two feet and the hills rise up to go and meet the streams; O Aton, keep me in attendance on thee, until thou preparest for me a burial of thine own bidding.

Akhnaton was so occupied with the sun that he did not see what mortals were doing on earth. He lost his empire and died young; Nefertiti returned to Thebes and the old religion; the multitudinous divinities came out of their hiding-places; Isis and Osiris reigned again; the temples of Akhnaton were utterly demolished; the name of the image-breaker was blotted out—in Egyptian annals he is referred to as "that criminal of El-Amarna."

Father Time is older and wiser than Egypt, and has reversed many verdicts first heard along the Nile. Today the world demands ultraviolet radiation: the treatment of disease by exposure to sunlight (*heliotherapy*) is one of the tenets of modern medicine. Numerous recent books and brochures, extolling the vital energy of the life-giving rays of the sun, open with a frontispiece of Akhnaton—and in more lands than he ever knew, the heretic king is hailed as the founder of heliotherapy.

Egypt was the medical center of the ancient world. The Biblical admission, "And Moses was learned in all the wisdom of the Egyptians," indicates the origin of Mosaic magic; and even the sarcasm of Jeremiah, "Go up into Gilead and take balm, O virgin daughter of Egypt; in vain dost thou use many medicines; there is no healing for thee," reveals that Egypt was noted for numerous remedies. Homer sang of "Egypt teeming with drugs, the land where each is a physician, skilful beyond all men." Herodotus described Egypt as the home of specialists: "Medicine is practised among them on a plan of separation; each physician treats a single disorder, and no more; thus the country swarms with medical practitioners, some undertaking to cure diseases of the eye, others of the head, others again of the teeth, others of the intestines, and some those which are not local." Diodorus Siculus explained: "The whole manner of life in Egypt was so evenly ordered that it would appear as though it had been arranged according to the rules of health by a learned physician, rather than by a lawgiver." Cyrus of Persia sent for an Egyptian oculist to take care of his sick mother, and the body-physician of Darius likewise came from the Nile.

Was antiquity's tribute to Egypt justified? Must we confirm or reverse the verdict? Authors yet unborn will some day add books, to those already existing, on the remarkable state of medical knowledge among the Egyptians. But the most surprising aspect of the matter, is that a people so capable, should have produced a medicine so barren. Egyptian medicine was non-progressive, and since it could not advance, it went backward with the centuries. The earlier papyri contain more medicine and less magic, while in the later scrolls the incantations are predominant.

Just as the Phoenicians who invented the alphabet, used it neither for science nor literature, but for their ledgers, so the Egyptians who opened the human body, neither observed nor dissected. In spite of their opportunities, they knew little anatomy, and the badly united bones and the abscessed teeth found in their mummies are evidence that their knowledge of surgery and dentistry was rudimentary. Century after century, millions upon millions of dead Egyptians were eviscerated by the embalmers—and the living Egyptians learned no pathology.

Since all wisdom was contained in the forty-two books of Hermes Trismegistus, the priest-physician could not question or modify the sacred writings: no blame attached to the practitioner if the patient died according to the hermetic rules, but if he deviated from the prescribed regulations and the case terminated fatally, then his own life was forfeit. The priest-physician was a hybrid that could not survive; the priest conquered the physician, and medicine succumbed in the enfolding arms of magic. Egypt will ever allure the imagination of men, but the very phrase, Egyptian science, carries an occult and ominous meaning.

Mother Egypt tended the cradle of civilization: her wonderful children possessed considerable empirical knowledge, but viewing nature through an inscrutable veil of mystery they could not investigate the laws of science or understand the principles of medicine. Egypt transmitted no scientific legacy to posterity; Sekhetenanch, the first physician mentioned in history, is but a name, Imhotep is a semi-myth, and we know nothing of their thoughts or methods. On Egypt's monuments, Pthah the creator still remains, and there the unwearying Neph sits at the potter's wheel, turning clay into men. But these gods are dead, and the men they mold are lifeless. From the pyramid fields, the silent Sphinx of Giza gazes eastward over the Nile valley, and has no message for the younger nations.

III

MEDICINE IN ANCIENT GREECE

IN the days when there was famine in Canaan, and Jacob—who was called no more Jacob, but Israel—sent his sons to Pharaoh to buy corn, Egypt was even then a land of antiquities. At the time that the Britons were staining their bodies with ochre and woad, the Great Pyramid was already an ancient monument. Egyptian sculptors, decadent with civilization, depicted skin-clad savages—these were Europeans. Centuries passed, and sunburnt barbarians, blue-eyed and red of hair, peered into the valley of the Nile. Slave-trading, women-stealing Phoenicians sailed everywhere, and the Greeks were beginning to ask questions. "You Greeks," said the tired Egyptians, "are mere children, talkative and vain. What do you know about the past?"

European civilization was bathed by the waters of the Mediterranean. Africa, Asia and Europe converge on the little island of Crete, whose inhabitants still point to the sacred cave where Zeus was born. It was here, too, that the grown Zeus raped Europa who became the mother of Minos. From time to time Zeus appeared before his son, instructing him how to govern the Minoans—a tale which bears a striking resemblance to the interviews which Jehovah later held with Moses. The Minoan civilization reaches back to about 4000 B.C., and has only recently been rediscovered—and under its age of bronze the stone age has been excavated. The Early, Middle and Later Minoan periods are of ceaseless interest. These pre-Greeks, who do not even belong to history, filled archives of clay tablets with hieroglyphic and linear scripts; the tribute of amazement is due the beauty of their ceramics before they knew a potter's wheel; the colors of their faïence figurines; their exquisite inlay work with gold and ivory; their votive offerings in front of a cross; the wall fresco of the Boy Gathering Saffron; the realistic drawings of insects and animals; the scenes and games carved on cups and vases; their masonry and plumbing which still endure—in the prehistoric Minoan palace of Knossos was found a fully-equipped sanitary bathroom and water-closet.

Literature begins with Homer about 1000 B.C., but in Homer's day the culture of Minoan Crete had already disappeared beneath a terrible new weapon—the iron sword. The legends which Homer knew and sang in those matchless hexameters, belong to the last phase of Minoan and Mycenean civilization. Greece had passed through its dark ages, and Homer stood at the door of a new era. Homer was a barbarian, and we have no evidence that he could even write, but he tutored the world. The founder of epic poetry depicted man in the raw: aside from placating the gods, the Homeric heroes are interested only in women and war. Homer never moralizes, and he is not indignant because the abduction of Helen caused the death of many brave men. In this respect he differed from the bored Persians who informed Herodotus: "We think that it is wrong to carry women off: but to be zealous to avenge the rape is foolish: wise men take no account of such things: for plainly the women would never have been carried away, had not they themselves wished it. We of Asia regarded the rape of our women not at all; but the Greeks, all for the sake of a Lacedaemonian woman, mustered a great host, came to Asia, and destroyed the power of Priam. Ever since then we have regarded Greeks as our enemies." In this one respect, the Persians were wiser than the Greeks.

Galen, in one of his lost treatises, set the pace by writing on the medical knowledge of Homer. Many authors have followed him, and since each was ambitious to improve on his predecessor, some were driven to declare that Homer must have been a physician. There is certainly no basis for this enthusiasm—Homeric medicine is really as meager as Biblical medicine—and it is only by commenting upon each word and magnifying every allusion that we are able to produce a tract on the subject. Nearly all of Homer's medical references are in connection with the wounds which the warriors so joyously inflict upon each other. An exception is the case of Thersites: "evil-favored beyond all men that came to Ilios, bandy-legged and lame on one foot, and his two shoulders were rounded, stooping together over his chest and above them his head was warpen and scant stubble grew thereon." This description of Thersites' deformity is certainly suggestive of rickets.

In the fourth *Iliad,* when the fair-haired Menelaus is wounded, he heartens his comrades by saying: "Be thou of good cheer, neither affright in any wise the host of the Achaeans. Not in a fatal spot hath the dart been fixed; ere that my flashing belt stayed it, and the kilt beneath, and the taslit that the coppersmith fashioned." "The lusty youth Simoeisius, as he strode amid the foremost, was smitten on the right breast beside the nipple and clean through his shoulder went the spear of bronze and he fell to the ground in the dust like a poplar-tree that hath grown up in the bottom-land of a great marsh. For his slaying waxed Odysseus mightily wrought at heart, and smote Priam's bastard son on the temple, and out through the other temple passed the spear-point of bronze, and darkness enfolded his eyes and he fell with a thud and upon him his armor clanked. . . . Then was Diores caught in the snare of fate, for with a jagged stone was he smitten on the right leg by the ankle; the sinews twain and the bones did the ruthless stone utterly crush; and he fell backward in the dust and stretched out both his hands to his dear comrades, gasping out his life; and there ran up he that smote him, Peiros, and dealt him a wound with the thrust of his spear beside the navel; and forth upon the ground gushed all his bowels and darkness enfolded his eyes, but as the other sprang back, Thoas of Aetolia smote him with the cast of his spear in the breast above the nipple and the bronze was fixed in his lung and Thoas came close to him, and drew his sharp sword and smote him therewith full upon the belly and took away his life."

In the fifth *Iliad*, the duels continue in full fury, and the rivals smite one another between the nipples and drive their spears through the breasts and shoulders of their rivals. Meriones pursued his rival, and when he had come up with him smote him in the right buttock, and the spear-point passed clean through even to the bladder beneath the bone—which shows an acquaintance with the symphysis pubis.

A knowledge of the large tendon at the nape of the neck which holds the head erect is revealed in Homer's next paragraph: "To him Phyleus' son, famed for his spear, drew nigh and smote him with a cast of his sharp spear on the sinew of the head; and straight through amid the teeth the bronze shore away the tongue at its base. So he fell in the dust and bit the cold bronze with his teeth."

Specimens of Homeric anatomy of violence are blows on the forehead above the base of the nose; on the throat beneath the chin; beneath the jaw under the ear; beside the shoulder where the collar-bone parts the neck and breast, where is the deadly spot; full upon the belly, the bowels gushing forth through the broken plate of the corselet; midway between the privy parts and the navel, where the pain is most cruel; on the hip where the thigh turns in the hip-joint into the lower belly; and upon the base of the leg where man's muscle is thickest. Mention is made of the vein that runneth along the back continually until it reacheth the neck; and of wounds of the windpipe where destruction of life cometh most speedily. The smitten heroes either recover rapidly when the spear-point or arrow-head is removed and healing herbs are applied, or they perish outright. Nothing is said of infection, suppuration, fever, gangrene, tetanus, concealed hemorrhage or healing by second intention. Homeric medicine is simple medicine, devoid of pathology.

The *Iliad* contains these references to the heart and blood: "and down ran the blood from his newly wounded arm"; "and he was gasping with painful breath, distraught in mind, and vomiting blood"; "but Patroclus in turn rushed on with the bronze, and not in vain did the shaft speed from his hand but smote his foe where the diaphragm is set close about the throbbing heart." Significant is the observation: "And he fell with a thud and the spear was fixed in his heart, that still beating made the butt thereof to quiver."

The passage in the *Iliad* most complimentary to medicine occurs in the eleventh book when Idomeneus speaks to Nestor: "For a leech is of the worth of many other men for the cutting out of arrows and the spreading of soothing simples."

Less blood is spilled in Homer's second epic—except at the end where the wily Odysseus locks the doors and kills all the wooers of his wife—and thus the *Odyssey* has fewer medical references than the *Iliad;* the fourth book of the *Odyssey* contains these lines: "Straightway Helen cast into the wine of which they were drinking a drug to quiet all pain and strife, and bring forgetfulness of every ill. . . . Such cunning drugs had Helen, drugs of healing, which Polydamna had given her, a woman of Egypt, for there the earth bears greatest store of drugs, many that are healing when mixed, and many that are baneful; there every man is a physician, wise above human kind."

We need not be surprised at Homer's extraordinary veneration of Egypt, since Greek authors long after his time regarded Egypt as the original source of wisdom and were always ready to acknowledge their intellectual indebtedness, even when they had far surpassed the Egyptians. Herodotus plainly states: "Indeed, well-nigh all the names of the gods came to Hellas from Egypt." It was a dangerous gift, but in time the Hellenic divinities became much more human than their Egyptian predecessors. Magic from Mesopotamia, with oracles and omens, and all the portents of Babylonian and Assyrian astrology invaded the Mediterranean lands, and would have overwhelmed any people less gifted than the Greeks.

It is interesting to note that although the *Iliad* and *Odyssey* swarm with gods and goddesses, Aesculapius was only a mortal in Homer's time. The first reference to him occurs in the second book of the *Iliad* where he appears as a minor chieftain from Thessaly: "these again were led by the two sons of Aesculapius, the skilled leeches, Podalirius and Machaon." In the next book he is mentioned as the peerless leech, and his son Machaon sucks out the blood from an arrow-wound and with sure knowledge spreads thereon soothing simples which of old the Centaur Chiron had given to his father with kindly thought. There is not the slightest intimation that Aesculapius was anything but a skilful physician, but just as the Egyptian Imhotep, who was originally an historical personage, in time evolved into a deity, so Aesculapius developed into the Hellenic god of medicine.

One of the earliest to raise Aesculapius above earthly beings was Homer's successor, the lost poet Arctinus of Miletus, who carried forward the unfinished epic of Troy, recounting such important episodes as the exploits of the Amazon Penthesileia, the last days of Achilles, the fatal dispute of Ajax and Odysseus, the introduction of the wooden horse, and the horror of the Laocoon. In a remarkable fragment, Arctinus relates that Aesculapius "endowed one of his sons with nobler gifts than the other; for while to Machaon he gave skilful hands to draw out darts, make incisions, and healing sores and wounds, he placed in the heart of Podalirius all cunning to find out things invisible, and cure that which healeth not"—a statement which not only first separates medicine and surgery, but emphasizes the physician's superiority to the surgeon.

His human parentage forgotten, Aesculapius was linked with Apollo, the ever-occupied and myriad-sided Olympian, god of innumerable realms, including the muses and medicine. Apollo sent pestilence on earth when mortals displeased him, and stayed the plague when he relented. He was physician to the other gods, and healed them with peony root. His talking raven detected Coronis, the beautiful nymph beloved by Apollo, under a tree with a youth of Thessaly; although warned by the gossiping crow not to tell, the raven informed his master of the unchastity of Coronis. Apollo grew pale and hot with jealousy, the laurel glided from his brow, and he sent an arrow into the bosom which had been so often pressed to his own. As her white limbs are drenched with her red blood he learns that she is pregnant with his child, but his lamentations and healing arts are in vain; after pouring fragrant incense on her unconscious breast and giving her the last embrace, he carries her with piteous groans to the funeral fires and delivers the child by caesarean section. This child was Aesculapius.

Abandoned on a hill-side, he was saved from starvation by a goat, and it has been pointed out that this is the first case of the artificial feeding of children. Apollo finally entrusted the medical education of his son to the Centaur Chiron, for the centaurs—part horse, part man—were also Apollo's children. Aesculapius grew up, learned and dignified; the Greeks could not help jesting even about sacred matters, and they spoke of him as "the bearded son of a beardless sire."

Aesculapius learned the art of medicine so well that he was accused by Pluto of depopulating Hades, and was slain by the thunderbolt of the angry Zeus who feared his skill in healing would make the children of earth immortal. Temples to Aesculapius as the specific god of medicine arose throughout Greece: those who sought the god, sacrificed a cock in his honor, and offered images of the diseased parts. Hearts, eyes, ears, limbs, abdominal viscera—sometimes the entire opened body if the patient did not know from what internal complaint he suffered—the generative organs, and even the placenta were manufactured in precious metals, costly stones, terra cotta or wax. While the cult of the healing gods lasted, the manufacture of votive offerings flourished.

Naturally craftier than the populace, the priests built the temples of Aesculapius in spots favored by nature—in the midst of a health-giving forest, by the side of a medicinal spring, on the brow of a lofty hill. The sight alone often served to bring the first smile of hope to the weary invalid—and patients who seemed too sick were not permitted to approach the sacred precincts. All the glories of Greek art were there—lovely Venus and laughing Bacchus, Zeus serene on his golden throne, and Aesculapius sorrowing for the ills of mankind. Fountains played in the shaded groves, and shelter-seats were arranged in semicircles of pure marble. And when hidden music floated over the southern flowers—the mingling of rhythm and perfume, the marriage of fragrance and melody—many sufferers raised their heads to repeat the prophecy of the Delphic sibyl: Oh, Aesculapius, thou art born to be the world's great joy.

Only after he had undergone a course in dietetics and hygiene, did the gates of the temple open for the pilgrim; but that night he lay at the foot of the statue of Aesculapius, awaiting and expecting a cure. At times, when the deep breathing of the patient was echoed back by the marble walls, the priests would steal noiselessly forth and bind a broken limb or anoint a wounded organ. Of course every temple rang with tales of wonderful cures. Who ever heard of a shrine that did not report miracles, and exhibit abandoned crutches and votive offerings as proof? The early Greek philosophers refused remuneration for their teachings, but Aesculapius demanded silver and gold for his services—at least so the priests claimed. Indeed, on one occasion, the god so far forgot himself as to say aloud to a patient, "Thou art healed, now pay the fee."

The assertion that Greek medicine originated in these healing shrines or Asklepions, shows a misconception of the essence of divine healing. Priestly medicine is infallible medicine: the god can never fail, and every case must be cured. Altogether different is the medicine practised by man: the diagnosis is difficult, the treatment uncertain, and often the end is death. Amid the ruins of broken inscriptions, the following *Cures by Apollo and Aesculapius* may still be read with wonder on the pillars of the temple at Epidaurus:

Cleo, pregnant five years. She being already five years pregnant came a suppliant to the god, and lay down to sleep in the sacred chamber; but she went out speedily, and got forth from the temple and bore a son, who immediately washed himself in the spring and walked about with his mother. Now, when this had happened to her, she wrote on a votive tablet: "Marvel not at the size of this tablet, but at the occurrence; five years Cleo was pregnant, she slept, and the god made her whole."

Euphanes, an Epidaurian boy. The patient incubated because of stone. The god seemed to stand and ask: "What will you give if I cure you?" and he said ten dice bones. The god laughed and said he would heal him, and when it was day he departed cured.

The cup. A porter on his way to the temple fell when ten furlongs from it. He rose and opening his sack found the contents were broken. Seeing that the cup his master drank from was smashed, he was in despair, and sitting on the ground tried to fit the pieces together. A passer-by seeing this, exclaimed: "Why, miserable man, waste time in trying to mend that cup; not even Aesculapius of Epidaurus could do it." The slave hearing this put the shards in his sack and went to the temple. On arrival he opened the sack and found the cup mended. He told the story to his master, who presented the cup to the god.

The lame Nicanor. As he sat wide awake a child stole his staff and ran; Nicanor rose and pursued him, and from that moment was cured.

Alcetas of Halice. He was blind and had a vision; the god seemed to open his eyes with his fingers and he saw the trees in the temple court. Day broke and he departed cured.

Heranus of Mytilene. This patient had no hair on his head, but much on his chin. Vexed by the ridicule of his neighbors, he incubated. The god anointed his head with a drug and made him have hair.

Not content with medical cures, the pillars relate instances of celestial surgery. A man from Torone drank a mixture of wine and honey into which his perfidious stepmother had put some leeches; his pain was so intense that he was obliged to visit the god, who opened his chest with a knife, took out the leeches, placed them in the patient's hands, sewed up the chest, and the Toronean was cured from that hour.

The Spartan girl Arete underwent an experience which does not befall everyone. She suffered from dropsy, and asked the god for relief. Aesculapius cut off her head, turned her upside down until the fluid ran out, and then replaced the head. As for Aristagora, she probably never stopped talking about her case. She had a worm in her belly, and slept in the temple of Troezen which was in her neighborhood. Aesculapius was absent at Epidaurus, but the priest had seen him work, and he cut off Aristagora's head. He was unable to put it on again, and in the morning plainly saw the head separated from the body. A messenger was sent to Epidaurus to consult the god. Aesculapius came, scolded his assistant, easily replaced her head, and opening her belly took out the worm and sewed her up again, and thenceforth she was healed.

Hermodius of Lampsacus was so feeble that he could not move. Aesculapius bade him stand up, walk outside the temple and bring back the largest stone he could find. He carried back a boulder which, as the inscription says, still lies upon the ground. It may be seen at Epidaurus today—mute testimony to ancient credulity.

Not all the Greeks could be fooled by such charlatanism, and in the sixth century B.C.—the period in which the wisdom of Zoroaster, Confucius, Buddha and Susruta illuminated the East—the Ionic philosophers looked at nature. In that early time there were already men who had outgrown the adult-infantilism of mankind, seeing the childishness of anthropomorphic polytheism, of the idea of creator and creation, of the dualistic dogma of god and the world, which views god not as the world but as outside of the world and as the maker of the world. In the presence of the Ionic philosophers, Olympian Zeus ceased to rattle his thunderbolts.

At the outposts of human knowledge, the first mind we meet is Thales—chief of the Seven Sages of Greece. We know little of the life of Thales of Miletus, except that on a narrow strip of land by the Aegean Sea, he became the father of science. By drawing angles and circles which he activated with theorems, he created geometry; by measuring the height of the pyramids by their shadows, he laid the base of physics; by predicting with accuracy an eclipse of the sun, he founded astronomy; by declaring that water is the origin of all things, he established Greek philosophy—Aristotle calls Thales the man who made the first attempt to establish, without myths, a physical Beginning. When Thales rubbed a piece of fossil resin and observed the amber attracting bits of cloth and feathers, he opened the story of electricity—and to this day children repeat the experiment of the great Ionian.

His friend Anaximander was the first evolutionist, teaching the transmutation of species, and that man himself developed from aquatic animals. He was the first who attempted to draw a map of the world. Anaximenes, who held the air to be the primary form of matter, infinite and in constant motion, believed in the eternity of matter. Xenophanes of Colophon, exiled from Ionia, brought philosophy to Elea in southern Italy. This Xenophanean fragment speaks volumes: "Yet men imagine gods to be born, and to have raiment and voice and body, like themselves. . . . Even so the gods of the Ethiopians are swarthy and flat-nosed, the gods of the Thracians are fair-haired and blue-eyed. . . . Even so Homer and Hesiod attributed to the gods all that is a shame and reproach among men—theft, adultery, deceit and other lawless acts. . . . Even so oxen, lions and horses, if they had hands wherewith to grave images, would fashion gods after their own shapes and make them bodies like to their own." Such men there were in the sixth century B.C.

To this period belongs the first physician of whom there is authentic information—Democedes of Croton, whose career occupies several lively pages of Herodotus. Democedes was not a scientific investigator like Alcmaeon, but a skilful practitioner serving various governments as a public physician; in attendance upon Polycrates, when that tyrant was duped, murdered and crucified in Asia, Democedes was taken prisoner. In spite of its extent, it seems that in those days no one could live in Asia without meeting Darius. During a hunt, while dismounting from his horse, Darius twisted his foot, the ball of the ankle-joint being dislocated from its socket; the leading physicians of Egypt, whom Darius kept near him, made conditions worse by their forcible wrenching, and by the eighth day his agony was intense. In this extremity the name of Democedes was mentioned: reduced to slavery, in chains and rags, Democedes was brought to Darius, who did not look any more regal than the wretched captive. It is difficult to appear majestic when your astralagus is out of place. The king asked the physician whether he knew anything about medicine, and Democedes said he did not, fearing that if he revealed his skill, he would never get back to Greece. Darius called for a whip, and Democedes confessed that his knowledge was not exact, but he had seen physicians work and knew a little. He applied Greek remedies and used gentleness instead of Egyptian violence, and the king was cured. Then the eunuchs conducted the doctor to the harem, telling the women that he saved the king's life. Each lady graciously gave him a vessel filled with staters, and the servant Sciton walked behind him, and collected a fortune by picking up the coins that fell to the floor.

The grateful Darius decided to impale the Egyptian physicians for being less skilful than a Greek, but Democedes begged the lives of his foreign colleagues and saved them. Democedes was given a fine house, and he ate at the king's table. Darius was ready to grant him every request, except what he most desired—permission to leave his service. "Mightily in favor with the king was Democedes," writes Herodotus and continues: "Not long after this, Atossa, Cyrus' daughter and Darius' wife, found a swelling growing on her breast, which broke and spread further. As long as it was but a small matter, she said nothing of it but hid it for shame; but presently growing worse, she sent for Democedes and showed it to him. He promised to cure her, but made her swear that she would requite him by granting whatsoever he requested of her; saying, that he would ask nothing shameful."

How Democedes, with the aid of Atossa, induced Darius to send a fleet against Greece; how he promised to act as the guide of the expedition; how he contrived to remove the steering gears from the ships and have the Persians arrested as spies as soon as they reached Grecian soil; how he escaped to Croton, and was pursued by the Persians who vowed the vengeance of Darius upon the town; how his countrymen protected Democedes who sent to his victimized patron the message that he was going to marry the daughter of Milon the wrestler—a name which Darius held in great honor—are matters which belong to intrigue rather than to investigation, and should be read in the unrivalled pages of Herodotus.

It is tempting to linger with the remarkable pioneers of the sixth century B.C.—even the mystic Pythagoras could not pass a blacksmith's shop, and hear the hammer on the anvil, without discovering a fundamental fact in physics—and yet this age was only the prelude to the chief epoch in the intellectual history of mankind. Many of the permanent names in art and literature, in philosophy and science, belong to the fifth century B.C. For all time to come, the test of culture will be our familiarity with these achievements, produced by a small group of people in the Classic Age of Greece. It is only necessary to mention the Parthenon of Phidias, the bronzes of Myron, the gold and ivory Hera of Polycletus, the vase-paintings of Euphronius, the Delphi frescoes of Polygnotus, the lyrics of Pindar, the dithyrambic fragments of Ion, the *Oresteia* of Aeschylus, the *Oedipus Rex* of Sophocles, the *Bacchae* of Euripides, the *Clouds* of Aristophanes, the *Kolakes* of Eupolis, the banter of Socrates, the *Dialogues* of Plato, the cosmical speculations of Anaxagoras, the astronomical discoveries of Meton, the paradoxes of the Eleatic Zeno, the dream-theories of Democritus, the anatomical researches of Empedocles, the general history of Herodotus, the Peloponnesian history of Thucydides, and the observations of Hippocrates, to realize the Hellenic bequest to human thought.

What we have salvaged from the legacy is imperishable, but we must never forget that only a small portion of the heritage has come down to us: many masterpieces have disappeared utterly, and only fragments remain of others—a piece of broken marble, or a few lines from a book that all antiquity venerated.

In the *Plutus* of Aristophanes occurs the first description of incubation—the act of sleeping in an Asklepion in order to be cured by the healing god—and a vulgar exposure of priestly quackery. The vase-painting of a Greek clinic, showing several patients surrounding a physician, and the kylix of Euphronius representing Achilles bandaging Patroclus, are landmarks in art and medicine. There are numerous medical sidelights in Plato, often of a humorous character. He was not a friend of the medical profession, though we owe to his *Gorgias* this splendid definition: "And I said of medicine, that this is an art which considers the constitution of the patient, and has principles of action and reasons in each case." It is difficult to realize that these ironic words about newfangled diseases occur in the Platonic *Dialogues:*

... men fill themselves with waters and winds, as if their bodies were a marsh, compelling the ingenious sons of Aesculapius to find more names for diseases, such as flatulence and catarrh; is not this, too, a disgrace?

Yes, he said, they do certainly give very strange and newfangled names to diseases.

Yes, I said, and I do not believe there were any such diseases in the days of Aesculapius; and this I infer from the circumstance that the hero Eurypylus, after he has been wounded in Homer, drinks a posset of Pramnian wine well besprinkled with barley-meal and grated cheese, which are certainly inflammatory, and yet the sons of Aesculapius who were at the Trojan war do not blame the damsel who gives him the drink, or rebuke Patroclus, who is treating his case.

Well, he said, that was surely an extraordinary drink to be given to a person in his condition.

Not so extraordinary, I replied, if you bear in mind that in former days, as is commonly said, before the time of Herodicus, the guild of Aesculapius did not practise our present system of medicine, which may be said to educate diseases. But Herodicus, being a trainer, and himself of a sickly constitution, by a combination of training and doctoring found out a way of torturing first and chiefly himself, and secondly the rest of the world.

How was that? he said.

By the invention of lingering death; for he had a mortal disease which he perpetually tended, and as recovery was out of the question, he passed his entire life as a valetudinarian; he could do nothing but attend upon himself, and he was in constant torment whenever he departed in anything from his usual regimen, and so dying hard, by the help of science he struggled on to old age.

The interview between the youthful Theaetetus and Socrates, as preserved by Plato, is droll and deathless:

Theaetetus: I can assure you, Socrates, that I have tried very often, when the report of questions asked by you was brought to me; but I can neither persuade myself that I have my answer to give, nor hear of any one who answers as you would have him; and I cannot shake off a feeling of anxiety.

Socrates: These are the pangs of labor, my dear Theaetetus; you have something within you which you are bringing to the birth.

Theaetetus: I do not know, Socrates; I only say what I feel.

Socrates: And did you never hear, simpleton, that I am the son of a midwife, brave and burly, whose name was Phaenarete?

Theaetetus: Yes, I have.

Socrates: And that I myself practise midwifery?

Theaetetus: No, never.

Socrates: Let me tell you that I do though, my friend; but you must not reveal the secret, as the world in general have not found me out, and therefore they only say of me, that I am the strangest of mortals, and drive men to their wits' end. Did you ever hear that too?

Theaetetus: Yes.

Socrates: Shall I tell you the reason?

Theaetetus: By all means.

Socrates: Bear in mind the whole business of the midwives, and then you will see my meaning better. No woman, as you are probably aware, who is still able to conceive and bear, attends other women, but only those who are past bearing.

Theaetetus: Yes, I know.

Socrates: The reason of this is said to be that Artemis—the goddess of childbirth—is not a mother, and she honors those who are like herself; but she could not allow the barren to be midwives, because human nature cannot know the mystery of an art without experience; and therefore she assigned this office to those who are too old to bear.

Theaetetus: I dare say.

Socrates: And I dare say, too, or rather I am absolutely certain, that the midwives know better than others who is pregnant and who is not?

Theaetetus: Very true.

Socrates: And by the use of potions and incantations they are able to arouse the pangs and to soothe them at will; they can make those bear who have a difficulty in bearing, and if they think fit, they can smother the embryo in the womb.

Theaetetus: They can.

Socrates: Did you ever remark that they are also most cunning matchmakers, and have a thorough knowledge of what unions are likely to produce a brave brood?

Theaetetus: No, never.

Socrates: Then let me tell you that this is their greatest pride, more than cutting the umbilical cord. And if you reflect, you will see that the same art which cultivates and gathers in the fruits of the earth, will be most likely to know in what soils the several plants or seeds should be deposited.

Theaetetus: Yes, the same art.

Socrates: And do you suppose that with women the case is otherwise?

Theaetetus: I should think not.

Socrates: Certainly not; but midwives are respectable women and have a character to lose, and they avoid this department of their profession, because they are afraid of being called procuresses, which is a name given to those who join together man and woman in an unlawful and unscientific way; and yet the true midwife is also the true and only matchmaker.

Theaetetus: Clearly.

Socrates: Such are the midwives, whose task is a very important one, but not so important as mine; for women do not bring into the world at one time real children, and at another time counterfeits which are with difficulty distinguished from them; if they did, then the discernment of the true and false birth would be the crowning achievement of the art of midwifery—you would think so?

Theaetetus: Indeed, I should.

Socrates: Well, my art of midwifery is in most respects like theirs; but differs in that I attend men and not women, and I look after their souls when they are in labor, and not after their bodies; and the triumph of my art is in thoroughly examining whether the thought which the mind of the young man is bringing to the birth, is a false idol or a noble and true birth. And like the midwives, I am barren, and the reproach which is often made against me, that I ask questions of others and have not the wit to answer them myself, is very just; the reason is, that the god compels me to be a midwife, but forbids me to bring forth. And therefore I am not myself at all wise, nor have I anything to show which is the invention or birth of my own soul, but those who converse with me profit. Some of them appear dull enough at first, but afterwards, as our acquaintance ripens, if the god is gracious to them, they all make astonishing progress; and this in the opinion of others as well as their own. It is quite clear that they had never learned anything from me; the many fine discoveries to which they cling are of their own making. But to me and the god they owe their delivery.

There is more of this dialogue, showing the method of Socrates—the method that finally led the old questioner to the law-courts. Unable to accept established beliefs without examination, he is accused of denying the gods of Athens and of corrupting the young—because he makes the sons wiser than their fathers. Five hundred men sit in judgment upon the barefoot citizen of the world. "Socrates is an atheist," declares Meletus —how often that cry was to echo down the ages against innovators!—and the majority vote for death. "The difficulty, O Athenians," replies Socrates, "is not to escape from death, but from guilt; for guilt is swifter than death, and runs faster. And

MEDICINE IN ANCIENT GREECE 45

I, being old and slow of foot, have been overtaken by death, the slower of the two. . . . It is now time that we depart, I to die, you to live; but which has the better destiny is unknown to all except the gods." It is obvious that the pot-bellied, snub-nosed philosopher will drink his hemlock like some rare wine. On the final day, near the setting of the sun, Socrates sits amid his disciples; a stranger, bringing a cup, enters the cell. "It is well my friend," says Socrates in his robust way, "but what is proper to do with it? for you are knowing in these affairs." The condemned man chaffs his executioner, but Plato's *Phaedo* must speak:

At the same time ending his discourse, he drank the poison with exceeding facility and alacrity. And thus far, indeed, the greater part of us were tolerably well able to refrain from weeping; but, when we saw him drinking, and that he had drunk it, we could no longer restrain our tears. From me, indeed, notwithstanding the violence which I employed in checking them, they flowed abundantly; so that, covering myself with my mantle, I deplored my misfortune. Crito, who was not able to restrain his tears, was compelled to rise before me. And Apollodorus, who, during the whole time prior to this, had not ceased from weeping, then wept aloud, and with great bitterness; so that he infected all who were present except Socrates.

Socrates, upon seeing this, exclaimed: What are you doing, excellent men? For, indeed, I principally sent away the women, lest they should produce a disturbance of this kind. For I have heard it is proper to die attended with propitious omens. Be quiet, therefore, and summon fortitude to your assistance. When we heard this we blushed, and restrained our tears. But he, when he found, during his walking, that his legs felt heavy, and had told us so, laid himself down in a supine position. At the same time, he who gave him the poison, touching him at intervals, considered his feet and legs. And, after he had vehemently pressed his foot, he asked him if he felt it. Socrates answered he did not. After this, he again pressed his thighs: and, thus ascending with his hand, he showed us that he was cold and stiff.

Socrates also touched himself, and said that when the poison reached his heart, he should then leave us. Now his lower belly was almost cold; when, uncovering himself (for he was covered) he said (which were his last words), Crito, we owe a cock to Aesculapius. Discharge this debt, therefore, for me, and don't neglect it. It shall be done (says Crito); but consider whether you have any other commands. To this inquiry of Crito he made no reply; but shortly after moved himself, and the man covered him. And Socrates fixed his eyes. Which, when Crito perceived, he closed his mouth and eyes. This was the end. . . .

The *History* of Herodotus, perhaps the most delightful book ever written, is the source of our knowledge of early medicine. Herodotus wrote with such ease that he has been accused of being uncritical, but modern scholarship confirms his trustworthiness. As the first of historians, it was necessary for him to rely much on hearsay instead of written authorities, but he is then careful to inform the reader: "for my part I do not believe the tale, but it is told." The following account of Babylonian customs, condensed from the first book, is characteristic of his narrative:

The wisest of these customs in my judgment is this: once a year in every village all the maidens as they come to marriageable age were collected and brought together into one place, with a crowd of men standing round. Then a crier would stand up and offer them for sale one by one, first the fairest of all; and then when she had fetched a great price he put up for sale the next comeliest, selling all the maidens as lawful wives. Rich men of Assyria who desired to marry would outbid each other for the fairest; the commonalty, who desired to marry and cared nothing for beauty, could take the ill-favoured damsels and the money therewith; for when the crier had sold all the comeliest, he would put her up that was least beautiful, or crippled, and offer her to whosoever would take her to wife for the least sum, till she fell to him who promised to accept least; the money came from the sale of the comely damsels, and so they paid the dowry of the ill-favored and the crippled. . . . And if the two could not agree, it was a law that the money be returned. Men might also come from other villages to buy if they so desired. This then was their best custom; but it does not continue at this time.

I now come to the next wisest of their customs: having no use for physicians, they carry the sick into the market-place; then those who have been afflicted themselves by the same ill as the sick man's, or seen others in like case, come near and advise him about his disease and comfort him, telling him by what means they have themselves recovered of it or seen others so recover. None may pass by the sick man without speaking and asking what is his sickness.

The worst Babylonian custom is that which compels every woman of the land once in her life to sit in the temple of love and have intercourse with some stranger . . . the men pass and make their choice. It matters not what be the sum of money; the woman will never refuse, for that were a sin, the money being by this act made sacred. After their intercourse she has made herself holy in the sight of the goddess and goes away to her home; and thereafter there is no bribe however great that will get her. So then the women that are fair and tall are soon free to depart, but the uncomely have long to wait because they cannot fulfil the law; for some of them remain for three years, or four. There is a custom like to this in some parts of Cyprus.

In the second book, Herodotus writes: "Now for the stories which I heard about the gods, I am not desirous to relate them; for I hold that no man knows about the gods more than another." If these simple words of the first historian had been heeded, the story of mankind would have been different. But in every land and age there have been men who claimed to have special knowledge about the gods, and the result has been written in blood.

Thucydides of the majestic prose, famed for his impartiality, investigated truth with such assiduity that his methods are wholly scientific. "So averse to taking pains are most men in the search for the truth," he says, "and so prone are they to turn to what lies ready at hand. And it may well be that the absence of the fabulous from my narrative will seem less pleasing to the ear; but whoever shall wish to have a clear view both of the events which have happened and of those which will some day, in all human probability, happen again in the same or a similar way—for these to adjudge my history profitable will be enough for me. And, indeed, it has been composed, not as a prize-essay to be heard for the moment, but as a possession for all time." These Periclean words reveal his insight into human nature: "for the dead are always praised—and even were you to attain to surpassing virtue, hardly would you be judged, I will not say their equals, but even a little inferior. For there is the envy of the living on account of rivalry, but that which has been removed from our path is honored with a good-will that knows no antagonism." His magnificent description of the plague of Athens is one of the earliest of medical classics, and ranks Thucydides as the first historian of epidemiology. It is most remarkable, that prior to any medical author, Thucydides wrote about infection, resistance and immunity.

In the 80th Olympiad, at about the same time that Thucydides was born in Athens—perhaps in the very year, 460 B.C.—Hippocrates was born at Cos, the little sea-girt island of limestone and wild olive which likewise mothered the poet Philetas and the painter Apelles. Aside from two inconsequential references by Plato, Hippocrates is not mentioned by any of his great contemporaries, and he had no Plutarch. His earliest biographers lived centuries after his time, and their accounts are trivial and mythical.

The incendiary remark that Hippocrates burned the temple of Cos or the library of Cnidos to conceal his plagiarisms, is as probable as the genealogical note that he was a direct descendant of Aesculapius. The story that Hippocrates met a girl one morning and addressed her as maiden, and met her later in the day and greeted her as woman, explaining to his disciples that he could tell by the change in her voice or the bulge of her neck that she was no longer a maiden, will hardly be credited by modern gynecologists who feel that a diagnosis of virginity is not so easy. The statement that Hippocrates halted the plague of Athens by lighting fires throughout the city, is contradicted by Thucydides' testimony that the physicians accomplished nothing. The belief that Hippocrates disdained an invitation to visit Persia during an epidemic, refusing to render aid to an enemy of his country, is obviously the invention of a Greek patriot. The incident of the Abderitans summoning Hippocrates to cure the madness of the laughing philosopher because he dissected animals, and the physician's reply, "Democritus is the wisest man among you," is too epigrammatic to be historical. The anecdote that he was asked to treat the Macedonian Perdiccas for consumption, and found the young ruler lovesick over his father's mistress, is similar to tales that have been told of various other physicians—stepmothers in antiquity must have been very attractive. The tradition that upon his tomb a swarm of bees settled, whose honey was effective in the thrush of children, is a sweet tale belonging to poesy and not to physic. Even the fact that the tomb was pointed out to travelers does not make it true. From the cradle to the grave, the life of the father of medicine is invested with legends; we know nothing about Hippocrates except that he was the greatest of physicians.

When we come to the writings of Hippocrates, our knowledge is equally dubious. The recent suggestion, that the Hippocratic collection represents the remains of the medical library of Cos, is gaining acceptance. Whatever view is taken—"according to Hippocrates," or "Hippocrates wrote," or "Hippocrates observed," means a contributor to the Corpus Hippocraticum. The ancient physicians, like the philosophers, wandered from city to city, studying and practising, and for these traveling physicians Hippocrates wrote *Airs, Waters, Places*, which is the first treatise on public health, medical geography, climatology, physiotherapy and balneology. It contains the earliest observations on urinary calculi, and the first account—a masterly one—of sexual impotence.

The treatise *On the Prognostics* will always be famous for the Hippocratic description of the signs of approaching death which we still call *facies Hippocratica:* nose sharp, eyes hollow, temples sunken, ears cold and contracted with their lobes turned outwards, skin tense and parched, face discolored, eyelids livid, mouth open, lips loose and blanched. There are valuable discussions of pain, fever, headache, pus and urine. The observation

—"A swelling in the hypochondrium [the abdominal region beneath the floating ribs] that is hard and painful is very bad, provided it occupies the whole hypochondrium; but if it be on either side, it is less dangerous when on the left"—is interesting as the first reference to appendicitis.

Herodicus, the teacher of Hippocrates, was a faddist; he believed in gymnastics in all circumstances, treating his feverish patients by making them indulge in promenades and violent wrestling. In *Regimen in Acute Diseases,* Hippocrates discarded his teacher. The keynote of Hippocratism is gentleness: no harsh measures, no drastic drugs, no unnecessary meddlesomeness. Venesection was performed when indicated, and the bowels were opened with enemas and suppositories. The chief remedies were barley gruel, hydromel, oxymel, and wine. The patient was made as comfortable as possible, and even his fussiness was respected. With faith in the restorative forces of the organism—in the healing power of nature—the master of the bedside waited, and watched as he waited. He looked at pneumonia and pleurisy, he knew pulmonary tuberculosis, and saw malaria in all its forms.

The *Epidemics* contain the first scientific case-histories, and they are much like the case-histories that we write on hospital-charts today and clip on the patient's bed. He describes the woman who lay sick by the Liars' Market, after a painful delivery; day by day, he puts down the symptoms as they occur; on the thirteenth day she vomited black, fetid, copious matters; rigor; later lost her speech; on the fourteenth day, nosebleed, then death. He tells of Silenus, who lived on Broadway: after fatigue, drinking and unseasonable exercise, he complained of pains in the loins, with heaviness in the head and tightness in the neck; acute fever on the second day; on the third, no power of restraining himself, but singing and much rambling laughter; same symptoms on the fourth; lucid intervals on the fifth; nothing passed from the bowels and urine suppressed on the seventh; on the eighth day, copious discharge after slight stimulus, but cold sweat all over, fitful sleep, coma and speechlessness; the symptoms continue, and on the eleventh day the coma becomes death.

Hippocrates writes down these fatal terminations without the faintest attempt at concealment. There is not the slightest inclination to emphasize his successes.

In writing of the consumptives, he says, "Many, and, in fact, the most of them, died; and of those confined to bed, I do not know if a single individual survived for any considerable time." Of the forty-two case-histories detailed in *Epidemics*, twenty-five end in death. If we compare these case-histories with the miraculous cures acclaimed at the temple of Epidaurus, both of which date from about the same period, it is obvious that there is no relationship between the priestly and secular medicine of Greece. If, as some assert, Hippocratism originated at the shrine of Aesculapius, it retained no trace of its celestial heredity. The scientist reports his results without emotion, and even in antiquity he was blamed for his lofty detachment, and his method was called a meditation on death. Today we regard those forty-two cases—with their sixty per cent mortality—as the foundation of clinical medicine; looking backward, we see that those ages which turned away from Hippocratism were the dark ages of medicine, and those ages which were guided by his fundamental principles were on the path that has led to modern medicine.

The essay on *The Sacred Disease* begins: "I am about to discuss the disease called sacred. It is not, in my opinion, any more divine or more sacred than other diseases, but has a natural cause, and its supposed divine origin is due to men's inexperience, and to their wonder at its peculiar character." With these opening words of his brief treatise on epilepsy, Hippocrates expels the gods from medicine. It was simply and quietly done, but marks the greatest revolution in the history of medicine. It enthroned the doctrine of the uniformity of nature, and Greek medicine became a science.

The compendium on *Dentition*, which consists of thirty-two paragraphs, may be regarded as the first treatise on the diseases of children. It exhibits, in condensed form, an extensive knowledge of the subject. The surgical books of Hippocrates, as *In-*

juries of the Head, Fractures, and *Articulations,* are highly technical, and of the first rank. Whether he discusses a compound fracture of the thigh-bone or a finger-joint dislocation, all subsequent surgery has profited by his genius. These works were neglected for centuries, as the surgeons were unable to follow the precepts or understand the operations.

The tract entitled *Physician* is devoted to rules of medical conduct: "The dignity of a physician requires that he should look healthy, and as plump as nature intended him to be; for the common crowd consider those who are not of this excellent bodily condition to be unable to take care of others. Then he must be clean in person, well dressed, and anointed with sweet-smelling unguents that are not in any way suspicious. This, in fact, is pleasing to patients. The prudent man must also be careful of certain moral considerations—not only to be silent, but also of a great regularity of life, since thereby his reputation will be greatly enhanced; he must be a gentleman in character, and being this he must be grave and kind to all. . . . In every social relation he will be fair, for fairness must be of great service. The intimacy also between physician and patient is close. Patients in fact put themselves into the hands of their physician, and at every moment he meets women, maidens and possessions very precious indeed. So towards all these self-control must be used. Such then should the physician be, both in body and in soul."

The *Aphorisms* have given rise to a library of commentaries. Hippocrates was a master of conciseness and often one of his lines has produced volumes of glossary. The Aphorisms are really the essence of the therapeutics and ethics of medicine. It would be impossible to estimate how frequently physicians of all lands and of all ages have quoted in their works the most famous of all the aphorisms: "Life is short, and the Art long: the occasion fleeting; experience fallacious, and judgment difficult. The physician must not only be prepared to do what is right himself, but also to make the patient, the attendants, and externals co-operate."

Equally remarkable is the treatise called *Precepts* in which the Hippocratic writer advises the physician not to begin by discussing fees and suggests that it is better to reproach a patient who has been saved, and refuses to pay, than to extort money from those who are at death's door. We detect a rare note of indignation as he continues: "For, in heaven's name, who that is a brotherly physician practises with such hardness of heart as not at the beginning to conduct a preliminary examination of every illness and prescribe what will help towards a cure, to heal the patient and not to overlook the reward, to say nothing of the desire that makes a man ready to learn? . . . Sometimes give your services for nothing, calling to mind a previous benefaction or present satisfaction. And if there be an opportunity of serving a stranger in financial straits, give full assistance to all such. *For where there is love of man, there is also love of the art.* For some patients, though conscious that their condition is perilous, recover their health simply through their contentment with the goodness of the physician. And it is well to superintend the sick to make them well, to care for the healthy to keep them well, but also to care for one's own self, so as to observe what is seemly."

Lacking the aids which we now deem essential, without any conception of contagion, or any knowledge of the pulse—in which respect he was behind the old Egyptian physicians—Hippocrates raised the art of medicine to heights which it has not attained again until recent times. For over two thousand years, Medicine, often straying after false speculations and lost in superstitions, has found the beacon of Hippocratism shining over the true path. Discovery after discovery only serves to confirm the truth of his method, for Hippocratic medicine, being essentially scientific medicine, is for all time. Within recent years his books have ceased to be used as texts in the schools, but he teaches the entire profession: the physicians of all nations ask for no other heritage than to be known as the children of Hippocrates.

We may sum up this epoch by saying that medicine, in the

enlightened sense of the term, originated in the Periclean age with Hippocrates. Medicine existed for centuries before him, and Hippocrates himself wrote a treatise entitled *On Ancient Medicine*, but we properly call him the Father of Medicine for the following reasons: By demonstrating that disease was not dependent upon supernatural causes, Hippocrates emancipated medicine from the gods; by his case-histories and bedside teaching, he founded clinical medicine; by his insistence, "Nature heals; the physician is only nature's assistant," he gave to medical practice its cardinal doctrine of *vis medicatrix naturae;* by his critical attitude toward potent drugs, he inaugurated an era in pharmacology; by discarding polypharmacy and drastic measures, and treating his patients with such "modern" procedures as proper diet, fresh air, change of climate and physiotherapy, he made medicine workable; by reporting his failures as well as his successes in treatment, he set a standard for all physicians to follow; by the principles in the *Hippocratic Oath*, he gave medicine its ethical basis.

There is much in the Hippocratic Oath that is puzzling to us, but it is still recited on the momentous day when the medical student receives his doctorate:

I swear by Apollo the physician, and Aesculapius, and Hygeia, and Panacea, and all the gods and goddesses, that, according to my ability and judgment, I will keep this Oath and this stipulation—to reckon him who taught me this Art equally dear to me as my parents, to share my substance with him, and relieve his necessities if required; to look upon his offspring in the same footing as my own brothers, and to teach them this art, if they shall wish to learn it, without fee or stipulation; and that by precept, lecture, and every other mode of instruction I will impart a knowledge of the Art to my own sons, and those of my teachers, and to disciples bound by a stipulation and oath according to the law of medicine, but to none others. I will follow that system of regimen which, according to my ability and judgment, I consider for the benefit of my patients, and abstain from whatever is deleterious and mischievous.

I will give no deadly medicine to any one if asked, nor suggest any such counsel; and in like manner I will not give to a woman a pessary to produce abortion.

With purity and with holiness I will pass my life and practise my Art. I will not use the knife, not even to cut persons laboring under the stone, but will leave this to be done by men who are practitioners of this work. Into whatever houses I enter, I will go into them for the benefit of the sick, and will abstain from every voluntary act of mischief and corruption; and, further, from the seduction of females or males, of freemen and slaves. Whatever, in connection with my professional practice or not in connection with it, I see or hear in the life of men which ought not to be spoken of abroad, I will not divulge, as reckoning that all such should be kept secret. While I continue to keep this Oath unviolated, may it be granted to me to enjoy life and the practice of the art, respected by all men, in all times! But should I trespass and violate this Oath, may the reverse be my lot!

If we accept 370 B.C. as the date of Hippocrates' death, then Aristotle was fourteen years of age at that time. Born in tiny Stagira on the Strymonic Gulf, at the edge of the Grecian world, he became the central figure of Greece. His father Nicomachus was physician to the second Amyntas, and the day came when a mightier king of Macedon—dynamic Pan-Hellenic Philip—summoned Aristotle to his court, not to heal, but to teach. Aristotle, as Plutarch tells us, was " the most famous and learned of philosophers," and with the passing centuries his reputation for wisdom was so great that it gave rise to the Aristotle-Phyllis legend.

According to the tale, Aristotle's pupil, the world-conquering Alexander, was himself enslaved by the exotic charms of the Indian maiden Phyllis. In the delights of the marriage-bed, the youthful ruler forgot his kingdoms and even neglected to annex others. Now Phyllis had been fed on the venom of serpents in the hope that Alexander would absorb the poison and die. The all-seeing Aristotle exposed the plot, whereupon Alexander, prudent for once, insisted on separate beds.

Phyllis was very angry, and decided to punish Aristotle by making him fall in love with her. She succeeded perfectly, and as proof of his devotion Aristotle offered to do anything she asked. She commanded him to get down on all fours, she put a bridle in his mouth, placed a saddle on his back, then mounting the philosopher she whipped him as he rode her around. Of course she had requested Alexander to watch the proceeding secretly, and Alexander was certainly surprised. He asked Aristotle for an explanation of his inconsistency, and received the answer: "If a woman can make such a fool of a man of my age and wisdom, is she not even more dangerous for those who are younger and less wise? To my precept I have added an example, and you may profit by both." Aristotle, as the horse of Phyllis, appealed to various artists; paintings, engravings, ivories and caskets tell the story of the philosopher's humiliation. Yet it is really a significant tribute to him, for it is nothing if an ordinary man succumbs, and legend chose Aristotle as Phyllis' victim because of his unequaled learning.

Had it been chronologically possible for Aristotle to have spent one year with Hippocrates, it would have done more for him than the twenty years he spent with Plato. For a man who was to devote his life to science, Plato was the worst teacher possible. The world owes an immense debt to Plato, but not as an interpreter of nature. Socrates did not concern himself with natural science, but he bubbled over with common sense, and his eternal questioning was the opening strain of the experimental method by which science has gained her victories. Plato did not ask questions—he answered them with a rhapsodizing dogmatism which was definitely unscientific. Aristotle, as a Platonist, was primarily a metaphysician; as an Hippocratist, he would have been primarily a scientist. We can forgive the many colossal errors of Aristotle only because of his many epoch-making observations.

Opposed to Aristophanes, who speaks in one of his plays of concussion of the brain; to Hippocrates, who recognized the primacy of the brain; and to the pre-Hippocratic physician Alcmaeon, who regarded the brain as the organ of thought, Aristotle believed the object of the brain was to secrete humors to cool the overheated heart. He wrote copiously on procreation, and nearly all that he remarked was incorrect, except the obvious fact that the semen, even in negroes, is white. He described five hundred species of animals, and since he dissected many of them, it is odd that he could not tell an artery from a vein. His account of the crocodile is borrowed from Herodotus, but the Halicarnassan nightingale—as Christodorus of Thebes called the first historian—was not a naturalist. Aristotle's certainty that fleas arise from filth, and that plant-lice are born from the dew which falls upon vegetation, was a biologic calamity. After reading interminable Aristotelian speculations, we sigh for a single experiment, especially when we find him giving credence to fables that some of his forerunners would have scorned. We are on the point of criticising him for such shortcomings, but then we remember that the history of morphology begins with the name of Aristotle.

Aristotle is the Father of Biology, though there were famous biologists before his time, and in the well-known passage of his *History of Animals,* in which he describes the mating of the octopus, he refers to his predecessors or contemporaries: "The octopus, the sepia and the calamary, have sexual intercourse all in the same way; that is to say, they unite at the mouth by an interlacing of their tentacles. When, then, the octopus rests its so-called head against the ground and spreads abroad its tentacles, the other sex fits into the outspreading of these tentacles, and the two sexes then bring their suckers into mutual connection. Some assert that the male has a kind of penis in one of his tentacles, the one in which are the largest suckers; and they further assert that the organ is tendinous in character, growing attached right up to the middle of the tentacle, and that the latter enables it to enter the nostril or funnel of the female."

In this same work, Aristotle devotes considerable space to bees, making the famous observation: "The little bees are more industrious than the big ones; gaudy and showy bees, like gaudy and showy women, are good for nothing." Such statements as "birds which are armed with spurs are never armed with lacerating claws; insects which bear a sting in the head are always two-winged, but insects which bear their sting behind are four-winged," show his gift for synthesis. His description of the placental development of the dog-fish, like many other of his observations, was not confirmed until recent times. We still separate fish into cartilaginous and bony, and divide animals into vertebrates and invertebrates, as Aristotle taught us to do.

How near he came to the general conception of evolution is apparent from these passages:

> Nature passes from lifeless objects to animals in such unbroken sequence, interposing between them beings which live and yet are not animals, that scarcely any difference seems to exist between two neighbouring groups owing to their close proximity. . . .
>
> In regard to sensibility, some animals give no indication whatsoever of it, whilst others indicate it but indistinctly. Further, the substance of some of these intermediate creatures is flesh-like, as is the case with the so-called Tethya and the Acalephae but the sponge is in every respect like a vegetable. And so throughout the entire animal scale there is a graduated differentiation in amount of vitality and in capacity for motion. A similar statement holds good with regard to habits of life. Thus, of plants that spring from seed, the one function seems to be the reproduction of their own particular species, and the sphere of action with certain animals is similarly limited. The faculty of reproduction, then, is common to all alike. If sensibility be superadded, then their lives will differ from one another in respect to sexual intercourse and also in regard to modes of parturition and ways of rearing their young. Some animals, like plants, simply procreate their own species at definite seasons; other animals busy themselves also in procuring food for their young, and after they are reared quit them and have no further dealings with them; other animals are more intelligent and endowed with memory, and they live with their offspring for a longer period and on a more social footing.

Aristotle's observations on the development of the chick were sufficiently important to create the beginning of embryology, although he did not have even a lens to aid him. As a result of his dissection of various animals, he created comparative anatomy. Aside from his work in logic, literature and philosophy, there is practically no field of science in which he did not blaze a trail—mechanics, physics, mathematics, astronomy, meteorology, geography, chemistry, botany, zoölogy, physiology and psychology—and in more than one of the paths he opened, there were no other footsteps for centuries.

Socrates could stand all day on one corner, Plato sat long and meditated, but Aristotle was so mobile that he walked as he lectured to his students at the Lyceum. That short body on its spindle legs, goaded on by the restless intellect, could seldom be still. It is doubtful if he wrote the books which appear under his name; some he dictated, and others seem to be collections of notes taken by his pupils; this "note-book theory" would also help to explain the juxtaposition of great descriptions and gross mistakes—students may misunderstand or misinterpret. Because of Aristotle's habit of walking among the Athenian youths as he talked to them, his disciples were known as peripatetics.

Aristotle's pupil, the physician Menon, wrote a history of medicine, and his feeding experiments are the first on record; the two most celebrated peripatetics were Theophrastus of Lesbos, and the mathematician and historian of science, Eudemus of Rhodes. That pedantic yet interesting grammarian, Aulus Gellius, whose *Attic Nights* are full of medical matters, refers to Aristotle as "a man skilled in all human knowledge"; in his thirteenth book, he relates that when Aristotle reached his sixty-second year, he was so sickly and weak of body that he realized his work would soon be over. Claiming that the domestic wines were too harsh for him, he asked for some foreign brands: testing the Rhodian, he said, "This is truly a sound and pleasant wine"; then tasting the Lesbian, added, "but this is sweeter." When he said this, continues Aulus Gellius, no one doubted that gracefully, and at the same time tactfully, he had by these words chosen his successor, not his wine.

We doubt this diplomacy, but Theophrastus indeed became Aristotle's successor, and like his master, took all knowledge for his province. Theophrastus was the first mineralogist and geologist, and if certain passages in his works are not interpolations, he was the first Greek to study the Romans and Jews.

Theophrastus is the most original figure in botanical history, and although a physician he was purely a scientific botanist, and did not study plants from the standpoint of therapy. Many of the ancient physicians acquired their knowledge by traveling in various countries, but as Theophrastus had 2,000 students to look after, he remained in Athens—in the library and the garden which his friend Aristotle had left him. Theophrastus was the Hippocrates of the vegetable kingdom: from chaos he created a science. In this garden the science of botany was born. In his will, Theophrastus asked to be buried in the garden in which he had labored for over half a century, but he charged his friends not to be at any superfluous expense either upon his funeral or his tomb. He left the garden, walks and adjoining houses to his friends, to be enjoyed by them in common as a sacred place, so that those who were interested in learning and philosophy would be able to visit one another familiarly and informally, and discourse together like comrades.

Diogenes Laërtius, of whose life we know nothing except that he devoted it to writing the lives of the Greek sages, informs us that when Theophrastus died, "the whole population of Athens, honoring him greatly, followed him to the grave." Not Theophrastus alone, but the classic period of Greek science, passed away in the third century B.C. The Greek genius, wearied at last, paused in its flight. Hellas became a memory, but a memory to which mankind returns, to drink again of the Pierian spring. The centuries can never exhaust that source: the more we take, the more remains. Even in this Machine Age, despite the false gods we worship, when we wish to bestow the highest possible praise upon an art and method and individual, we say they are Greek.

IV

GREEK MEDICINE IN ALEXANDRIA

"WELL, then," says the biographer of Alexander, "as a place where master and pupil could labor and study, Philip assigned them the precinct of the nymphs near Mieza, where to this day the visitor is shown the stone seats and shady walks of Aristotle. . . . Moreover, in my opinion Alexander's love of the art of healing was inculcated in him by Aristotle preëminently. For Alexander was not only fond of the theory of medicine, but actually came to the aid of his friends when they were sick, and prescribed for them certain treatments aand regimens, as one can gather from his letters."

We hesitate to disagree with Plutarch, but the seven years Aristotle spent with Alexander were wasted on Alexander. His real teacher was his terrible mother Olympias, who had his father assassinated, tortured and killed men, and murdered a woman and her infant by dragging them slowly over a bronze vessel filled with fire. From this mother Alexander learned that the people have no rights, and a hundred Aristotles could not have tamed him. Before he reached his majority, as heedlessly as a boy sets his foot upon an ant-hill, he began his world-conquering career, wiping out ancient cities, scattering races and selling whole populations into slavery. Fearless and high-spirited, ever at the head of his troops, the first to plunge into a stream or leap a ditch or scale a wall, Alexander was irresistible. His victories were unparalleled, and Europe, Africa and Asia lay in his youthful hands.

Along the Nile he fought no battles, for Egypt, enslaved by a Persian madman, hailed Alexander as an emancipator. But in Egypt, Alexander also lost his reason. Vague whisperings of Olympias, hitherto unregarded, were now remembered: he was not really the son of Philip, for Zeus Ammon in the form of a serpent had shared his mother's couch, and Alexander was the offspring of this embrace. Superstitious, in dread of omens—he was badly frightened when his pet ass kicked a fine lion to death —surrounded by soothsayers, he crossed the desert to consult the Egyptian priests, and was astonished to hear himself addressed, O son of Zeus. Alexander enriched the priests—gifts which they had anticipated—and thereafter demanded to be adored as a divinity, although at times he suffered from diarrhea. In saner moments he admitted he was human, saying that sleep and sexual intercourse, more than anything else, made him feel he was mortal. Apelles, foremost of painters, depicted Alexander holding the thunderbolts, but during a great peal of thunder which terrified all, Anaxarchus asked Alexander: "Couldst thou, the son of Zeus, thunder like that?" Instead of rebuking the philosopher, Alexander smiled. On another occasion Anaxarchus pointed to Alexander's wounded finger with the remark, "Behold the blood of a mortal, not of a god."

Capricious and conceited, Alexander the Great was utterly unreliable. His closest associates could not foretell what would arouse his fury or his laughter. With his own hands, in wine or in frenzy, he destroyed friend, companion and faithful follower, and his subsequent loud lamentations did not prevent recurrences. At times fair, generous and noble, at other times he was treacherous and cruel. He cannot be blamed for being suspicious of his attendants, yet on receiving warning that his physician, Philip the Acarnanian, was about to poison him, he placed the letter under his pillow, and as the unsuspecting physician entered the royal chamber with the medicine, Alexander gave him the letter. "It was an amazing sight," says the incomparable Plutarch, "and one well worthy of the stage—the one reading the letter, the other drinking the medicine, and then both together turning their eyes upon one another." It was the letter, and not the medicine that was poisoned, and Alexander recovered. But this tale recalls another: the flatterer Hephaestion, being sick with fever, was instructed by the physician Glaucus to be temperate in his diet; when the physician went off to the theater —Alexander had imported three thousand artists from Greece— Hephaestion sat down to table, and feasted and drank heavily. The fool killed himself, and Alexander expressed his sorrow by slaughtering men wholesale, by cutting off the tails of all his mules, and by crucifying the physician.

Because of such things the life of Alexander makes depressing reading, despite its daring and unexampled splendor, despite even its glimmerings of internationalism: Alexander married the daughter of Darius, and induced the Greeks to take Persian brides—the wedding of Europe and Asia. Yet if he had any purpose in view, except to increase his own power and glory, it was lost in the intoxication of blood. Wherever he sailed or marched, he carried death with him, and young Lucan spoke truly of young Alexander: "Goaded by the impulse of destiny, he rushed through the peoples of Asia, mowing down mankind; he defiled distant rivers, the Euphrates and the Ganges, with Persian and Indian blood; he was a pestilence to earth, a thunderbolt that struck all peoples alike, a comet of disaster to mankind."

He had the curiosity of a child who is always ready to see something new or odd, but this must not be translated into scientific interest. Pliny exaggerated—which was easy enough for Pliny—when he wrote: "Alexander the Great, fired by desire to learn of the natures of animals, entrusted the prosecution of this design to Aristotle. . . . For this end he placed at his disposal some thousands of men in every part of Asia and Greece, and among them hunters, fowlers, fishers, park-keepers, herdsmen, bee-wards, as well as keepers of fish-ponds and aviaries in order that no creature might escape his notice. Through the information thus collected he was able to compose some fifty volumes." Alexander in oriental costume, executing Aristotle's relative, the upright philosopher and historian, Callisthenes—because he scorned his deification—had indeed forgotten his tutor. Theophrastus eulogized his martyred friend, and Seneca declared that the death of Callisthenes constituted the eternal crime of Alexander. It is significant that in the copious writings of Aristotle, there is no line in praise of Alexander.

Since Alexander did everything both ways, he was not only a destroyer but a builder of cities. Characteristically, one city was named after his dog, another after his horse, and one after himself. According to the tradition, while the site for the new city was being discussed, Alexander had a dream in which an old man with hoary locks quoted from the *Odyssey:*

> Now there is an island in the much-dashing sea,
> In front of Egypt; Pharos is what men call it.

Hastening to Pharos, Alexander exclaimed that Homer was a great architect, and the ground beneath his feet became Alexandria. A long causeway later joined this island to the mainland, but Alexander did not pass through his city again until nine years later, and then he was dead. He died in Babylon, as the result of a prolonged debauch—there was suspicion of poisoning, among those accused of instigating the deed being Aristotle—and the body of the young conqueror was brought back for burial in Alexandria.

At once that colossal artifice, the empire of Alexander, collapsed; his bewildered army was likened to a blinded Cyclops; his generals carved kingdoms for themselves, and butchered each other without shame; so none might be successor of the great adventurer, Cassander killed Alexander's mother, wife, natural child and legitimate son. Cassander, when he first came to Babylon and saw the Asiatics prostrating themselves before the Macedonian god, laughed uproariously until the offended Alexander seized him with both hands and dashed his head against the wall. Without restraint, Cassander could now laugh at the dead lion whose progeny he destroyed. The world-dominions of Alexander, gained by the sword, fell to pieces beneath the daggers of assassins.

Alexander's chief monument is the city he founded and forgot—Alexandria. In the division of the spoils, the shrewdest of his generals, Ptolemy Soter, possessed himself of Egypt. He had been conspicuous in the conquest of Afghanistan and India, and wedded a Persian princess at Alexander's desire. The Ptolemies became so intimately identified with Egypt, that we are apt to forget they were Macedonians. We read of the Egyptian dark-skinned Cleopatra: we know little about her skin, but we do know she did not have a drop of Egyptian blood in her. The Ptolemies were extremely consanguineous, and married only each other. As for the first Ptolemy, according to contemporary gossip he was the half-brother of Alexander; if not, he could have been, for Ptolemy's mother had been the mistress of Alexander's father. Macedon was a part of the Hellenic world, but geographically it stood on the outskirts of Greece, and culturally was admittedly barbaric—hence its sensitiveness to Greek opinion. Ptolemy, as a Macedonian, ran true to tradition: since triumphant Macedonia always paid intellectual homage to Athens, Ptolemy began transforming Alexandria into a second Athens.

His successor, Ptolemy Philadelphus, of frail physique, but equally enthusiastic over his various mistresses and the glory of Hellenic culture, actually made Egypt's capital the center of Greek learning and the playground of the world. The early Ptolemies were noted for their collections of books and women; the finest houses in the town were owned by courtesans, and when the rhetorician Dio Chrysostom sat down to describe immorality in Alexandria, he had abundant data. The third of the line, Ptolemy Euergetes, confiscated every book that tourists brought to Egypt—returning to the owner a copy of the work—and he secured, by purchase or trickery, the original manuscripts of the classics from the Athenian archives.

When a king is the librarian of his nation, the results are astonishing. Moreover, the Ptolemies monopolized the manufacture of papyrus-paper for which all Greece clamored. The Alexandrian Library grew until it contained three-fourths of a million papyrus-rolls. Not nearly so many volumes had been written at that time, and it has been conjectured that many of these papyri were duplicates which were sold to individuals or to smaller libraries outside of Egypt—thus the Ptolemies were the first international publishers. Of course the scholars of all nations made their home in the Alexandrian Library, and the Ptolemies gave them dinners which are still famous. The first editions of Homer, Hippocrates and Aristotle were edited at Alexandria—Aristotle's private library was believed to be the nucleus of the Alexandrian Library. The Ptolemies held conferences with Egyptian priests, and welcomed Buddhists from India. There were more Jews in Alexandria than in Jerusalem, and since they were forgetting their Aramaic, seventy Alexandrian Jews translated the Scriptures into Greek. Scientists, physicians, philosophers, poets, philologists, geographers, chronologists, bibliographers, grammarians—and many charlatans—found a haven in Alexandria. The catalogue of the library, compiled in 120 books by Callimachus, formed the basis of a history of Greek literature.

A visitor to Alexandria, conducted through the library buildings by Zenodotus or Apollonius, or their assistants, walking through the lofty halls embellished with the statues of famous men, passing the students and countless scribes at work amid the unending papyri, must have been amazed to learn that there was still more to see—the Alexandrian Library was only a part of the Alexandrian Museum. There had never been anything like it before. It was not a Museum as we employ the term, but a university which at one time enrolled fourteen thousand matriculants. The lecture-halls for the well-paid professors and the eager students were supplemented with extensive gardens for botanists, menageries for zoölogists, observatories for astronomers, laboratories for chemists and physicists, while the anatomical school for physicians was equipped with dissecting-rooms. Evidently didactic instruction was coördinated with practical demonstration, and the first modern university is the University of Alexandria, established in the fourth century B.C.

Anatomy and physiology, the first of the basic and experimental sciences born of medicine, were cradled in Alexandria —but drew their sustenance not from Egypt, but from Greece. During the centuries that this medical school flourished, it was unrivaled. "It is sufficient as a recommendation," wrote Ammianus Marcellinus, "for any medical man to be able to say that he was educated at Alexandria." Several of these pupils acquired practice and fame, though none of the Alexandrians approached in importance the founders of the school—Herophilus and Erasistratus. These two physicians stand out as the first who publicly dissected the human body—and it has been whispered down the ages that the Ptolemaic zeal for science furnished condemned criminals to these investigators who were thus enabled to contrast dissection with vivisection. The first who made this statement was Celsus: "They procured criminals out of prison by royal permission, and dissecting them alive, contemplated, while they were yet breathing, the parts which nature had before concealed."

Herophilus was born at Chalcedon, and Erasistratus came from the Homeric island of Chios, where Glaucus of old learned how to weld iron. Both Herophilus and Erasistratus were thus Asiatic Greeks, and both were pupils of the Egyptian-trained Chrysippus of Cnidus, who avoided drastic medicines, stopped hemorrhages by bandaging of limbs, and rejected venesection because blood is the food of the soul. Herophilus studied also under Praxagoras of Cos, who advanced diagnosis by attention to the pulse, and is remembered as the first who differentiated veins and arteries. Erasistratus was said to be the grandson of Aristotle and the pupil of Theophrastus. The discovery of a catheter for the relief of urinary retention is sometimes credited to Herophilus, sometimes to Erasistratus; in fact, it is difficult to separate their discoveries. It is one of the calamities of culture that their writings are lost. They survive only in extracts— usually quoted by authors for the purpose of refuting them.

Pliny, Plutarch, Aulus Gellius, Galen, Sextus Empiricus, Oribasius, and Caelius Aurelianus have preserved passages.

Examples of the sayings of Herophilus include: "He is the best physician who knows how to distinguish the possible from the impossible." "Medicines are nothing in themselves, if not properly used, but the very hands of the gods, if employed with reason and prudence." "To lose one's health renders science null, art inglorious, strength effortless, wealth useless and eloquence powerless." They deserve a place beside the Hippocratic aphorisms, or Sophocles' "Sleep is the physician of pain," and "Death is the supreme healer of maladies."

The much-traveled Diocles of Carystus, dissector of animals and occasionally of human material, was acclaimed the greatest physician after Hippocrates: today he is not even a torso, he is a fragment. We know, however, that he wrote the first Greek herbal and the first book entitled *On Anatomy;* he is to be grouped therefore with Alcmaeon of Croton, the discoverer of the optic nerves, and with Diogenes of Apollonia, the investigator of the blood vessels, as among the forerunners of Herophilus. Because Herophilus was the first who regularly dissected the body of man and studied it systematically, he is known as the Father of Anatomy.

Herophilus carried forward the work of his teacher Praxagoras in distinguishing between arteries and veins, and also elaborated his teacher's view on paralysis of the heart as a cause of sudden death. Herophilus is the earliest of the commentators on the Father of Medicine, and it has been pointed out that he revered Hippocrates so much that when obliged to disagree with him, he avoided mentioning his name; Hippocrates was unfamiliar with the pulse, the importance of which was first emphasized by Praxagoras, but Herophilus was the earliest sphygmologist: the first to study the rhythmical tides produced in the arteries by the beating heart. He had no instrument corresponding to a watch, and his leaking water-filled glass-cistern (*clepsydra*) must have been of dubious value, yet he mastered the pulse-beat in health and illness, comparing its variations to the musical scale, causing Pliny to write: "To detect its exact harmony in relation to age and disease, one needs to be a musician and even a mathematician to understand the pulse according to Herophilus." A goat rises from the ground by two actions: first there is a great heave of its hind legs, followed by a lesser one of its fore limbs; there is a condition of the pulse in which the examining finger feels two beats, the second being weaker than the first, and Herophilus named it the goat-leap pulse (*pulsus caprizans, dicrotus*), by which it is still known.

Finding that the first part of the small intestine was about twelve fingerbreadths long, he called it the duodenum; around the neck of the bladder where the urethra begins in the male, he found a gland which he named the prostate, and in the female he described the ovaries and the oviducts; in his studies on the structure of the eye, he delineated the ciliary body, vitreous humor, retina and choroid, and this new knowledge enabled him to improve the operation for cataract. His researches on the liver, pancreas, and salivary glands, his discovery of the hyoid bone, his understanding of the unique nature of the pulmonary artery, and his separation of the nerves of sensation from those of motion, attest the master of anatomy. He noted the chyle and lymph, and aside from his work and that of his contemporary Erasistratus, the subject of the lacteals was closed for two thousand years. Anatomically, he gave the profession a new brain: he described its coverings (*meninges*), discovered the groove (*calamus scriptorius*) at the bottom of the fourth ventricle, and the venous sinuses, including the meeting-place of the blood-currents forming the whirlpool known as the winepress of Herophilus (*torcular Herophili*).

No man of his time devoted so much attention to the anatomy of the female, the problems of childbirth, and the diseases of women; he taught his students the various causes of a difficult delivery, invented an embryotome, and wrote a famous textbook for midwives. His prominence in this field has linked the name of Herophilus with that of Agnodice: he instructed her in obstetrics, and she returned to Athens to practise the art. As the

Athenians, continues the tale, forbade women and slaves to engage in medicine, she disguised herself in male attire, but her identity becoming gradually known, she was consulted by many women whose modesty shrank from the glance and touch of a male physician. After her patients were sufficiently numerous to arouse the jealousy of the legitimate physicians, she was arraigned on the charge of corrupting females. At the trial she confounded her accusers by revealing her sex, but was then pronounced guilty of practising contrary to the laws. Here the wives of important Athenians came to her aid, declaring how much she had done for them—and when the Athenian women banded together, their husbands retreated. Agnodice was acquitted, and the unjust law was repealed. A pretty story, and a doubtful one. The learned fabulist Hyginus started it—in a moment when he forgot that the mother of Socrates and the sister of Pyrrho were midwives, and that in the *Hippolytus* of Euripides, the nurse advises Phaedra: "If thou hast some ailment which thou dost not care to reveal to men, here are women who are competent to treat the condition properly."

We learn from Sextus Empiricus, physician and historian of Greek scepticism, that Herophilus was also noted as a general surgeon; at the court of Ptolemy, Herophilus could not avoid meeting Diodorus Cronus, one of the foremost of the Megarian sophists. Diodorus Cronus drove the philosophers of antiquity nearly crazy attempting to solve his syllogism: "The impossible cannot result from the impossible; a past event cannot become other than it is; but if an event, at a given moment, had been possible, from this possible would result something impossible; therefore the original event was impossible." Equally provocative of sleepless nights was another quibble of Diodorus on the non-existence of motion: "If a body moves, either it moves from a place where it is, or from a place where it is not; but it does not move from the place where it is, because it would not then be there, and it does not move from the place where it is not, for a body cannot move from a place where it is not. Therefore nothing moves."

Philosophers are subject to the ordinary accidents of mankind, and it so happened that the subtle Diodorus dislocated his arm, and sent in haste for Herophilus. There must have been malice in the heart of Herophilus as he spoke to Diodorus: "Either the bone of your arm moved itself from the place where it was, or from the place where it was not. According to your principles, it could not have moved from one or the other place. Therefore it has not moved." A philosopher in pain ceases to be a philosopher, and Diodorus begged for surgical instead of dialectic treatment.

Any faculty is fortunate to count an Herophilus on its staff, but the medical school of Alexandria at the same time possessed another investigator equally gifted. Herophilus' younger colleague, Erasistratus, had such a flair for the function of things that he is remembered as the Father of Physiology. When he placed some birds in a jar, and weighed them after feeding and digestion, calculating their visible and invisible excreta, he gave physiology its first respiration calorimeter and its first experiment in metabolism. He concerned himself with such problems as muscular action producing movement, the superior intelligence of man as manifested in his deeper cerebral convolutions, the cause of the pulse and hemorrhage, and the processes of nutrition and secretion. He gave the trachea its name, and studied how it was closed by the epiglottis.

Herophilus accepted the humoral pathology of Hippocrates: the doctrine that disease is the result of disturbed or abnormal conditions of the four fluids or humors of the body—blood, phlegm, black bile, yellow bile. Depending on the predominating humor, a man's temperament was either sanguine, phlegmatic, melancholic or choleric. The theory is gone, but the terms survive. Erasistratus rejected the entire humoral pathology, and even black bile—the dreaded *atra bilis* of ancient pathology—did not frighten him. He believed disease was due to excess of blood producing *plethora;* oddly enough, for these conditions he did not prescribe blood-letting—as a follower of Chrysippus, he was opposed to all violent evacuations—but treated the affected part by diminishing the local blood supply. The theories of Erasistratus, as has happened with hypotheses before and since, often hindered him in his quest for truth, but his connection of plethora of the liver with dropsy of the abdomen was so brilliant an observation that it remains a landmark in pathology today, though we translate the terms into cirrhosis of the liver with ascites.

He was interested in the problems of hunger, and described abnormal hunger (*boulimia*). Aulus Gellius who often spent whole days with Favorinus—the physician's delightful conversation holding his mind enthralled, so he attended him wherever he went, as if actually taken prisoner by his eloquence—informs us that Favorinus expounded to him the views of Erasistratus. Later, Aulus Gellius, who could never see a volume without reading it, came across the first book of Erasistratus' *Distinctions*, and was delighted to find the very passages which Favorinus had quoted: "I reasoned therefore that the ability to fast for a long time is caused by strong compression of the belly; for with those who voluntarily fast for a long time, at first hunger ensues, but later it passes away. . . . And the Scythians also are accustomed, when on any occasion it is necessary to fast, to bind up the belly with broad belts, in the belief that the hunger thus troubles them less; and one may almost say too that when the stomach is full, men feel no hunger for the reason that there is no vacuity in it, and likewise when it is greatly compressed there is no vacuity."

Erasistratus' refusal to tap the abdomen in dropsy, on the ground that removal of the fluid did not remove the cause of the disease and that the fluid would form again, was characteristic of his sagacity. He abandoned many drugs, and advocated exercise, rest, proper diet and the vapor bath—in these respects being an Hippocratist despite himself. Complaining that the physicians of his time neglected hygiene, he wrote a treatise on the subject which makes him one of the pioneers of preventive medicine. He insisted that venesection lowers the resistance of the patient, and had the profession followed him,

GREEK MEDICINE IN ALEXANDRIA

the history of medicine would have been less bloody. When Erasistratus saw a bleeding artery, he tied it: much to the detriment of mankind this simple method was forgotten, and in comparatively recent times the ligature was reintroduced as a new discovery. The flaxen thread is the most important instrument known to surgery.

Erasistratus, by his researches on the cerebrum, cerebellum and cerebral cavities, paralleled those of Herophilus, and surpassed him in his work on the heart and vascular system. Erasistratus observed the arteries are empty in the dead, but bleed when injured during life; he explained the hemorrhage by the escape of vital air or the *pneuma* into the wounded vessels, and since, he argued, nature abhors a vacuum (*horror vacui*), blood immediately flows from the veins into the arteries filling up the empty spaces. This pneumatic theory, which considered the normal arteries to contain life-giving air or spirits instead of blood, was developed by Erasistratus from the doctrines of Strato and Praxagoras; the pneumatic theory was interesting enough as the forerunner of the oxygen theory, but it prevented Erasistratus from discovering the circulation of the blood. That he stood on the threshold of the right path is remarkable enough; he compared the heart's action to a blacksmith's bellows, knew it contracted and dilated by its innate force, named the tricuspid valve and understood the function of the semilunar valves, described the tendinous cords (*chordae tendineae*) that stretch between the ventricular walls, realized that arteries and veins communicate through invisible orifices (*synanastomoses*) which we now call capillaries, and for twenty-two hundred years he seems to have been alone in his belief—finally proven by mathematical physics—that the pulse progresses as a wave.

There is a story about Erasistratus which we should believe, despite its familiar stepmother motive, for it is told by Plutarch, Appian and Lucian, and is noticed by Galen. The scene takes place at the court of Seleucus Nicator, the diplomatic soldier who at one time held the lost empire of Alexander, except Egypt, within his grasp. He succeeded Alexander as master of Babylon, and established a great city on the Tigris not far from Bagdad —and Hellenism reigned in Babylon until Rome laid Seleucia in ruins. Alexander, in his Asiatic enthusiasm, had given the oriental princess Apama to Seleucus, and the blood of Macedonia and Persia mingled in their offspring, Antiochus Soter. In his latter years, Seleucus married the youthful Stratonice, daughter of that notorious Demetrius the Besieger who filled Greek temples with courtesans, and oppressed the Athenians with excessive taxes, commanding them to give the money to his mistresses, so they could buy soap. Stratonice was beautiful, and no one was more aware of it than Antiochus. He knew it was wrong to be in love with his stepmother, and he attempted in vain to subdue his unnatural passion. Melancholy possessed him, he neglected his person, and refused to eat. The royal archives of that period reek with parents who slew their children and children who slew their parents, but the relationship between Seleucus and Antiochus was one of true affection. The father summoned various physicians to examine his afflicted son, but they could find no evidence of disease, and did not know what was amiss. The mighty Seleucus saw the hopes of his house tumbling, and he wept like a peasant, and at last asked for Erasistratus.

Even Erasistratus was baffled in the beginning, but one day while examining Antiochus, he felt a sudden leaping of the patient's pulse, and looking around for the cause, saw that Stratonice had entered the room. He thus learned the secret of Antiochus, and revealed the situation to Seleucus, who immediately arranged a marriage between the son and stepmother. Erasistratus received an enormous fee, Seleucus saved his dynasty, Antiochus carried on his father's work, Stratonice became the queen of Upper Asia, and apparently every one was satisfied except Galen—who had nothing to do with the matter.

Galen scornfully remarks that he cannot understand the diagnosis of Erasistratus, since there is no such thing as a lover's pulse. It should be remembered that Galen was a chronic critic of Erasistratus, and abuses him as if he were a contemporary. In speaking of Erasistratus' theory of urination, Galen exclaims:

"It may be seen then, how false is this hypothesis—by Zeus, I cannot call it a demonstration!—of Erasistratus." In his treatise on the *Natural Faculties,* Galen scolds Erasistratus for his plethora, for his horror vacui, for claiming that the spleen is a useless organ, for rejecting the idea of the innate heat of the body, for not reading Hippocrates' splendid study *On the Nature of Man,* for declaring that peristalsis is due to contractions of the stomach instead of the intestines, and for unscrupulously attacking others. Galen could never write long without working himself into a state of indignation, and in the second book of this diatribe he says that "the high and mighty Erasistratus affected to despise thousands of the ancient physicians and philosophers."

At times Galen quotes Erasistratus in derision, and unwittingly saves a passage which arouses our deepest admiration. For example: "Imagine the heart to be, at the beginning, so small as to differ in no respect from a millet-seed, or, if you will, a bean; and consider how otherwise it is to become large than by being extended in all directions and acquiring nourishment throughout its whole substance, in the way that, as I showed a short while ago, the semen is nourished. But even this was unknown to Erasistratus—the man who sings the artistic skill of Nature! He imagines that animals grow like webs, ropes, sacks, or baskets, each of which has, woven on its end or margin, other material similar to that of which it was originally composed." Little did Galen realize that he was quoting Erasistratus' anticipation of the cell-theory!

The adherents of Herophilus and Erasistratus formed rival schools, and at one time their disputations made much noise. Long after the masters rested from their labors, the disciples expounded their doctrines, not with the scalpel, but with the tongue—and gave early evidence that argumentation without experimentation remains sterile. A scientist should not be a good orator. The result of dialectic is more dialectic. The Herophileans and the Erasistrateans talked themselves into oblivion.

Weary of the battle of words, the Empirics arose in Alexandria. "We know that honey tastes sweet," they said, "but we do not know what the sweet taste is." "The farmer and the pilot are not trained by disputations, but by practice." "The important question is not what causes disease, but what dispels it." "Diseases are not cured by talk, but by drugs."

The spiritual father of the School of Empirics was Pyrrho of Elis, the central figure of Greek agnosticism—see the *Pyrrhonian Sketches* of Sextus Empiricus—but its actual founders were Philinus who thought he was the enemy of all dogmas; Serapion who, in his efforts to avoid wrangling, abused all physicians from Hippocrates down; and Glaucias, the proud inventor of the Empiric Tripod: individual observations, made accidentally or by design—*autopsia;* records of the observations of others—*history;* and in unknown diseases, drawing conclusions from similar diseases—*analogy.* Since a tripod is apt to be unsteady, a fourth leg was attached: inference of previous conditions from present symptoms—*epilogism.* For example, in examining a case of insanity, if the physician found a scar on the head, he was justified in regarding the injury as the cause of the disease. The empirics never searched for the general laws or the hidden causes and essential nature of disease, and they deemed superfluous all investigation in anatomy, physiology and pathology. Little wonder that their tripod, even with its additional leg, has been badly upset. Modern medicine knows no greater term of reproach than empiricism.

It seems very strange, but it has happened again and again, that when a school determines to be practical, and concern itself exclusively with the treatment of disease, it is no more productive than a rival school of theorists. Medicine, lacking fundamental principles, and approaching the bedside with a knife in one hand and a drug in the other, is striking in darkness. Without theory, medicine is a collection of scattered facts which do not recognize each other; with theory, the isolated facts acquire unity which is science. The misfortune of medicine is not that most of its theories were wrong, but that they remained intrenched after they ceased to be useful. A working hypothesis should not outlast the generation which gave it birth.

In its day, Alexandrian Empiricism was a needed corrective, and had the Serapions been able to avoid the human propensity of going to extremes, they would have saved their doctrines from the fatal blight of sectarianism. But when Philinus declared, "The anatomical knowledge which I derived from Herophilus has been useless to me in treating the sick," the decline of Alexandrian medicine had begun. These early Empirics, however, were more deserving than their subsequent reputation: they advanced the practice of obstetrics, and their management of fractures, dislocations and herniae proved their surgery of high rank. In their hands, bandaging became one of the fine arts, and when they applied the capeline bandage, the patient looked as if he were wearing a beautiful ornament. Ammonius found that in many cases the stone in the bladder was too large for ordinary extraction, and he solved the difficulty by inventing the lithotrite to crush the calculus. The name of Amyntas is associated with a dressing for fracture of the bridge of the nose.

Alexandria, because of its geographical position and political importance, was the commercial center of the world, and now Egypt teemed with more drugs than in the days of Homer. The Empirics were such zealous advocates of medicaments that poets sang of poisons, and monarchs hunted for prophylactics. Plutarch writes of the last king of Pergamus: "And Attalus Philometor used to grow poisonous plants, not only henbane and hellebore, but also hemlock, aconite, and dorycnium, sowing and planting them himself in the royal gardens, and making it his business to know their juices and fruits, and to collect these at the proper season." Justin adds, that in his playful moments, Attalus distributed fruits to his friends: some of these fruits were natural, and some were poisoned.

As a royal toxicologist, Attalus is overshadowed by the dominating Mithridates Eupator of Pontus. In his youth, Mithridates fled to the mountains to escape the funeral that his mother planned for him. He grew to gigantic stature and strength, and his capacity for food and drink surpassed that of all other men; none could ride so fast, none was so swift of foot, none could wield his weapons, nor love so many women, as Mithridates the Great. He mastered twenty-two languages to address the nations without interpreters; in his prime he spoke Latin with the sword, and in one day butchered one hundred thousand Romans who were living in Asia. Incidentally, he murdered his mother, brother, several of his numerous children, his sister-wife and his harem. The latter act was probably dictated by jealousy, as he wished to prevent his concubines from falling into the hands of his foes.

Mithridates was a practical botanist, and *Mithradatea, Eupatoria* and *Scordion* were named in his honor. He learned about poisons by experimenting upon his relatives, criminals and himself; he even kept data. Mithridates was surrounded by enemies, and to avoid a pharmacologic accident, he had a personal interest in knowing the effects of poisons and their antidotes. In time he developed the "universal antidote" of antiquity, mingling it with the blood of Pontine ducks who thrived on toxic substances, and by gradually increasing the dosage, his poison-saturated body was protected against all poisons. Eventually cornered, he took the deadliest drugs in vain; he was living proof of immunity, and only by calling for the spear of a Gallic soldier was he able to end his life. This is an oft-told tale, and yet we do not believe it; but as Plutarch remarks on another occasion, "At any rate, so the story runs."

The legend was wonderful propaganda for the universal antidote, which under the name of *mithridate* or *theriac* became the most famous of all drugs, and made the fortune of pharmacists. There were court physicians whose sole duty was to prepare this remedy for their rulers. Nor was this an easy task, for seemingly the entire contents of many apothecary-shops—aside from hunting vipers in deserts—went into its composition. As sagacious a scientist as Galen believed in this universal panacea, and manufactured it with his own hands; he considered himself a benefactor when he published "The hundred-ingredient antidote

I use, and which I compounded for the emperor, suitable for all deadly poisons." Added to, subtracted from, multiplied and modified, the formula of Mithridates, the first toxicologist, not only survived for eighteen centuries, but it was stamped with municipal seals and took its place in the official pharmacopeias.

At the court of Mithridates lived the rhizotomist Crateuas, who dedicated his writings to the king. The rhizotomists or herb-gatherers were usually members of the lower classes, illiterate and superstitious, without any pretense to botanical knowledge. "As he stands in comparison with the carpenters, laborers and tradesmen," said Galen, "so the true physician stands in comparison with his servants, the rhizotomists, ointment-makers, cooks, plaster-spreaders, poultice-makers, administrators of clysters, bleeders and cuppers." Nevertheless, at least one of the rhizotomists deserves to be remembered with gratitude, for Crateuas not only collected herbs, but described them and drew them, thus becoming the founder of plant illustration.

The literature of Alexandria underwent a fate similar to its medicine. The idylls of Theocritus and the mimes of Herondas —he who wrote the *Visit of the Women to Aesculapius*—were jostled by the sharp note of the partisan and the heavy accent of the pedant. Apollonius and Callimachus started a dispute about Homer, and Apollonius called Callimachus a crow, and Callimachus insinuated that Apollonius was an ibis. This literary feud over the long-departed Homer became so personal that swarming Alexandria could not hold them both, and Apollonius moved to Rhodes. In its day, Lycophron's *Alexandra* was greatly admired: its poetry was submerged beneath erudition which required scholia and glosses for every line; the allusion to Helen as the "Aegean bitch," is one of the few references that can be understood without marginal explanation. Scholarship gave way to the scholasticism which was to bear such bitter fruit in the ages to come. Learning began to preen its feathers in bookish Alexandria, and friendships were broken over a footnote. There were men who grew round-shouldered beneath the weight of asterisks, and the town's wits inaugurated the still-prevalent custom of joking about the absent-minded professor. Aratus, under the influence of the Alexandrian school of literature, composed *Phenomena,* a poem so technical that it needed a commentary by Hipparchus, founder of trigonometry and discoverer of the precession of the equinoxes.

In mathematics and astronomy, in physics and mechanics, Alexandria outdistanced all nations. The lighthouse which Sostratus raised in the harbor, towering hundreds of feet in air, was one of the wonders of the world. Centuries afterwards, it was overthrown by an earthquake, and today not one of its stones remains on the spot, but the passing generations have not erased the work of Euclid. Every school child who has pondered over his theorems, will admit the justice of his reply to Ptolemy, as preserved by Proclus: "Sire, there is no royal road to geometry." Euclid's *Elements of Geometry* is one of the most-edited and best-studied books of the present day. The Euclidian axioms are as inexorable as the laws of nature. Euclid's work on light is the earliest landmark in the theory of optics.

Among those who wrote commentaries on Euclid, none excites our curiosity more than Hero of Alexandria. The wizard of mechanics, he could make objects dance by means of steam, and open temple doors without touching them; he had a magic jar from which wine flowed or stopped at will; he described siphons, water-organs, fire-engines, mirrors which distorted the spectator, a lamp which trimmed itself, and coin-in-the-slot machines; he constructed automata which were almost alive— statues which poured libations upon the altar, dogs which could drink, birds which sang, and serpents that hissed; there was little about cogwheels or pulleys that he did not know, and as we walk our streets today we see builders utilizing the mechanical devices originated by the ingenious Alexandrian. He was the father of surveying, which he enriched with instruments; his knowledge of astronomy enabled him to compute the distance between Rome and Alexandria.

Hero's fountain, by which a jet of water is supported by condensed air, is a stock experiment in pneumatics; the first steam-engine that man ever saw, revolved in Alexandria, and Hero was its inventor. His experimental demonstration that the angle from which light is reflected from a surface is equal to the angle of incidence, was an important contribution to optics. Hero's syringe, formed of a metal cylinder with a well-fitting plunger, is the parent of air pumps and hypodermic syringes.

Between the time of Euclid and Hero there intervenes the noble and imposing figure of the founder of hydrostatics, the supreme scientist of Alexandria, one of the greatest intellects, not only of antiquity, but of all times—Archimedes. This mathematical giant amused himself by devising a Planetarium which showed the movements of the planets and their eclipses; the sand-reckoner, by which he could compute the number of grains in the universe; and the loculus, which is the earliest puzzle on record. Contrived in a sterner mood, his engines at Syracuse worked such havoc among the attacking Romans, that whenever they saw a bit of rope or a stick of timber projecting over the wall—Plutarch relates this in his life of Marcellus—they fled in panic. The Screw of Archimedes is still employed in Egypt to raise water. These machines brought renown to Archimedes, but his lofty soul regarded them as vulgar and due to necessity; he was more proud of his discovery of the relationship between a volume of the sphere and its circumscribing cylinder. In his hands the lever accomplished such wonders, that Archimedes declared, "Give me whereon to stand, and I will move the world."

No accident in physics is better known than the story told in graphic detail by Vitruvius: stepping into his bath, Archimedes noted that as his body was immersed, the water ran over; instead of being annoyed at this law, he was transported with joy, and rushed naked through the streets, crying Eureka! Eureka! The interrupted bath of Archimedes is immortal, for he had discovered the method for the determination of specific gravity. Never was so important a discovery made in so undignified a manner.

The physicians and surgeons of Alexandria were too alert

to neglect the mechanical improvements of Archimedes; they found uses for his burning mirror and endless screw; the trispaston, which Archimedes invented to drag ships on shore, was adapted by Pasicrates to reduce dislocations—no gymnasium was complete without it. Heraclides, the most gifted of the Empirics, treated injuries of the hip with an apparatus believed to have been of Archimedian derivation.

Archimedes met his fate in the spirit of Socrates. Relying on his invincible engines, the Syracusans grew careless; treachery accomplished the rest, and Rome entered the fallen city. A warrior found the mathematician drawing figures in the sand. "Do not disturb my circles," said Archimedes, and the soldier, untrained in geometry, killed him. The act was symbolic of the conquest of Greece by Rome. The great days of antiquity were over. A baser nation, but armed with stronger weapons, had triumphed. Alexandria indeed survived, but in accumulating humiliation. Rome, which despoiled all it touched, elected athletes as members of the Museum.

Rome turned its thumb down on the work of Herophilus and Erasistratus. Alexandria, which had introduced human dissection, went back to the pig. Rome, which would not attend a circus unless human blood was spilled, blunted the scalpel. Those ages which destroyed life for amusement, or took it at the least provocation, were the most stringent in protecting the cadaver. In the coming centuries, with fatal results, medical students studied anatomy at the reading-desk instead of the dissecting-table. Not until recent times were there authorities as enlightened as the Ptolemies. The practical Romans were better plumbers than the Greeks—their aqueducts are still working; otherwise, the legacy of Rome is largely evil. But we cannot wipe out the crimson chapters of history: Rome now ruled the world, and Greek science slowly left the ebbing Nile to dwell beside the flowing Tiber. As we cross the Mediterranean, let us not forget the land where the human body was first properly studied, and whenever we put on a dissecting-apron, let us remember our first alma mater, the long-vanished University of Alexandria.

V

GREEK MEDICINE IN ROME

In the midst of an epidemic, Apollo was the first of the healing gods of Greece to enter Rome. Aesculapius, as a dutiful son, followed from the temple of Epidaurus to the *insula Tiberina*, and this Island of Aesculapius, known also as the Island of the Epidaurian Serpent, developed into the first public charity hospital: the masters sent sick and worn-out slaves there as to a city of the dead. The custom found favor with the thrifty Romans, and the sanctuary was overcrowded with outcasts—until a law was passed, liberating every slave who recovered on the Island of Aesculapius. This made the Romans more careful.

Native deities, especially goddesses, were as numerous as plebs on the Janiculum. Febris was goddess of the malarias of the Roman marshes; Scabies, goddess of itch; Angina, goddess of quinsy; hydrogen sulphide issuing from the earth was believed to be Pluto's breath, wherefore the people of the valley worshiped Mefitis, goddess of stench. The divinities of childbearing evidently gave a Roman bride little privacy. Juga was present throughout her entire courtship; Domiducus watched her as she was conducted to her husband's home; Cinxia loosened her girdle; Virginensis saw the breaking of the maidenhead; Pertunda supervised the first coition, which was pleasant only if Volupia willed it; after conception, Fluonia stopped the monthly flow, and Mena, goddess of menstruation, went elsewhere; Rumina made her breasts swell, Alemona fed the embryo, and Ossipaga hardened its bones; Antevorta presided over head presentations, and Postvorta over breech presentations; Intercidona guarded the navel, and Partula fastened the binder; Vagitanus opened the infant's mouth for its first cry, and Educa taught it to suckle. The Fates hovered about, and if anything went wrong, Opigena, the divine midwife, was invoked. No wonder the noble Romans gave the mother little credit for her share in bringing a child into the world.

The Greek physicians found it more difficult than the Greek divinities to establish themselves on the seven hills. Cato, the dominant Roman of three generations, stood as a bulwark in the path of Greek learning. Cato the Censor was the embodiment of Roman virtue. He bought boys, and after training them for a year, sold them at profit, which was an example of frugality. When his old horses and slaves could no longer work for him, he turned them adrift, which was applauded as economy. Suspicious of harmony among his slaves, he deliberately provoked them to dissension and to spy upon one other, which was declared the height of prudence.

The exponent of honest poverty, he loaned out his money at exorbitant interest, and by shrewd investments in ships and lands, in hot springs and forests, acquired riches that could not be ruined by Jupiter. While the Forum rang with praise of Cato because he preferred water and vinegar to wine, and would not have the walls of his tenants' cottages plastered, he was flogging or murdering a servant who had made a mistake at table. He rose before dawn to devote himself to the public welfare, and asked for no reward except the privilege of interfering with the private lives of citizens. He hated Greek literature, and wrote so much about its dangers that he became the founder of Latin prose. A far-seeing statesman, he set in motion the forces which destroyed Carthage. Averse to sexual passion, he supervised the coition of his dependents. Preaching purity, Cato the Censor was detected in his own home in the act of corrupting a slave-girl.

The apostle of continence, in his old age he took a young bride. Such was the man without a vice, who made virtue loathsome.

Cato the Censor wrote to his son: "I shall speak of those Greeks in their place, Marcus my son. I shall prove what I have found at Athens that it is good to look into their literature but not to study it deeply. Theirs is a most worthless and intractable race, and believe that I speak this as a true prophet: wherever that nation shall bestow its learning it will corrupt all things, more especially if it sends its doctors hither. They have sworn to slay all foreigners by medicine, and this very thing they do for pay so that trust may be reposed in them, and their work of destruction may be easy. Us also they call barbarians, and they degrade us even more than others by the name of bumpkins. I forbid you any dealings with doctors."

Cato, as *paterfamilias*, was the physician of his household and barnyard. He survived his own treatment, but lost his wife and son. He stood his sick cows up on their hind legs, poured remedies down their throats and recited incantations. His medical library was a receipt-book of folk lore, and the cabbage his panacea. In his famous work on agriculture (*De re Rustica*), he wrote: "Cabbage is good for everything. . . . And this further: keep the urine of one who is wont to eat cabbage. Warm it. Immerse the patient in it. You will soon cure him by this treatment. It has been tried. Also if you wash small children with this urine, they will never become weakly. . . . And if there is any bruise it will break it up and heal it if you apply mashed cabbage. And if any ulcer and cancer arise in the breasts apply mashed cabbage, it will heal it." Cato's instructions in dislocation or fracture were as follows: "Split a divining-rod up the middle, apply it to the body, trim off fragments of wood, bind them to the injured parts, and do not fail to sing, *Huat hanat huat ista pista sista domiabo damnaustra et luxato*." With such gibberish, Cato the Censor kept Hippocrates at bay.

By giving some of their slaves a medical education, the Romans avoided the necessity of employing foreign medici— and no physician is as convenient as a resident physician. If the slave engaged in outside practice, the fees he collected belonged to his owner; if requested to let his knife slip in the wrong place, or mix a poison for his master's enemy, it was not etiquette to refuse. This explains why a medical slave sold for a higher price than even a eunuch, and it likewise explains why medicine was not considered a fit occupation for a Roman gentleman. It is understandable that the best-established Greek physicians were the least tempted to exchange their honors at home for the uncertainties of an unfriendly land, and there must have been truth in Pliny's complaint that the newcomers were adventurers who abused their position by seeking legacies and adulteries. When they grew sufficiently numerous to compete with each other, we may well imagine such a scene as Theodorus Priscianus later described: "While the patient, racked by his pains, tosses himself to and fro on his bed, doctors in crowds rush in, each one of whom is only concerned to fix the attention of the rest upon himself, and cares but little for the condition of the patient. In a spirit of emulation like that displayed in a circus or at a pugilistic contest, one endeavors to gain extraordinary fame by his oratory or his dialectics, another by the artistic building up of theses—a structure which his adversary soon levels with the ground."

Rome may have been prejudiced against medicine as a profession, but Latin laymen certainly found medicine of interest. There is a question in Quintilian, which though designed as a problem, is revealing: "A man, having three sons, a philosopher, a politician, and a physician, divides his property into four parts and leaves the extra share to the one most useful to the State. Which should have it?" "I am of opinion," writes the Roman author of *Attic Nights*, "that it is a disgrace not merely for a doctor, but for every independent man who has been well brought up, to be ignorant of those things which concern the human body and of the means for preserving health which Nature lays open before our eyes. I have on this account given all the time I could spare to the study of medical works, since it was in them that I hoped to find the best instruction." The veterinary medicine in Virgil, the military medicine in Lucan, the pharmacology in Persius, and the anthropology in Tacitus are frequent subjects of commentary; volumes may be compiled by extracting the medical references in Cicero and Seneca, in Horace and Ovid. Juvenal's query, "Who wonders at goiter in the Alps?" is seldom omitted in any book on the thyroid. The student of sexual perversions and psychopathology will find inexhaustible founts in the poems of Catullus, Ovid, and the Neronic Petronius, the biographies of Suetonius, the annals of Tacitus, the sham-smashing satires of Juvenal, and the skin-stripping, blood-drawing, bone-piercing epigrams of Martial.

Rome was a brothel, with emperor or empress as chief whoremonger. Julius Caesar gave his virginity to King Nicomedes, and was henceforth known as the Queen of Bithynia. In the pursuit of venery, Caesar was as unscrupulous as in political bribery, or in butchering countless provincials for the sake of plunder; he debauched not only the wives, but the sons and daughters of his friends and foes, becoming known throughout the world as the bald adulterer—which is why he insisted on wearing the laurel-crown—and giving rise to the elder Curio's remark that he was "every woman's man, and every man's woman."

Those who knew the circumstances said that if the young Octavian had not allowed himself to be corrupted by his conquering uncle, he would never have become Augustus. Noted for his austerity, Augustus exiled Ovid because of his amatory poems, and banished the females of the imperial family because they were chronic prostitutes—he sadly called them his three ulcers—yet Suetonius writes: "Augustus could not dispose of the charge of lustfulness and they say that even in his later years he was fond of deflowering maidens, who were brought together for him from all quarters, even by his own wife."

His successor, Tiberius, issued an edict against general kissing, and busied himself with public morals, but his own lust and cruelty were notorious to his contemporaries, who said that he thirsted not for wine but for blood. He devised exquisite torments for his subjects, and the Stairs of Mourning were crowded daily. Those who wished to die, were commanded to live; those who begged for life, were tortured and destroyed. In the seclusion of his villa at Capreae, with the obscene poems of the Greek poetess Elephantis as his guide, Tiberius indulged in unmentionable orgies, concluding with the agonized death of his numerous victims, male and female. One of his mildest tricks was to make men drink copious draughts of wine, and then suddenly tie up their private parts. No day passed without executions, and it was his delight to watch the dying bodies thrown into the sea, where the waiting marines broke the bones with boathooks and oars. Large and strong, he thrived on human blood, and reached extreme old age with undiminished appetites.

Then came Gaius Caesar, surnamed Caligula—a name at which all humanity will never cease to shudder. He banished sexual perverts from the city, but every perversion involving blood was his passion. All who served him met a bloody death; some he killed because he wished their estates, and others because of their virtues. He destroyed many in secret, and assumed surprise that they did not visit him. He insisted that death be made painful and lingering, so the victim would feel he was dying. After living in constant incest with all his sisters, he prostituted them to others, and later denounced them as adulteresses. He ordered human beings to be thrown to wild beasts to be devoured, or to be torn to pieces by his attendants, and he watched as their bowels were dragged through the streets. Here is a passage from Suetonius about Caligula: "He forced parents to attend the executions of their sons, sending a litter for one man who pleaded ill health, and inviting another to dinner immediately after witnessing the death, and trying to rouse him to gayety and jesting by a great show of affability. He had the manager of his gladiatorial shows and beast-baitings beaten with chains in his presence for several successive days, and would not kill him until he was disgusted at the stench of his putrefied brain. He burned a writer of Atellan farces alive in the middle of the arena of the amphitheater, because of a humorous line of double meaning. When a Roman knight on being thrown to the wild beasts, loudly protested his innocence, he took him out, cut off his tongue, and put him back again."

A mushroom, which passed through the skillful hands of Agrippina, was the last delicacy tasted by Claudius; at the age of seventeen, Nero stepped over the poisoned corpse to the world's throne, calling the mushroom the food of the gods. Nero's incest with his wanton mother, and his subsequent murder of her whose last words were "Smite my womb, it bore Nero"; his seduction of the vestal virgin Rubria; his marriage-ceremonies with the boy Sporus whom he castrated for the purpose; his playing the woman's part with his freedman Doryphorus, "going so far as to imitate the cries and lamentations of a maiden being deflowered"; the large estates with which he rewarded his professional poisoner, Locusta; his blood-gluttony which could not be appeased; his fiddling and singing at the burning of Rome; the poets and philosophers who opened their veins at his command; his designs for the wholesale destruction of his people—have held the ages fascinated by the stark horror of naked crime.

Fate drove the hesitant Galba against Nero, and after the latter's death Galba was Caesar for seven months; his decency was his doom, and the abandoned Otho used Galba's bewildered old head for a stepping-stone; in three months, Vitellius appeared on the scene, and Otho performed the one good act of his life by dying on a suicide's dagger. Between Vitellius and Vespanian broke out the civil warfare of which Tacitus has written in a pen dipped in blood:

> Horrible and hideous sights were to be seen everywhere in the city: here battles and wounds, there open baths and drinking shops; blood and piles of corpses, side by side with harlots and the compeers of harlots. There were all the debauchery and passion that obtain in a dissolute peace, every crime that can be committed in the most savage conquest, so that men might well have believed that the city was at once mad with rage and drunk with pleasure.

And all this blood was the baptism of Domitian. In the beginning of his reign he became famous as an insect-hunter, spending whole days in catching flies and stabbing them with a sharp-pointed stylus. Later he demanded bigger game, and amused himself by inserting fire in the privates of men, and killing them after dreadful torture and mutilation. He too occupied himself with public morals: enforced the laws against adultery, abolished the liberty of the stage, deprived courtesans of the use of litters and the right to receive inheritances and legacies, punished a Roman knight for pardoning an erring wife, expelled a senator for dancing, and buried vestal virgins alive for unchastity. Having improved the public morals, he placed his own conduct above the law, as we learn from Suetonius: "He was excessively lustful. His constant sexual intercourse he called bed-wrestling, as if it were a kind of exercise. It was reported that he depilated his concubines with his own hand and swam with common prostitutes."

So run the annals of Rome, etched deep by Clio's graphium. Against this lurid background, Greek medicine reached its second climax before its ultimate fall—always handicapped by the prohibition of human dissection. Senator and slave were never free from torture and death at the imperial whim, and more than one emperor's head rolled at the feet of his praetorian guard—but all were safe from anatomical investigation.

The first Greek physician who settled in Rome was appropriately named Archagathus, which means a good beginning. Some fortunate operations caused the Romans to forget their prejudices, for the Senate purchased a taberna for Archagathus in the crowded Acilian crossway, and conferred citizenship upon him. Intoxicated with unexpected success, Archagathus now indulged in such burning and cutting that only the undertakers continued to smile upon him, and his title of wound-curer (*Vulnerarius*) was changed to executioner (*Carnifex*). All this we learn from Pliny, who quotes it from the old Roman compiler, Cassius Hemina; no Greek author mentions Archagathus, and Pliny is never above suspicion.

One day a long funeral procession, with torches raised over the anointed and spice-sprinkled corpse, was winding its dolorous way through the streets of Rome. A physician who was returning from the suburbs to the city, happened to be passing, and professional instinct caused him to approach the body. Unseen by the mourners, he managed to touch the dead man, and certainly no one saw the dead man move. With lagging feet, and in silence broken only by weeping, they came nearer the pyre. Suddenly the loud commanding voice of the physician startled all: "I am Asclepiades, and I say take this funeral feast from the pyre to the table." Some turned in anger and mockery upon him—were they the heirs already in possession of the inheritance?—but others insisted that the physician be heeded. While the discussion continued, Asclepiades brought the body to his house, applied restoratives which reëstablished respiration, and the supposed corpse participated in his own funeral festivities.

The name of Asclepiades is undoubtedly suggestive of Aesculapius, and this sensational incident must have made the multitude believe they were closely related. Asclepiades, a native of Prusa in Bythia, which is in Asia Minor, began his career by teaching rhetoric. He found he could not make much money as a rhetorician, but it helped him enormously in medicine. In fact, Asclepiades had enough of the charlatan in him to make him a popular practitioner. He started out by abusing his predecessors, and reversing all medical rules; this attracts attention.

Did others attribute disease to a disturbance of the humors? The opposite of humoralism is solidism, and thus Asclepiades declared that disease is due to constriction or relaxation of the solid particles. We ceased to suffer from *atra bilis,* only to be afflicted by *strictum et laxum.* Did Hippocrates say, "Nature is the healer of disease?" Then Asclepiades said, "Not only is nature useless, it may even be harmful. A natural healing power, curing diseases by design, is a delusion. The physician must actively interfere with nature. It is the physician's duty to cure safely, quickly, pleasantly"—and here we have the origin of the classic phrase: *tuto, cito et jucunde.*

Democritus made the atom famous, but Asclepiades was the first who built a system of pathology on the atom. Health signifies that the atoms in the pores are present in such proportions that their movement is unimpeded, and disease is the result of a disturbed movement of the atoms. The atomic materialism of Democritus was the foundation of the philosophy of Epicurus, which in its turn was the inspiration of Lucretius' *On the Nature of Things*—the supreme product of Latin genius. "It is a hard task," wrote Lucretius, "in Latin verses to set clearly in the light the dark discoveries of the Greek, above all when many things must be treated in new words, because of the poverty of our tongue and the newness of the themes." The Greek-inspired Roman succeeded so well in his discussion of the first beginnings, that *De rerum natura* is as significant a contribution to science as to letters and philosophy, and is of primary importance in anthropology, biology, medicine and psychology.

Whether dealing with the formation of the world, the size of the sun and stars, the cause of the moon's light, the origin of human life and primitive man, the first steps of civilization, the mortality of the soul and its connection with the body, the swerve of the infinity of atoms, the porousness of solid things, the permanence of matter and motion, the folly of the fear of death, the special senses and physiological functions, the law of plague and disease; whether hurling his hexameters at superstition and supernaturalism, or exposing the lightning that strikes the innocent and spares the guilty, or describing with deepest pathos the action of a cow over her lost calf, we feel in the presence of Lucretius one of the loftiest spirits of antiquity, which the clashing centuries can never dim.

His poem in six books, concluding with the Thucydidesian plague of Athens, was never finished, but it ranks as the culminating flower of Epicurianism and the greatest nature-poem of all times. Must we accept the strange tale that Lucretius was poisoned by a love-philtre and killed himself in his prime? We know so little of the life of Lucretius. He was contemporaneous with Asclepiades, and if the physician had been able to save the poet's life until his reed was worn, it would have been his greatest achievement.

Asclepiades has much to his credit: he was the first who definitely divided diseases into acute and chronic; the first who opened the dark cells of the insane, treating the mentally afflicted with sunlight and gentleness, with music and song; he was familiar with the psychic complications of pneumonia and pleurisy; his definitions of frenzy, lethargy and catalepsy could go in a dictionary; his description of malaria places him among the great clinicians.

This ex-rhetorician was a foreigner, but he knew his Romans. His most frequent prescription called for wine, either pure or diluted with sea-water; in the post-febrile state, he permitted luxurious meals; even when treating baldness, he looked after the diet; he popularized bathing and massage, and introduced swinging beds and hanging baths; no patient received a bitter medicine from him, but many were told they must take up walking, riding or dancing—to set the stagnant atoms in motion; in some cases he prescribed plenty of sleep, and in others sexual intercourse, which was then regarded as gymnastic exercise. The Romans hailed him as a heaven-sent messenger, and he has been called the Father of Fashionable Physicians.

Pliny's criticism discredits Pliny rather than Asclepiades: "There is, however, one thing, and one thing only, at which we have any ground for indignation—the fact, that a single individual, and he belonging to the most frivolous nation in the world, a man born in utter indigence, should all on a sudden, and that, too, for the sole purpose of increasing his income, give a new code of medical laws to mankind." So suave was Aesclepiades that Crassius and Mucius were his friends, and Atticus and Cicero his eulogists. Mithridates invited him to his court, but the tactful Asclepiades sent his books instead.

Asclepiades had many disciples, the most conspicuous being Themison of Laodicea, who molded the solidist pathology into a system: disease is the result of rigidity, dependent upon contracted and narrow pores (*status strictus*), or of relaxation due to loose and wide pores (*status laxus*); this was too simple to be satisfying, since both conditions may occur in one disease, and therefore a mixed condition was recognized (*status mixtus*). The treatment was obvious: large pores should be reduced, and small pores enlarged—the principle that contraries are cured by contraries (*contraria contrarius curantur*).

Themison considered his doctrines a middle way or method between the dogmatists and empiricists, and was responsible for the formation of another medical sect—the Methodic School. Themison is quoted by Seneca, Pliny, Soranus, Galen, Caelius Aurelianus, and Dioscorides, who relates that Themison was once bitten by a mad dog, and therefore could not write on rabies without developing the symptoms; Celsus mentions Themison several times, summing up his doctrines with characteristic impartiality.

Themison did not escape a thrust from the terrible pen of Juvenal. It occurs in the midst of a devastating picture of Old Age extending over several appalling pages: "Besides all this, the little blood in the old man's chilly frame is never warm except with fever. All kinds of diseases dance around him in a troop. If you were to ask their names, I could sooner tell you how many lovers Hippia had; how many patients Themison has killed off in a single autumn; how many partners Basilus has cheated; how many wards Hirrus has corrupted; how many embraces tall Maura has submitted to in a single day." The world respects Juvenal because he was so magnificent a hater, but we must not expect the satirist who coined the expression of matrimonial halter, and greeted a rake's announcement that he had found a girl of old-fashioned virtue with the exclamation, "O physicians! open the middle vein, he is mad!"—to spare the medical profession.

Themison liked to quote the Hippocratic aphorism, "Life is short and the art long," and then boast that he had reversed it. But the weaver's son, Thessalus of Tralles, most notorious of the Methodics, shortened it still more—he guaranteed to teach the medical art in six months to all who wished to be physicians, and previous experience was not necessary. Dyers, rope-makers, butchers and tanners, cooks and cobblers crowded his heels, eager to exchange their former occupations for the practice of medicine—did not the doctor Stertinius earn six hundred thousand sesterces per annum?

Pliny speaks of Thessalus as "a man who swept away all the precepts of his predecessors, and declaimed with a sort of frenzy against the physicians of every age; but with what discretion and in what spirit, we may abundantly conclude from a single trait presented by his character: upon his tomb, which is still to be seen on the Appian Way, he had his name inscribed as the *Iatronices*—the Conqueror of the Physicians. No stage-player, no driver of a three-horse chariot, had a greater throng attending him when he appeared in public." How Galen raged when he passed the Via Appia and saw that mausoleum! If Thessalians were standing around, he raised his voice. . . . "Thessalus, impudent, insolent, stupid, barbarous, asinine. Yes, that worthless son of a weaver, whose only education was the gossip of the women's wool-spinning room. You asses of Thessalus. . . ."

The name of Thessalus has descended to posterity as the model of a quack. He had a natural talent for therapeutics, but unfortunately for medicine, his arrogance was remembered and his merit forgotten: Thessalus taught his pupils at the bedside, and by bringing them into actual contact with disease, he stands out as a founder of the polyclinic. This practice is alluded to in one of Martial's best-known epigrams:

Languid I lay, and thou camest, O Symmachus, quickly to see me;
Quickly thou camest and with thee a hundred medical students:
The hundred pawed me all over with hands congealed by the north wind.
Ague before I had none, but now, by Apollo, I have it.

Of the three great Roman encyclopedists, Marcus Terentius Varro, the Sabine savant, is the earliest. The brutal Marc Antony deprived him of his library, but the old polymath died with his pen in his hand. His comprehensive work—it was in forty-two sections—on Antiquities has perished along with his book on medicine, but as soon as we open Pliny, Plutarch, Aulus Gellius and Macrobius, and note their frequent citations, we realize that Varro is one of the standard sources of knowledge. He knew that the earth is shaped like a great egg, and at eighty he wrote a book on farming (*Rerum rusticarum*) which contains these remarkable lines on microörganisms: "Small creatures, invisible to the eye, fill the atmosphere in marshy localities, and with the air breathed through the nose and mouth penetrate into the human body, thereby causing dangerous diseases." That Varro knew this, is a mystery; that posterity did not know it, is a misfortune.

Varro, as an adherent of Pompey, found himself in conflict more than once with Julius Caesar, but instead of following the prevalent custom and destroying him, Caesar utilized his scholarship, and some of Varro's books are dedicated to the dictator. While Julius Caesar was enough of an internationalist to grant citizenship to certain Greek physicians, their status was not definitely improved until the reign of his successor. Augustus suffered from a disease which his contemporaries were as unsuccessful in relieving as posterity is in diagnosing. It is undetermined whether the imperial malady was liver trouble or gout or constipation, but it is on record that several physicians exhausted their arts in vain. Standing on the brink of fame, they passed into oblivion. Then Augustus summoned to his sick-room his former slave, the well-educated Antonius Musa, a Greek who had studied medicine in order to take care of his sick father.

When a monarch is the patient, medicine becomes melodramatic; if a remedy is not forthcoming the physician is disgraced; if a cure is effected, the physician is elevated to the nobility. As the illness of Augustus had not yielded to warm baths and hot fomentations, Musa boldly reversed the treatment, and drenched the world's *princeps civitatis* with draughts of cold water, and made him eat lettuce. Augustus recovered, and his gratitude was immense: not only did he endow Musa with money and grant him citizenship, but he invested him with the gold ring of knighthood, and sponsored a public subscription which erected the statue of Antonius Musa in brass, by the side of the God of Medicine in the Aesculapian temple which adorned the island in the Tiber. Cold douching became one of the cardinal principles of balneology, and Horace informs us that the myrtle groves and warm sulphur springs at Baiae were deserted for the chilly fountains of Elusium. The astute and fortunate freedman now acquired the most unforgettable clientele in history, for among the immortal invalids who sought health at the hands of Musa were Marcus Agrippa, Maecenas, Virgil and Horace.

Of Musa's pharmaceutical works, only a few fragments remain, and these fragments are not precious. Various remedies, with his name attached, were quoted by Galen and employed for generations, but have disappeared with the rising tide of pharmacologic skepticism. He introduced into therapeutics the lettuce—of which he was an ardent champion—and chicory and endive; his brother Euphorbus was medical adviser to the gifted King Juba of Mauritania, who discovered near Mount Atlas the medical plant which he graciously named Euphorbia in honor of his physician—at least so the anecdotist Pliny says. Antonius Musa certainly holds no rank among the great physicians of antiquity, but he is of historic interest because his popularity with the masters of his day acted as an antidote to the warning of Cato: "I forbid you to have anything to do with physicians."

Menecrates, physician to the emperor Tiberius, labored industriously over his 155 works, including a treatise on pharmacology, but he is now remembered for his early use of escharotics, as the first who suggested that in prescriptions the capricious signs for weights be discarded in favor of actual figures, and as the inventor of the famous Diachylon Plaster, which was celebrated—along with tooth-powders—in iambic verse by one of the rhyming physicians of the period, Servilius Damocrates.

In the reign of Tiberius, we meet the second of the encyclopedists, Aurelius Cornelius Celsus. Since Celsus is believed to have been a Roman patrician, it is inferred he was not a practitioner, and the ever-quoted Pliny names him among the *auctores* instead of the *medici*. Yet the breadth of his vision, his impartiality of outlook, the serenity of his judgment, and the vivacity of his observations, combined with the elegance of his Latinity—he was called *Cicero medicorum*—have combined to make his work one of the imperishable monuments of antiquity. An accident is sometimes propitious: nearly the whole of his all-embracing encyclopedia has disappeared, except *De re medicina*, which survives to keep green the name of Celsus.

The opening passage is characteristically Celsian: "As agriculture promises food to the healthy, so medicine promises health to the sick. There is no place in the world where this art is not found: for even the most barbarous nations are acquainted with herbs, and other easy remedies for wounds and diseases. However, it has been more improved by the Greeks than any other people." We cannot discuss the history of *Chirurgia* without quoting Celsus' qualifications of a surgeon: "A surgeon ought to be young, or at any rate, not very old; his hand should be firm and steady, and never shake; he should be able to use his left hand with as much dexterity as his right; his eye-sight should be acute and clear; his mind intrepid, and so far subject to pity as to make him desirous of the recovery of his patient, but not so far as to suffer himself to be moved by his cries; he should neither hurry the operation more than the case requires, nor cut less than is necessary, but do everything just as if the other's screams made no impression upon him."

Celsus is notable for the classic description of inflammation, familiar to every medical student: redness, swelling, heat and pain (*rubor et tumor, cum calore et dolore*). His reference to "pus discharging from the ear, leading to insanity and death," is an early recognition of meningitis. His "distemper seated in the large intestine principally affecting that part where I mentioned the caecum to be, accompanied by violent inflammation and vehement pains, particularly in the right side," is an unsurpassed description of a disease which was supposed to be discovered in modern times—appendicitis. He was the first to mention that a vessel may be ruptured within the cranium, without fracture or depression; the first to use such terms as heart disease (*cardiacus*) and insanity (*insania*); and the first to describe circular amputation by a single sweep of the knife. He considered amputation "the last sad remedy," permissible only in gangrene; circular amputation is still known as Celsus' operation.

Other eponyms are in dermatology, for Celsus described forty skin diseases: severe acute papular eczema (*lichen agrius*) is called Celsus' papules, anesthetic leprosy is Celsus' vitiligo, the soft chancre is known as Celsus' chancre, suppurating ringworm of the scalp is called Celsus' kerion, and the ever-famous condition of patchy baldness (*alopecia areata*) is not less distressing because it bears the classic name of Celsus' area. He was a pioneer in the history of medicine, and in such diverse fields as dentistry, laryngology, ophthalmology, lithotomy and plastic surgery—reparative work was needed by those Jews who wished to hold office among the Romans and could not do so if they lacked a prepuce.

The Hippocratic writers treated hemorrhage by cold, pressure, styptics, and finally the actual cautery; nowhere do they refer to the ligature. Taking a hint from the Alexandrians, Celsus gives us the first satisfactory account of arresting hemorrhage, for after mentioning dry lint, cold sponge, compression, vinegar, corrosives and caustics, he writes, "Finally, if the bleeding continues it will be necessary to grasp the vessel from which the blood is escaping, to ligate it above and below the wounded part, and then divide the vessel between the two ligatures in order that it may retract."

Celsus is one of the mysteries of medicine: if he was a physician, we cannot understand why he apologized for using certain anatomical terms; if not a physician, it is still more difficult to understand how he acquired his technical knowledge. Another reason why some do not consider him a practitioner is rather curious; it is due to "the delicacy of his censure in condemning others." If his work is only a compilation from the Greek, it is nevertheless in a class by itself—never before or since has there been so original a translation. Aside from the Hippocratic writings, Celsus is the most ancient medical classic extant, and will never grow old.

An enthusiastic collector of formulae—which he derived from the most varied sources, by all sorts of methods, including bribery—was Scribonius Largus, whose book on the compounding of medicines may be regarded as the earliest of pharmacopeias. *De compositione medicamentorum* was received with favor by the emperor Claudius, whom Scribonius Largus accompanied on his expedition for the conquest of Britain. Scribonius likewise acted as physician to Claudius' third wife, the loving Messallina, who was always ready to doff the purple robes of office to appear naked in the public brothel. Scribonius describes in detail, the ingredients of the tooth-powder that Messallina employed. The relationship between this medicus and the warm-blooded spouse of Claudius was evidently strictly professional, in which respect the discreet Scribonius differed from his colleague Vettius Valens, who not only prescribed for his young empress, but committed adultery with her—until the day of discovery.

This little intrigue is characteristic of the mad period in which royal ladies set the pace in salacity, and wives poisoned husbands for pastime, and parents and children debauched and murdered each other. In the thick of this welter of darkness and gore, when the monstrous boy Nero was permitted to destroy a Seneca, it is pathetic to hear the voice of Scribonius Largus proclaiming the sanctity of human life. Scribonius possessed a noble conception of the duties of the medical profession, and his book is not only the first pharmacopeia, but a code of ethics.

Scribonius Largus, then, deserves a wreath as one of the few practitioners of his age who honored the Hippocratic Oath, as the first who presented an accurate method of obtaining opium, and as the first who suggested the repeated application of the electric ray-fish in headache and facial neuralgia, which is probably the earliest use of electricity in therapeutics.

Dioscorides, an army surgeon in the service of Nero, in which capacity he traveled extensively, everywhere on the lookout for medicines, is the greatest of medical botanists. In the sense that Hippocrates is the Father of Medicine, and Theophrastus the Father of Botany, Dioscorides is the Father of Materia Medica. Dioscorides came from a province in Asia Minor, and spoke Greek with an accent, but he wrote so clearly that many of his descriptions of ancient plants enabled these plants to be recognized in modern times. His work on materia medica is a limitless storehouse from which all subsequent ages have drawn information.

Opium was known long before his time, but Dioscorides was the first who distinctly praised it. He pointed out that it allays pain, induces sleep, is useful in chronic coughs, and in overdoses occasions a deep and terrible lethargy. He distinguished the juice of the capsules from the extract of the entire plant, and described how the capsules should be incised. He explained how to prepare lard for medicinal purposes, and his method of preparing elaterium has been only slightly modified in recent times. He knew the therapeutic applications of linseed, and gave the technic of making vinegar of squills. He was the first to mention ginger, aconite and ammoniacum, and the first who discussed the therapeutics of aloes. He gave mercury its name of hydrargyrum, or fluid silver. He recommended aspidium for tape-worm. He refers to the astringent properties of iron, and advocated its use in uterine hemorrhage. He knew also that all oaks are astringent. He was the first who indicated means for detecting adulterations in drugs. An enthusiastic student counted 958 remedies in Dioscorides, and of course he overlooked some. As a birth-controller, Dioscorides seems to have been neutral, for while he mentions medicines for the prevention of conception, he likewise specified remedies for promoting the birth of children.

The third of the encyclopedists, Pliny the Elder, disliked Greece and resented its culture, yet was constrained to say, "My object is to treat of all those things which the Greeks include in the Encyclopedia," and amid his official duties for the Roman emperors he followed Greek culture with a fidelity that makes his name a symbol of the unwearied student. We learn from his nephew and heir, Pliny the Younger, that the uncle began work long before daybreak, that he extracted from all he read, saying there was no book so bad as not to contain something of value, that he listened to the reading of his secretaries even while he was rubbed in the bath, as he deemed all time wasted that was not employed in study. Larcius Licinus offered him a fortune for his material, but Pliny would not have parted with it for the Golden House of Nero.

Pliny studied so hard that he had no time for reflection. He swallowed huge chunks of knowledge raw, he gulped it down whole, for that capacious palate could not discriminate between fact and fable. He verified nothing, he rejected no story that was interesting. He was convinced that men who compose books are scholars and not liars, and what was good enough for them was good enough for him. Did not Mutianus say he knew an elephant who could write Greek? If Mutianus, who was three times consul, believed it, why not Pliny? Does not Mucianus speak of shell-fish stopping a vessel in full sail because it was freighted with boys of noble birth who were sent off by Periander to be castrated? Why not insert this in the section on fish? Was it not stated that the lion could tell by the peculiar odor of the panther that the lioness had been unfaithful, and avenged himself with the greatest fury, so that the female when guilty of a lapse, washes herself or else follows the lion at a considerable distance? This was too good to lose, and we can picture Pliny seizing it with avidity for his chapter on lions.

Pliny had been a commander of cavalry, and knew a good deal about horses, even mentioning hermaphrodite horses; he claims that if horses are tricked into committing incest, they will kill themselves or the groom; he quotes King Juba's remark that Queen Semiramis was so enamored of a horse as to cohabit with it; forgetting a previous statement that only man sheds tears, he speaks of weeping horses. Perhaps his most remarkable horse-story is in connection with Apelles: during a pictorial contest, this artist found that his rivals were likely to get the better of him through intrigue, and decided to appeal from the judgment of his fellow-men to the true authorities. Accordingly, horses were shown the various portraits of themselves, which they passed by without notice, but when they came to the picture that Apelles painted, they began to whinny; and it has always been the case since, continues Pliny, whenever this test of his artistic skill has been employed.

Pliny ate eggs, and saw egg-shells; he gathered information about eggs until he was able to describe twenty-two remedies derived from eggs; then he wrote: "Of such strength is an eggshell, that if it is set upright and not inclined to one side, no force or weight can break it." Aulus Gellius, who says Pliny was considered the most learned man of his time, quotes these words from him: "Yawning during childbirth is fatal, just as to sneeze after coition produces abortion." Such is the result of closing one's eyes and immersing one's self in erudition.

In his book on man, Pliny, after assembling his notes from Herodotus, Aristotle, Varro, Isigonus, Nymphodorus, Apollonides, Megasthenes, Crates of Pergamus, Beeton and many others, especially Ctesias, evidently wishes to prepare us for some stories that are coming, for he asks: "Who, for instance, could ever believe in the existence of the Negroes, who had not first seen them? Indeed, what is there that does not appear marvellous, when it comes to our knowledge for the first time?" Following this warning, he tells us of various races of man: of the Arimaspi, who have but one eye in the middle of the forehead and carry on a perpetual conflict with the gold-guarding Griffins; of the Illyria who have two pupils in each eye; of another tribe who are without necks, and have their eyes in their shoulders; of the Triballi, who can kill an enemy by fixing their gaze upon him; of the inhabitants of Abarimon, whose feet are turned backwards; of the Monocoli, who have only one leg, but are able to leap with surprising agility; of the Thibii, who cannot drown in water; of the Scyritae, who have no nostrils, but holes in their faces; of the Astomi, who have no mouths, but subsist by inhaling odiferous fruits and flowers; of the Pandore, whose hair is white in youth and black in old age; of men born with long tails; of others, who have ears so large as to cover the whole body; and of Indians who have connections with animals, the offspring being half man and half beast.

These wonders uplift the soul of Pliny, who exclaims, "Nature, in her ingenuity, has created all these marvels in the human race, with others of a similar nature, as so many amusements to herself, though they appear miraculous to us. But who is there that can enumerate all the things that she brings to pass each day, I may almost say each hour? As a striking evidence of her power, let it be sufficient for me to have cited whole nations in the list of her prodigies. Let us now proceed to mention some other particulars connected with Man, the truth of which is universally admitted." Then follows an equally chimerical catalogue, interesting and multifarious, but with scant relationship to truth. It must not be thought however, that Pliny is invariably preposterous. His science is usually addled, but his interjections are often admirable, as witness: "But it is the belly, for the gratification of which the greater part of mankind exist, that causes the most suffering to man. It is for its sake, more particularly, that avarice is so insatiate, for its sake that luxury is so refined, for its sake that men voyage to the shores even of the Phasis, for its sake that the very depths of the ocean are ransacked. And yet, with all this, no one ever gives a thought how abject is the condition of this part of our body, how disgusting the results of its action upon what it has received!"

As a collector of data, he had few equals. Of his voluminous writings, only the thirty-seven books of his Natural History remain, and his nephew, in the letter to Baebius Macer, was not far wrong when he described it as "a work remarkable for its comprehensiveness and erudition, and not less varied than Nature herself." Since the younger Pliny, in the epistle to Sura, relates in detail a full-fledged ghost-story—including a haunted house, silence, rattling of chains and bones—and says he believes it, he probably found nothing amiss with the Natural History. It is impossible to give an idea of these volumes—thousands of pages of useful information, mixed with the absurdest nonsense ever written under the auspices of science, interlarded with many excellent comments. Had the mind of Pliny been of a higher type, his Natural History would not be a treasure-house of endless curios. His errors no longer misinform us, and the items remain to charm the succeeding generations.

Pliny is inimitable. He had no qualifications for science, except industry and enthusiasm. He is so anxious to give us information, that he lies without limit. His discussion of menstruation is characteristically Plinian:

It would indeed be a difficult matter to find anything which is productive of more marvellous effects than the menstrual discharge. On the approach of a woman in this state, must will become sour, seeds which are touched by her become sterile, grafts wither away, garden plants are parched up, and the fruit will fall from the tree beneath which she sits. Her very look, even, will dim the brightness of mirrors, blunt the edge of steel, and take away the polish from ivory. . . .

Over and above these particulars, there is no limit to the marvellous powers attributed to females. For, in the first place, hailstorms, they say, whirlwinds, and lightning even, will be scared away by a woman uncovering her body while her monthly courses are upon her. The same, too, with all other kinds of tempestuous weather; and out at sea, a storm may be lulled by a woman uncovering her body merely, even though not menstruating at the time. As to the menstrual discharge itself, a thing that in other respects, as already stated on a more appropriate occasion, is productive of the most monstrous effects, there are some ravings about it of a most dreadful and unutterable nature.

Of these particulars, however, I do not feel so much shocked at mentioning the following. If the menstrual discharge coincides with an eclipse of the moon, or sun, the evils resulting from it are irremediable; and no less so, when it happens while the moon is in conjunction with the sun; the congress with a woman at such a period being noxious, and attended with fatal effects to the man. At this period also, the lustre of purple is tarnished by the touch of a woman: so much more baneful is her influence at this time than at any other. At any other time, also, if a woman strips herself naked while she is menstruating, and walks round a field of wheat, the caterpillars, worms, beetles, and other vermin, will fall from off the ears of corn. Metrodorus of Scepsos tells us that this discovery was first made in Cappadocia; and that, in consequence of such multitudes of cantharides being found to breed there, it is the practice for women to walk through the middle of the fields with their garments tucked up above the thighs. In other places, again, it is the usage for women to go barefoot, with the hair dishevelled and the girdle loose: due precaution must be taken, however, that this is not done at sun-rise, for if so, the crop will wither and dry up. Young vines, too, it is said, are injured irremediably by the touch of a woman in this state; and both rue and ivy, plants possessed of highly medicinal virtues, will die instantly upon being touched by her.

Much as I have already stated on the virulent effects of this discharge, I have to state, in addition, that bees, it is a well-known fact, will forsake their hives if touched by a menstruous woman; that linen boiling in the cauldron will turn black, that the edge of a razor will become blunted, and that copper vessels will contract a fetid smell and become covered with verdigrease, on coming in contact with her. A mare big with foal, if touched by a woman in this state, will be sure to miscarry; nay, even more than this, at the very sight of a woman, though seen at a distance even, should she happen to be menstruating for the first time after the loss of her virginity, or for the first time, while in a state of virginity.

Icetidas the physician pledges his word that quartan fever may be cured by sexual intercourse, provided the woman is just beginning to menstruate. It is universally agreed, too, that when a person has been bitten by a dog and manifests a dread of water and of all kinds of drink, it will be quite sufficient to put under his cup a strip of cloth that has been dipped in this fluid; the result being that the hydrophobia will immediately disappear. This arises, no doubt, from that powerful sympathy which has been so much spoken of by the Greeks, and the existence of which is proved by the fact, already mentioned, that dogs become mad upon tasting this fluid.

Another thing universally acknowledged and one which I am ready to believe with the greatest pleasure, is the fact, that if the doorposts are only touched with the menstruous fluid all spells of the magicians will be neutralized—a set of men the most lying in existence, as any one may ascertain. I will give an example of one of the most reasonable of their prescriptions—Take the parings of the toe-nails and finger-nails of a sick person, and mix them up with wax, the party saying that he is seeking a remedy for a tertian, quartan, or quotidian fever, as the case may be; then stick this wax, before sunrise, upon the door of another person—such is the prescription they give for these diseases! What deceitful persons they must be if there is no truth in it! And how highly criminal, if they really do thus transfer diseases from one person to another! Some of them, again, whose practices are of a less guilty nature, recommend that the parings of all the finger-nails should be thrown at the entrance of ant-holes, the first ant to be taken which attempts to draw one into the hole; this, they say, must be attached to the neck of the patient, and he will experience a speedy cure.

It is odd to hear the gullible Pliny, after immersing his readers in the deepest sorcery, raising an indignant voice against magicians.

It was Pliny's destiny to devote himself to what he thought he disliked. Had he been asked his opinion of the medical profession, and especially of Greek physicians, he would have drawn his toga around him with disdain as sadness clouded his eyes. Horace was not the only Roman who said "Captive Greece has taken captive her rude conquerer." Pliny complains in more prosaic but equally emphatic terms: "Yes, avow it we must—the Roman people, in extending its empire, has lost sight of its ancient manners, and in that we have conquered we are the conquered: for now we obey the natives of foreign lands, who by the agency of a single art have even out-generalled our generals. More, however, on this topic hereafter."

Pliny liked to remind his readers that for six hundred years the Romans knew no physicians, and he also liked the epitaph he found on a tomb-stone: "He died by reason of the confusion of the doctors." Pliny wrote, "The dignity of the Roman does not permit him to make a profession of medicine, and the few Romans who begin to study it are venal renegades to the Greeks."

But Pliny was fonder of medicine than he knew, otherwise he would not have devoted so much attention to it. Nearly all parts of the *Naturalis historia* are of some medical interest, while several of its books are exclusively medical. The debt of medicine to Pliny is simply incalculable. He has preserved for us all the old systems of medicine as he understood them, with countless anecdotes and details that no one else would have dreamt of putting on paper. The names of scores of physicians survive in the pages of Pliny alone. In a single one of the thirty-seven books he discusses: whether words are possessed of any healing efficacy; remedies from the wax of the human ear, hair, teeth, blood, excretions, and the dead; remedies obtained from sneezing, from the sexual congress, woman's milk and spittle; remedies from foreign animals—nineteen from the crocodile; remedies to be adopted against enchantments, poisons, baldness, toothache, tonsillitis, pains in the neck, spitting of blood, stomach and liver complaints, tapeworm and trouble in the colon, gout and diseases of the feet, epilepsy, jaundice, melancholy, lethargy, phthisis, asthma, dropsy, erysipelas, hemorrhage, ulcers, carcinomatous sores and broken bones. This learned layman never hesitates; he knows every detail about medicine—did he not read it, and cannot he cite his authorities? The *Naturalis historia* is a portentous jest, but it is certain that from the first century A.D. to the present time, no one has written a history of medicine without cribbing from Pliny.

We cannot write about history or geography, science or medicine, literature or art, without quoting Pliny—and it is never necessary to believe him. Babbling, garrulous, credulous Pliny—how indispensable he is! Whoever has not pored long hours over his Pliny, has missed one of the greatest delights that reading affords. Few works of antiquity are more instructive, fewer still are so entertaining. Better that Pliny should have been saved, than that the Colosseum should still be standing. Had the

Naturalis historia of Pliny perished with the rest of his works, much of the savor of antiquity would have been lost.

The character of Pliny deserves our highest admiration. It is strange that one so lost in superstition and overwhelmed by magic should not have believed in a future life—he states plainly that after death the soul has no more existence than it had before birth—but he worked until his last day. Unequipped to investigate science, he nevertheless was a martyr of science. The world knows how Pliny died, for the nephew told the historian Tacitus who informed posterity. On the twenty-fourth of August 79 A.D., Pliny was in command of a fleet at Misenum. He had bathed and lunched and was engaged in study when his attention was directed to an unusual cloud. His habitual curiosity was immediately aroused, and calling for his shoes, he ascended a hill. The younger Pliny declined to accompany him, and remained at home reading a volume of Livy. Pliny breathed heavily as he climbed, for he was fifty-six and fat. It was more than a cloud that Pliny saw—it was a volcanic force. He could have escaped, but he could not desert a scientific phenomenon. The sea ebbed, cities rocked and mountains slipped; day was darker than night, and pumice and sulphur blotted out the sun; life stopped as the volcano spread for the inhabitants an eternal blanket of ashes.

On the third day they found Pliny near Pompeii, his body fully clothed, and without a sign of injury. But a vapor from Vesuvius had blocked his windpipe, and now he slept with Empedocles who long ago had disappeared in the crater of Mount Etna. The name of Pliny is imperishable, and the concluding words of his *Naturalis historia* constitute his own best epitaph: "Farewell, Nature, parent of all things, and in thy manifold multiplicity bless me who, alone of the Romans, has sung thy praise."

The prolix Galen complains of the Syrian Archigenes of Apamea: "It should have been the special duty of Archigenes, who appeared on the scene next in order after a series of the most illustrious physicians, to infuse more light into medical teaching. Unfortunately, he did the very opposite; for we who have grown old in the exercise of the art, and should therefore find it easy to comprehend what is written about medicine, are at times unable to understand what he says. Such being the true state of affairs, I now propose to undertake what Archigenes failed to accomplish." From the surviving fragments, however, we wish we had a little less of Galen and a little more of Archigenes. Elsewhere, even Galen speaks highly of him, and it is now claimed that much of Aretaeus and Aëtius is derived from Archigenes. The ancients had admirable qualities, but their utter disregard of quotation-marks has wrinkled the brow of posterity.

Archigenes wrote the best contemporary account of leprosy; distinguished between primary and secondary symptoms in disease; attempted to locate the pathology by the variety of pain; suggested classification of mineral waters according to their composition; and found time—in the intervals of using the vaginal speculum and prescribing hair-dyes for the fashionable ladies—to become the author of the most elaborate of the ancient treatises on the pulse. As a member of the Pneumatici—a sect which took its name from the *pneuma* or vital spirit, and was founded by Athenaeus of Cilicia—this was expected from Archigenes, for the pneumatists were subtle, and it has been said that although they discovered new diseases, they established more varieties of fever than exist in nature. Archigenes was one of the great surgeons of his era, operating in cancer of the breast and womb, and amputating limbs, with employment of the ligature, in a manner that we consider modern.

Surprisingly enough, Archigenes, thrice-mentioned by Juvenal, escapes unscathed from those grim hands, but the satirist has branded with eternal infamy the name of another great surgeon—Heliodorus. Shocked translators omit the passage in which Juvenal depicts Heliodorus castrating robust young slaves so their lustful mistresses may use them with impunity: "matron and maid, the sex has turned all whore; to escape abortion they love the eunuchs, but only such as have been gelded at manhood's age; all that the navel-string could give is present except the beard—and that's the barber's loss, not theirs." History cannot be written by prudes.

Had his writings survived, Heliodorus would be a famous figure. The fragments saved by the devotion of Oribasius, and later by Nicetas—on probing injuries of the skull, bandaging, torsion of blood-vessels, flap and circular amputations, operative treatment of hernia and stricture, and resections—are ample evidence of a great surgeon. One passage, which incidentally reveals the surgeons of that time as operating with needless rapidity, exhibits Heliodorus as a pioneer of the ligature: "Amputation above the elbow or knee is very dangerous owing to the size of the vessels divided. Some operators in their foolish haste cut through all the soft parts at one stroke, but it seems to me better to first divide the flesh on the side away from the vessels, and then to saw the bone, so as to be ready at once to check the bleeding when the large vessels are cut. And before operating, it is my habit to tie a ligature as tightly as possible above the point of amputation."

Another surgeon who lives only in fragments is Antyllus. We grope through the centuries, reading the works of his successors, grateful to Oribasius, seizing upon the few lines in Paulus Aegineta, invading the vast *Continens* of Rhazes for a reference, always hoping for additional information about Antyllus. The scalpel of Antyllus opened new frontiers for Greek surgery. He operated on the opaque crystalline lens without injuring the humor, relieved suffocation by cutting into the windpipe, repaired or restored defective organs with the neighboring skin and connective tissue, removed diseased portion of bone without disturbing its continuity, and extracted bones in their entirety while preserving the joint.

This master of major surgery did not neglect the little things which count for so much: when he mentions plasters or ointments, he tells how to prepare and spread them; if he speaks of wet or dry cupping, he describes the bronze, horn and glass vessels; if he recommends the natural or artificial leech, he explains how it should be applied; if he discusses abscesses, he points out the lines of incision; when necessary to probe a fistula, he shows how to make a bougie from rolled papyrus; when he visited a patient he regulated the temperature and lighting of his home, instructed him whether or not to indulge in gymnastics, told him what to eat and drink, how to bathe, and even how to lie in bed.

Antyllus was the creator of arterial surgery, and was the first to distinguish aneurysm caused by pathological dilatation and aneurysm forming after trauma of the artery. When he treated a circumscribed distention of the arterial wall by ligating the aneurysm above and below the pulsating sac, followed by opening the aneurysm and evacuating its bloody contents, he projected his name to the present time, for the method of Antyllus is still pictured in the textbooks and defined in the dictionaries.

Soranus of Ephesus in Asia Minor—nearly all the leading Greek physicians of the Roman empire came from Asia Minor—stands out as the first specialist in diseases of women and children. Like most of the famous physicians of the time, he studied in Alexandria, and settled in Rome. His work on Diseases of Women, written for midwives, was composed in Greek, which was still the language of medicine in the reigns of Trajan and Hadrian. Soranus, a determined foe of superstition, begs the midwives not to make their practice dependent on their dreams; if he had any success in this line, his pupils were wiser than those of later generations. Soranus belonged to the School of Methodics, and Caelius Aurelianus called him "chief among the leaders of our sect" (*methodicorum princeps*).

There was little about the female genitalia that Soranus did not know, and after his description of the anatomy of the womb, there was no longer any excuse for confusing the vagina and the uterus. He popularized the vaginal speculum, and his obstetric chair or labor-stool was the parent of numerous offspring. Instead of hastening the expulsion of the fetus by manhandling the mother in the traditional manner—shaking her, rolling her, making her run up and down stairs, or jolting her on a ladder—he instituted gentleness in the lying-in chamber. He knew that conception can be prevented by closing the mouth of the womb with cotton or ointments, that the *os uteri* opens during coitus and menstruation, that the woman conceives most readily following the menstrual period, and that sterility occurs in men as well as women—which some modern gynecologists seem to forget. He described all afflictions to which female flesh is heir, from the viscid vaginal discharge and excessive accumulation of gas, to hysteria and nymphomania.

His pediatric section is noteworthy, and the minuteness with which he catalogues the qualifications of a wetnurse—he knew that an infant may thrive at the breast of one woman and not of another—must have gained for him the confidence of mothers. Medicine cannot always divorce itself from patriotism, and Soranus preferred Greek nurses in order that the suckling might early become accustomed to the most beautiful of languages. No modern pediatrician is more meticulous about the removal of the vernix caseosa, the baby's bath, clothing, feeding habits and bowel movements, teething and tonsillitis, than Soranus. If the infant had diarrhea, Soranus gave astringents to the nurse; if it suffered from constipation, it was the nurse who took the laxatives. Soranus could diagnose the child's condition from the varieties of its cries, and he even described baby-carriages.

Living in Rome, he found it necessary to inform the ladies that by tampons saturated with a decoction of galls, they could reduce the vagina to virginal size; it may seem strange that a man of his extensive experience, familiar with every detail of female anatomy, had never seen a hymen and was unaware of its existence—but this merely proves that Martial and Juvenal were right. As a concluding refrain for the work of Soranus, we may quote this passage from Juvenal: "These poor women, however, endure the perils of childbirth, and all the troubles of nursing to which their lot condemns them; but how often does a gilded bed contain a woman that is lying in? So great is the skill, so powerful the drugs, of the abortionist, paid to murder mankind within the womb. Rejoice, poor wretch; give her the stuff to drink whatever it be, with your own hand: for were she willing to get big and trouble her womb with bouncing babies, you might perhaps find yourself the father of an Ethiopian; and some day a colored heir, whom you would rather not meet by daylight, would fill all the places in your will."

Aretaeus the Cappodocian, a Greek physician of a Roman province in Asia Minor, described diseases in admirable Ionic. This one sentence is the complete biography of Aretaeus; all else about him is surmise. Even the age in which he lived is in dispute, for Clio celebrates the birthdays of the destroyers, rather than of the healers, of men.

It is a delight to read Aretaeus; he is seldom superstitious, his mind is not heavy with befuddled theories, and he does not indulge in any of those mystical speculations which disfigure the pages of so many of his successors. No doubt the strangest passage Aretaeus ever wrote was his fantastic account of the uterus: "In the middle of the flanks of women lies the womb, a female viscus, closely resembling an animal, for it is moved of itself hither and thither in the flanks, also upwards in a direct line to below the cartilage of the thorax; and also obliquely to the right or the left either to the liver or spleen; and it likewise is subject to prolapsus downwards, and in a word, is altogether erratic. It delights in fragrant smells, and advances towards them; and, it has an aversion to fetid smells, and flees from them: and, on the whole the womb is like an animal within an animal."

No medical author surpasses Aretaeus in his vivid portrayal of disease. When he describes consumption, we must not read the symptoms twice to make the diagnosis. We hear the hoarse chronic cough, the clearing of the throat, the blood and pus spat up; we notice the sweats, the pallor, the cadaverous aspect; we see the bony fingers, the thickened joints, the curved nails, the sharp and slender nose, and the prominent Adam's apple; we see the narrow chest, the lips drawn over the teeth, the muscles of the arm gone, the ribs sticking through the skin, the shoulder-blades projecting like wings of birds, and the eyes hollow and brilliant.

His description of tetanus, epilepsy, hysteria and asthma have been especially praised, but his picture of satyriasis is as powerful as any: "Satyrs, priests of Bacchus, in the paintings and statues, have the phallus erect, as the symbol of the divine performance. It is also a form of disease, in which the patient has erection of the genital organ, the appellation of satyriasis being derived from its resemblance to the figure of the god. It is an unrestrainable impulse to connection; but neither are they at all relieved by these embraces, nor is the tentigo soothed by many and repeated acts of sexual intercourse. Spasms of all the nerves, and tension of all the tendons, groins, and perineum, inflammation and pain of the genital parts, redness of countenance, and a dewy moisture. Wrapped up in silent sorrow, they are stupid, as if grievously afflicted with their calamity. But if the affection overcome the patient's sense of shame, he will lose all restraint of tongue as regards obscenity, and likewise all restraint in regard to the open performance of the act. Raving with his obscene imagination, he cannot contain himself; tormented with thirst, he vomits much phlegm, and the foam sits on his lips as in a lascivious goat, and he has a smell like that animal." Strangely enough, the author of the above had no knowledge of nymphomania, and even denied its existence. Yet he lived after Valeria Messallina!

In his writings we find the first satisfactory description of diphtheria. He is now famous as the author of the first systematic account of diabetes. He correctly called it a species of dropsy, and paints with realistic strokes the patient's fiery thirst, his imperative desire to pass water, his dry mouth and parched skin; it is a wonderful malady, he says, a melting down of the flesh into urine.

Aretaeus seems to have understood the direction of the blood-flow in the veins; if so, he knew more than the physicians of subsequent centuries. He distinguished between the paralyses of motion and of sensation, and knew that injuries to the brain produce paralysis on the opposite side. He divided mental disturbances into mania, melancholia, and settled insanity—not a bad classification. He described lead colic, and other disturbances due to lead poisoning. In obstruction of the urethra by vesical calculus, he employed the catheter. He removed stone by incising below the scrotum, and cutting inward to the neck of the bladder until there was an escape of urine and calculi. He deserves credit for his efforts to found pathology upon an anatomical basis. One of his greatest claims to our consideration is that he was the first to employ, so far as we know, the beginnings of inspection, palpation, percussion and auscultation—the four features of physical diagnosis.

He had few queer notions. It is true, in conformity with the custom of his age, he was too fond of venesection, but he always warned against excess of bloodletting, claiming it was better to err on the side of chariness. He believed castor was a remedy in all diseases of the nerves, and that white hellebore would vanquish any case of gout. For this we must not blame him severely, for there is scarcely a practitioner who has not at least a couple of old standbys by which he swears.

An idea of the nicety of his observations may be gained from a random passage; in discussing methods of procuring sleep he writes: "Gentle rubbing of the feet with oil, patting of the head, and particularly stroking of the temples and ears is an effectual means; for by the stroking of their ears and temples wild beasts are overcome, so as to cease from their anger and fury. But whatever is familiar to any one is to him provocative of sleep. Thus, to the sailor, repose in a boat, and being carried about on the sea, the sound of the beach, the murmur of the waves, the boom of the winds, and the scent of the sea and the ship. But to the musician the accustomed notes of his flute in stillness; or playing on the harp or lyre, or the exercise of musical children with song. To a teacher, intercourse with the tattle of children. Different persons are soothed to sleep by different means."

Here is a bit of psychology which every medical man will endorse: "This is a mighty wonder, that in hemorrhage from the lungs, which is particularly dangerous, patients do not despair, even when near their end. The insensibility of the lungs to pain appears to me to be the cause of this; for pain even when slight makes one fear death. In most cases pain is more dreadful than pernicious, whereas the absence of it, even in serious illness, is unaccompanied by fear of death and is more dangerous than dreadful."

Aretaeus' caution and scepticism may be sensed from these remarks on the treatment of epilepsy: "It is told, that the brain of a vulture, and the heart of a raw cormorant, and the domestic weasel, when eaten, remove the disease; but I have never tried these things. However, I have seen persons holding a cup below the wound of a man recently slaughtered, and drinking a draught of the blood! O the present, the mighty necessity, which compels one to remedy the evil by such a wicked abomination! And whether even they recovered by this means no one could tell me for certain. There is another story of the liver of a man having been eaten. However, I leave these things to be described by those who would bear to try such means."

One of the mysteries of medicine is the absence of any Hippocratic reference to infection, although at least two of his contemporaries—the historian Thucydides and the orator Isocrates—wrote that certain diseases are communicable; casual allusions to contagion are scattered in the writings of Lucretius, Virgil, Dion Cassius of Utica, Dionysius of Halicarnassus, Livy and Plutarch. The encyclopedist Varro visualized invisible infecting organisms, and according to Ovid: "Bodies rot on the ground, blasting with their stench, and spreading contagion far and near. No one can control the pest, which fiercely breaks out upon the very physicians, and their arts do but injure those who use them. The nearer one is to the sick and the more faithfully he serves them, the more quickly is he himself stricken unto death." The poet vividly indicated, in the magnificent description from which these lines are taken, that the disease passed from animal to animal and spread by contact from man to man, but the profession remained silent, still believing in atmospheric influences, and dreading miasma instead of infection. Aretaeus is the earliest medical author to allude to the doctrine, and was the first to distinguish between conveyance of disease by actual contact (*contagion*) and transmission of disease at a distance (*infection*).

There is a vague foreshadowing of endocrinology in this passage: "For it is the semen, when possessed of vitality, which makes us to be men, hot, well braced in limbs, hairy, well voiced, spirited, strong to think and to act, as the characteristics of men prove. For when the semen is not possessed of its vitality, persons become shriveled, have a sharp tone of voice, lose their hair and their beard, and become effeminate, as the characteristics of eunuchs prove."

There is another sentence which should be quoted, as it will arouse a response from every physician who has been called at the last moment or when there was no hope for recovery: "If you give a medicine at the height of the dyspnea, or when death is at hand, you may be blamed for the patient's death by the vulgar." What a world of reserve and dignity is in this simple remark! The shoulders of Aretaeus the Cappadocian were broad enough to wear becomingly the mantle of Hippocrates.

Many centuries ago Aretaeus knew the knack of driving a point home by a good story. Wishing to illustrate that the gout may intermit, he relates that a person subject to gout won the race in the Olympic games during the interval of the disease. And he closes his chapter on melancholy thus: "A story is told that a certain person, incurably affected, fell in love with a girl; and when the physicians could bring him no relief, love cured him. But I think that he was originally in love, and that he was dejected and spiritless from being unsuccessful with the girl, and appeared to the common people to be melancholic. He then did not know that it was love; but when he imparted the love to the girl, he ceased from his dejection, and dispelled his passion and sorrow; and with joy he awoke from his lowness of spirits, and he became restored to understanding, love being his physician."

Aretaeus shows himself a true physician by his concern and sympathy for the patient, in small matters and great: "Inunctions are more agreeable and efficacious than fomentations; for an ointment does not run down and stain the bed clothes—a thing very disagreeable to the patient—but it adheres, and being by the heat of the body, is absorbed. Thus its effects are persistent, whereas liquid preparations run off." Aretaeus uttered this noble phrase, rarely equaled and never bettered: "When he can render no further aid, the physician alone can still mourn as a man with his incurable patient: this is the physician's sad lot."

In Galen's time, the Syrian satirist, Lucian of Samosata, came to Rome in search of an oculist. Lucian was the wittiest sceptic of the ancient world, a warrior against superstition charging with unsurpassed Greek at the gods, pouring unquenchable laughter over the ghosts of his day. The question which Lucian asked of another, "What business had he to be the only sane man in a crowd of madmen?"—explains why Lucian's exposure of imposture was foredoomed to failure. Lucian's references to doctors and diseases are numerous, and his *Life of Alexander the Paphlagonian* is the classic chapter in the annals of quackery. Alexander was strikingly handsome, and according to Lucian, "while in the bloom of his youthful beauty, he traded quite shamelessly upon it." In maturity and old age, to man and to woman, Alexander's charm remained irresistible.

Trained by a medical charlatan, he realized that "fat-heads" —to use his own descriptive expression—could be shorn profitably in Aesculapian pastures. In Apollo's temple on the Bosporus he secreted brass tablets, which were discovered to bear the information that Aesculapius would appear in Alexander's birthplace; at night, in the mud of the foundation of the new shrine, Alexander hid a new-born reptile in a blown goose-egg, sealing the breakage with wax and white lead. How he found this sacred egg and exhibited the nascent god to the populace; afterward showed them a Macedonian serpent which he claimed was the fully-grown Aesculapius; established an oracle and was consulted by all the world; furnished mysterious answers which could be interpreted only by his own interpreters at additional cost; set up a far-reaching espionage system in Rome itself, so that he knew who planned to visit him and for what purpose; how every trick was swallowed and every deceit added to his fame; how he grew fabulously wealthy by blackmail; how the few who protested against his frauds were stoned by his orders; how he increased his prestige during the great plague; how Marcus Aurelius requested and followed Alexander's advice with disastrous results—are all matters which must be read in Lucian's animated pages.

Lucian, under an assumed name, sent a closed packet to Alexander; he declared on the outside that it contained eight questions; and he paid eight fees. Occupied with his followers, and rarely encountering unbelief, Alexander neglected his forged seals and heated needles, and returned eight meaningless answers. Lucian smiled as he received the replies, for he had asked only one question: "When will the villainies of Alexander be exposed?" It was a rash inquiry, for when the deceiver learned that he had been deceived, Lucian narrowly escaped with his life. It is a sad reflection that it required gangrene of the leg to terminate the long and successful career of this necromancer. Medals from the joint reigns of Marcus Aurelius and Lucius Verus, in commemoration of Aesculapius and Alexander the Paphlagonian, have survived; when these coins crumble to dust, new Alexanders will arise and find new victims, for the disease of credulity is incurable—yet the words of Lucian are eternal: "The historian's one task is to tell the thing as it happened."

In the year 162, a stranger entered Rome—it was Clarissimus Galen (130-200), native of Pergamum in Mysia, Asia Minor. Pergamum was celebrated for its shrine to the healing god, and according to Lucian, Jupiter complained that his altars were deserted since Apollo set up his oracle at Delphi, and Aesculapius opened shop at Pergamum. The school of medicine and library of Pergamum made even Alexandria envious, and the second Ptolemy, to prevent Pergamum from adding manuscripts to its archives, was ignoble enough to decree that no more papyrus be exported from Egypt. The Pergamenians took splendid revenge by turning the skin of sheep and goats into parchment (*per-*

gamena), and nearly all the extant classical manuscripts are written, not on papyrus, but on parchment. Pergamum gloried in these books until Marc Antony, who never read anything except Cicero's name on the list of the proscribed, stole the entire library as a gift for Cleopatra.

Galen, the best-educated and most gifted physician of the second century—and of the centuries to come—could not be content in the provinces or in fallen Alexandria. Aware of his power, and consumed with ambition, he hungered and thirsted for the center of the world's stage. He longed for an opportunity to diagnose the disease of a senator or praetor—and thus win fame and fortune at a stroke. Among his first patients at home was Eudemus, a peripatetic philosopher of renown. The wife of the consul Boethus was sick, Galen cured her, and received the consul's friendship, four hundred gold pieces, and a reputation. A noble Roman matron, the wife of Justus, could not sleep; her case baffled all the physicians; but Galen traced her insomnia to her love for the dancer Pylades.

It was not long before Galen became the most distinguished practitioner in Rome. He was called the wonder-worker—Paradoxopoeus. Galen did not accept the title with blushing cheek and downcast eye. The conceit which enabled him to say, "Whoever seeks fame need only become familiar with all that I have achieved," was thick enough to protect him from embarrassment at any compliment. Not only did the boastful Galen praise himself unceasingly, but he mocked all his rivals with a scornful tongue; he called them fools and asses, and told them they did not know anything.

"I have done as much to medicine," wrote Galen, "as Trajan did to the Roman Empire, in making bridges and roads throughout Italy. It is I alone that have pointed out the true method of treating diseases: it must be confessed that Hippocrates had already chalked out the same road, but as the first discoverer, he has not gone so far as we could wish; his writings are defective in order, in the necessary distinctions; his knowledge in some subjects is not sufficiently extensive; he is often obscure after the manner of the ancients, in order to be concise; he opened the road, but I have rendered it passable." Some figures of antiquity appear hardly human: the white-robed Plato, broad of brow and ever-thoughtful, slowly pacing down the shadeful aisles of the Academic Grove, seems more like a personification of philosophy than a man, but Galenus had qualities like our next-door neighbors.

The leaders of Roman society requested Galen to establish a course of lectures on Anatomy and Physiology, which he gladly did, illustrating them with experiments on goats and pigs. The élite crowded to these demonstrations, and were pleased to be informed that they possessed more common sense than the physicians. At Alexandria Galen had been fortunate enough to witness two human skeletons, and he strongly urged all who intended to study osteology to go to Africa. But at his lectures a human skeleton was never exhibited, for the good reason that there was not a single one in all Rome. So bloodthirsty were the Romans of this period, that neither the populace nor the fashionables could enjoy a holiday unless contending ranks of gladiators were butchered for their sport, but they recoiled with horror at the notion of permitting a scientist to examine the murdered corpse. In this respect the Romans resembled a small and persecuted sect—despised by Galen—which was just rising into prominence at this time, but which was later to overrun all Europe and forbid dissection on the ground that it was impious to mutilate the image of God, and yet showed no hesitancy in crushing the bones or burning the bodies of thousands of heretics. The psychology of inconsistency is tragically interesting.

For four years Galen resided at Rome, writing many of the works which have perpetuated his name: he worked as hard as he bragged. "There are many physicians," declared Galen, "like the athletes, who would like to win prizes in the Olympic games, and yet will not take the pains necessary to gain them. For they are loud in their praises of Hippocrates, and place him in the highest rank among physicians; yet never think of imitating him themselves. It is certainly no small advantage on our side to live at the present day, and to have received from our ancestors the arts already brought to such a degree of perfection; and it would seem an easy thing for us, after learning in a short time everything that Hippocrates discovered by many years of labor, to employ the rest of our lives in investigating what still remains unknown."

In the year 166 it was practically certain that he was to be admitted into the imperial court. Yet it was at this very time that he secretly left the capital. Galen claimed he so acted because he feared his envious rivals had decided to assassinate him. But the truth seems to be that he left Rome because an epidemic had come. Rome, with its usual intrigues, was bad enough; but Rome, with an eastern pestilence added, was too much for the Pergamene physician. Galen was too selfish to die for others. In those days there were real plagues: this one spread over Europe, infected everything in its wide path, and remained for fifteen years, slaughtering men and animals by the million, terrorizing the world into a mad-house and a morgue. Aesculapius must have been sleeping.

Galen set his face toward home, studying all the way; from the copper mines of Cyprus he collected medicinal ores, Balm of Gilead at Palestine, asphalt from the Dead Sea, and many drugs in Phoenicia. At last he stood once more in the fertile valley of Pergamum; he remained there about a year. But the Greeks and Romans had a habit of recalling their famous sons almost as soon as they were out of sight. Half the illustrious men of Athens and Rome were exiled and invited to return. The emperor Marcus Aurelius summoned Galen to his side. Marcus Aurelius was at Aquileia, preparing to wage war against the Marcomanni, though he would much have preferred to be in his study, writing his *Meditations*. When Galen arrived in the camp, the flesh-fed plague was thinning the army, and the emperor and his soldiers fled back to Rome. On setting out a second time against the enemy, Marcus Aurelius desired Galen to be his companion, but the physician informed his ruler that in a dream Aesculapius had warned him to remain at Rome and attend the emperor's children. And sure enough, little Commodus soon became sick, and Galen performed the doubtful service of saving a creature that became one of the most infamous of the hideous Roman emperors. But Faustina, the mother of the monster, was pleased, and she thanked Galen heartily, and crooned into the ear of her child that one day he would wear the purple.

Upon the decease of Demetrius, Galen was appointed court physician, but he had considerable time for scientific work, as his chief duty consisted in preparing for Marcus Aurelius a costly treacle, the supposed antidote against all poisons: in the days of imperial Rome such precautions were not superfluous.

In 175 Marcus Aurelius succeeded in subduing the fierce Marcommani, and returned to the capital. Of course a triumphant emperor must be feasted, and the Romans were champion gluttons with extraordinary alimentary canals, but the scholarly Aurelius was really a transplanted Greek whose ordinary stomach gave way under the endless courses. Poor Marcus needed all his stoic philosophy to keep him from groaning, and he sent for several physicians. A physician's function is to administer medicines, and they did so, but their drugs did not avail. Galen was sent for, but we must allow him to relate the incident in his characteristic style:

Hereupon I was summoned also to spend the night in the palace, a messenger coming to fetch me, by order of the emperor, just as the lamps were being lighted. Three physicians had seen him in the morning and at the eighth hour, and two had felt his pulse, whilst to all did it appear the beginning of an attack. I, however, remained silent; then the emperor, perceiving me, asked why I had not, like the others, felt his pulse. I replied: Two have already done this, and from their experiences upon the journey with thee are better able to judge of its present condition. As I said this he called on me to feel him, and as the pulse, taking into consideration the age and constitution of the patient, seemed to me inconsistent with an attack of fever, I declared that none was to be feared, but that the stomach was overloaded with nourishment which had been coated with phlegm. This diagnosis called forth his praise and he thrice repeated: Yes that is it, it is exactly as thou sayest; I feel that cold food is disagreeing with me. He then asked me what was to be done. I answered him frankly that if another than he had been the patient, I should, following my custom, have given him wine with pepper. With sovereigns like thyself, however, I said, physicians are in the habit of employing the least drastic remedies, therefore it must suffice to apply wool saturated with warm spikenard upon the abdomen. The emperor replied that warm ointment on purple wool was his usual remedy for pain in the stomach, and called Peitholaus to apply it while he bade me depart. No sooner had I gone than he demanded Sabine wine, threw pepper into it and drank, after which he said to Peitholaus that now at last he had a physician and a courageous one, repeating that he had tried many but that I was the first of physicians and the only philosopher among them.

On fevers, and everything connected with febrile affections, whether ephemeral, bilious, putrid, hectic, tertian, quatran or quotidian, Galen was the chief fountain-head of wisdom. Regarding the plague, however, he had little to say; perhaps his conscience was pricked, for he had only to open Thucydides to see how Grecian physicians perished at their posts during the epidemic at Athens. Such homely subjects as corns and callosities, burns and blisters, coughing and sneezing, a bruised nail, headache, toothache, baldness, bleeding of the nose, loss of eyelashes, wrinkles and freckles, Galen treated with sense and skill. He wrote good descriptions of jaundice, colic, dropsy, asthma, coryza, dysentery; and on such diverse maladies as diseases of the teeth and wounds of nerves, erysipelas and emphysema, he was the chief authority. As far as we know he was the only one of the ancients who wrote a treatise on feigned diseases; he wrote seventeen chapters on the pulse; he was among the first to realize the importance of predisposition to disease; he based his prognosis upon diagnosis; he paid much attention to secretions and excretions; it is claimed that his ophthalmic collyria could be consulted with advantage by present-day oculists; he knew that phthisis was infectious, saying, "It is a matter of experience that those who sleep in the same bed with consumptives fall into consumption, also those who live long with them, eat and drink with them, or wear their clothes and linen."

In obstetrics Galen did not distinguish himself; Galen spoke of the two uterine cavities, the right for the male fetus, and the left for the female—which leads us to suspect that he never examined a woman's womb. Galen, however, did make some meritorious investigations into the causes of sterility. He was a prolific writer on pharmacy; he wrote so much about plasters that if he had been an ordinary worker he would not have had time for anything else. The preparation of medicines by physical means is still called galenical pharmacy. As a writer on materia medica he cannot rank with Dioscorides, but he was second to him alone. It has been calculated that Galen's materia medica consisted of 540 plants, 180 animal, and 100 mineral substances.

Medicine is not an isolated branch of learning; it is a part of general culture, and the therapeutic tree cannot flourish in the soil of corruption. We get an insight into the temper of this period when we remember that the medicaments most in demand were cosmetics, antidotes, and abortifacients. The pure principles of Hippocratism were polluted by a variety of wrangling sects, while hosts of uneducated and irregular practitioners dabbled in medicine without restraint by law. The well-trained physician found himself in competition with the impudent quack. Everyone had secret formulas, and the most successful practitioners were those who prescribed the most fantastic drugs. Even physicians who had intended to practise decently, were forced to enter the mountebank's booth in the market-place and advertise the wonders of their panaceas. Economic pressure caused medicine to wallow in the scum of intrigue and falsehood—and crime. Hippocrates died in Thessaly, but six centuries later Hippocratism perished at Rome.

Galen looked with scorn and disgust at his colleagues. He said that between the robbers and the physicians there is this difference: the robbers commit their misdeeds in the mountains, while the physicians commit theirs in the capital. Yet in the midst of this degradation, Galen founded experimental physiology, made a vast number of discoveries, and wrote innumerable important treatises—which proves that there must have been some intelligent physicians even at that time, because Galen was not the man to write for himself alone. But when we examine his pharmacology, we see that he did not escape the infection of the age. The Galen that turned toward Hippocrates, blamed Dioscorides for attributing too many virtues to the same medicine, but the Galen that leaned toward his contemporaries was a prop of rampant polypharmacy. He was an authority on hygiene, but he pandered to the fashions of the day by preparing complicated concoctions—although we are duly grateful to him for inventing cold cream. Galen was a giant among dwarfs, but sometimes he stooped to the level of the dwarfs.

Today, whoever speaks of anatomy, pays tribute to Galen; the *platysma myoides,* says the modern anatomist, but this muscle was first named and described by the Pergamene physician. The frontalis muscle, the popliteus, the two muscles of the eyelids, the six muscles of the eyeball, the muscles of the spine, the muscles of each lateral cartilage of the nose, the maxillary group of muscles, with many muscles of the head and neck, both extremities and the body proper, were comprised in the Galenian myology, and in many instances the names which he suggested have been retained unto the present time.

He divided the vertebrae into cervical, dorsal and lumbar, and gave a correct account of the number and the situation of each. He named the bones and sutures of the cranium, and knew the squamous, styloid, mastoid and petrous portions of the temporal bones; the sphenoid, the ethmoid, the malar, the maxillary and nasal bones were familiar to him. In these descriptions Galen made few errors. The moderns have made little change in his osteology.

The science of blood-vessels and lymphatics (*angiology*) was the weakest point in the Galenic structure of anatomy, but even here he built better than his contemporaries, for in opposition to the prevailing views of the age, he proved that the arteries convey, not air, but blood. He was the first to describe, with some correctness, the aorta, the jugular vein, and the three coats of arteries. We are not in the habit of thinking that the capillary connection between the arteries and veins was known in antiquity, but let us not be startled at anything that we find among the Greeks: Hippocrates used the word *circulation,* though of course not in its present sense, and Galen knew anastomosis. In *De usa partium* Galen wrote: "The arteries and veins anastomose with each other throughout the whole body, and exchange with each other blood and spirits by certain invisible and exceedingly minute passages." His description of the thoracic contents is good—except that he thinks the heart is not a muscle because it acts continuously, while all muscles alternate their work with rest.

Galen's contributions to neurology were noteworthy. He knew that the brain is the central organ of the nervous system, and that the spinal cord is an offshoot, but he made the mistake of thinking that the nerves of sensation arise in the former, and the nerves of motion originate in the latter. His method of demonstrating the brain was a masterpiece of minuteness, and he traced several of the cranial and spinal nerves with accuracy. "If the spinal cord," wrote Galen, "be divided lengthwise from above downward by a straight section through the median line, none of the nerves going to the intercostal muscles are paralyzed, either on one side or the other, nor any of those going to the loins or the lower limbs." We agree with him that the motor fibers do not cross the cord, but we wait to hear what he will say as to the effect on sensibility; but he was silent, and seventeen centuries passed before the answer came that a longitudinal section of the cord in the median line, while it does not interfere with motion, destroys sensibility. Galen made a series of cross-sections, severing the cord between each of the vertebrae, —one of the most important experimental demonstrations of antiquity.

Of all the old dietitians, and it must be remembered that the ancient physicians paid much attention to food—Athenaeus being enthusiastic enough to remark that a good physician ought to be a good cook—Galen was the most distinguished. He stood high as a hygienist; he was the man to consult on questions of baths and gymnastics; his work among the gladiators made him a leading authority on exercise. Galen regularly indulged in wrestling before entering his bath, until a dislocated collar-bone caused him to decide that walking and "small ball exercise" were more suitable sports for a philosopher. Galen trained Commodus, and the young emperor regarded himself as the incarnation of Hercules—in his statues, Commodus wears the lion-skin and club of the Hellenic hero. He did not, however, wrestle barehanded with the Nemean lion, but from behind a secure screen shot his arrows at uncounted thousands of wild animals; safe in impenetrable armor, and wielding the secutor's sword, he fought in the gladiatorial arena against the naked retiarius whose weapons were harmless, and slaughtered an army; brandishing the club of Hercules, he crushed great numbers of men dressed as sons of Earth, who before their death were permitted to pelt him with rocks of sponge. A veritable giant of sexuality, he prostituted hundreds of women of all known varieties, and perverted men and boys, from his leading senators and ministers of state down to young freedmen and slaves.

It was probably in protest against the influence of Commodus, that Galen in the brief reign of Pertinax, wrote his *Exhortation to the Study of the Arts, Especially Medicine*—a vigorous address to students against the quest of riches, and the professions of gentlemen by birth, male prostitute and athlete. After quoting Euripides: "A thousand evils afflict Greece, and not one greater than athletics"; and Hippocrates: "The extreme development which athletes acquire is deceiving," Galen relates an anecdote about Phryne, the Athenian hetaira, about whom so many stories have been told. On one occasion, her lawyer, anticipating an unfavorable verdict, obtained her acquittal by exposing her bosom to the judges; at the festival of Poseidon, casting off her garments and stepping into the sea with dishevelled hair, she served as the model for the Venus Anadyomene of Apelles, and the Cnidian Venus of Praxiteles;

acquiring riches by the sale of her beauty, she offered to rebuild the Theban walls at her own expense, provided she were permitted to inscribe upon them, "Destroyed by Alexander, restored by Phryne the courtesan." Here is Galen's passage:

The story of Phryne appears apropos. At a banquet the game of "follow-the-leader" was inaugurated, consisting in each commanding in turn whatever he or she wished. Seeing the women's faces painted with orcanette, white lead and rouge, Phryne ordered "hands in water of the finger bowl, touch cheek and wipe immediately with napkin." She began by doing it herself. The faces of the others smeared with streaks were made repellent, Phryne only became more radiant—she alone possessing a natural beauty without need of detestable artifice. As true beauty exists only apart from ornamentation, we will examine the profession of athlete to see if it possesses in itself some utility for the state, or for the individual. There are in nature goods of the mind and goods of the body. Athletes enjoy none of the former, since they are too ignorant to appreciate even that they have a mind. In the amassing of their great quantity of flesh and blood their mind is lost in the vast mire. Receiving no stimulation to develop, it remains as stupid as that of brutes.

Galen follows this with another passage which, with advantage, might be nailed upon every modern stadium:

If by the will of Jupiter all living beings were brought together in harmony, and if the herald of Olympus called both men and animals to a contest in the same arena, no man would receive a crown. The horse would take it on the long course called the dolichos; the hare in the stadium; the antelope in the dialus. No mortal could enter into competition with the animals in quickness of foot. O light-footed athlete! What a miserable showing you make!

A descendant of Hercules himself would not prove strong as an elephant or a lion. The bull would triumph over the pugilist and if the ass, adds the poet, was allowed to combat with his heels he would be a victor. In the learned annals of history then would have to be written that man had been conquered in the pancratium by the ass, and it would probably be recorded in these words:

"Twenty-first Olympiad, Mr. John Ass—the Laurel Crown."

Galen was not always so discerning, as is apparent from these supercilious reflections:

> You would have me learn many languages, but I feel that it is enough to know one, a language which is so essentially singular and unique, and yet so suited for the use of all, so dulcet-toned, and so expressive of man's human needs. But if you wish to learn the language of barbarians, you had better clearly understand that some of these resemble the noises made by swine or frogs, or jackdaws or crows, inasmuch as they are without form or grace, and unfitted for the tongue, mouth or lips. For some of these people speak for the most part from the depths of their throats, just as if they were snoring, or they use their lips and sibilate, or they pitch the voice, or speak in a dull monotone, or they speak with gaping open mouth and roll the tongue about, or else they hardly open the mouth at all, and would seem to have tongues that are motionless and inert as if they were tied to the mouth.
>
> And would you then neglect the Grecian language, so very pleasant and so expressive of man's deepest feelings, a language, too, in which so much grace and beauty abound? Would you prefer to acquire your medium of expression from methods of speech that are as unsuitable as they are ugly? It were much better to learn one language, and that the most perfect of all, than to acquire six hundred debased tongues. . . . You do not wish, Sir, to learn the language of the Hellenes, well, be a barbarian if you will. . . .
>
> I wrote these instructions not for the use of the Germans, nor for any other race of savage or barbarous men, no more than I write for bears or goats or lions, or for any other wild beasts. But we address ourselves to the Greeks and to those other peoples who, although by birth barbarians, strive to emulate the manners and customs of the Hellenes.

Men always fall hardest when they are most certain of their superiority. Little did Galen think that his barbarous Germans would conquer the invincible Roman Empire, and still less did he imagine that his chief editors and commentators would be German scholars!

Galen was an explorer, but the lands that lie beyond the seas did not interest him like the unknown regions of the body;

he did not crave to discover distant kingdoms, for locked within the cranium he found ample treasures; he blazed no path in primitive forests, but all through its winding labyrinths he followed the trigeminal nerve, slowly discovering the secrets that were strewn along its tortuous way. Galen adored the mechanism of the body; he was filled with wonder at the perfection of its parts. He claimed that in writing anatomy he was really celebrating the Creator; again and again the great Pagan physician breaks forth into paeans of praise: "In writing these books I compose a true and real hymn to that awful Being who made us all; and, in my opinion, true religion consists not so much in costly sacrifices and fragrant perfumes offered upon his altars, as a thorough conviction of his unerring wisdom, his resistless power, and his all diffusive goodness."

An extract like the following illustrates Galen's interest and delight in the body: "In the inner cavity of the larynx there is a structure of peculiar formation, which we have already shown to be the principal organ of the voice. It resembles the mouthpiece of a reed-pipe, especially when seen either from above or from below. Instead, however, of comparing the glottis with the tongue of reed instruments, it would be more appropriate to compare them with the glottis. For the works of Nature are both earlier in time, and more perfect in construction, than those of art; and, as the glottis is the work of Nature, while the reed-pipe is the production of art, it is possible that the latter might have been made in imitation of the glottis by some clever artist, able to understand and copy the structure of natural objects."

His teleological proclivities are seen in passages such as these: "In my view there is nothing in the body useless or inactive; but all parts are arranged to perform their offices together, and have been endowed by the Creator with specific powers." We regret that we cannot share Galen's convictions in these respects. Man is compelled to perform the lowest and highest functions in life with the same organ, and was it nice on Nature's part to place the womb between the bladder and the rectum? St. Augustine was no physiologist, but he was vilely correct when he said that we are born between urine and feces.

Teleology was indeed a rotten spot in Galenism. Wise Anaxagoras had said that adaptation to function disproves teleology, but Plato and Aristotle believed in design in nature, and Galen followed them, and erected the most elaborate teleological system ever known. Hippocrates approached questions with an open mind, but Galen came with his dogmas, and sought to make his observations fit into the mold of preconceived notions. His practical work was invaluable, but most of his theoretical digressions are tedious and worthless. He wrote volumes of nonsensical assumptions, and seemed to suffer from an Asiatic imagination. It often happened that he was prevented from interpreting his results correctly because of his predilection for *a priori* reasoning.

Hippocrates left medicine free, but Galen fettered it with hypotheses. Hippocrates related his failures, and used to say, "I do not know," but Galen always imitated an oracle. "Science and Faith," said Hippocrates, "are two things: the first begets knowledge, the second ignorance"; but Galen sought to mix the observations of Hippocrates with the metaphysics of Plato. Galen abhorred doubt; his mind craved for finalities. Galen admired Euclid's method of proving things, and he tried to make medicine as exact a science as geometry; it is difficult to decide which was the greater—the absurdity or the audacity of the attempt. In his system everything was explained; everything was catalogued and tabulated. He answered all questions, he solved all problems. There seemed nothing left for others to do except to say, Amen. And so it was. Galen was the last of the Greeks and when he spoke no more, the voice of the ancient world was hushed. Galen was the final star that shone in the twilight of antiquity, and when his effulgence was extinguished, there settled over Europe a darkness that was not lifted for many centuries.

VI

ARABIAN MEDICINE IN THE MIDDLE AGES

At the time that Galen kept on thundering in numerous treatises against empirics and methodics and other sects in medicine, Celsus wrote the *True Word* which, aside from a scornful notice by Tacitus, is the earliest literary attack on a new sect in religion—Jews who called themselves followers of Christus. Galen, in one of his bibliographical lists, mentions an *Epistle to Celsus the Epicurian,* and Lucian dedicated his *Life of Alexander the Lying Prophet* to Celsus. Galen's Celsus, Lucian's Celsus, and the anti-Christian Celsus are probably the same Celsus; he is therefore not the medical Celsus of the preceding century—chronology may be dull, but it is a splendid preventive of errors.

The second century Celsus is also of scientific interest, for Lucian refers to his "excellent treatises against the magicians." Celsus, who regards the Jews as slaves escaped from Egypt, traces their origin to "the first generation of lying wizards," and says they are "blinded by some crooked sorcery, or dreaming dreams through the influence of shadowy specters." He accuses the Jews and their Christian progeny of practising magic, adding that Egyptian jugglers in the market-place can perform better tricks. Evidently, miracles are miracles only to those who believe them. After repeating the assertion that Jesus, the illegitimate son of the Hellenic-Roman officer Josephus Pandera and the Jewess Miriam, was raised in Egypt where he imbibed the black art, Celsus assails the doctrine of incarnation: "Why should man consider himself so superior to the ant and the elephant as to assume that God appeared in human form? And why should God choose to show himself to mankind as a Jew?" He compares the followers of the new sect to a synod of worms on a dunghill or a council of frogs in a marsh croaking, "For our sakes was the world created." Indignation sweeps through his pagan blood as he says that, like all quacks, they gather their converts among women and children, slaves and idlers. There is no Lucianian laughter in Celsus. "I speak bitterly," he declares, "because I feel bitterly." The contempt of Celsus for the disciples of Moses and Jesus is profound, but fear creeps along the lines of his argument, as he pleads: Why renounce Hellenism for the fables of Genesis? Why not adopt the philosophy of Plato or Epicurus? Why be disloyal to Marcus Aurelius?

The fate of these polemics has been very different. The sects against which Galen contended have long been replaced by others, and the sect which Celsus tried to reason out of existence has long dominated mankind. Celsus' book had little influence: his countrymen agreed with him, and saw no reason for excitement; and those whom he controverted were not yet powerful enough to exterminate him. The work of Celsus would have disappeared utterly, had not Origen, seventy years later, quoted most of it in his *Reply to Celsus*. Origen's famous answer was written in 248, when Rome was celebrating the thousandth birthday of the largest and longest-lasting empire that the world had known. The golden eagles led triumphant cohorts from the Atlantic to the Euphrates; the legions that planted their standards in Britain, carried them across to Assyria; the javelin which humbled the Danube and the Rhine, vanquished Ethiopia and Arabia. Yet that millennial celebration was delusional—the giant who had fattened on the blood of all races was sitting at his own funeral feast. Generation after generation he was to shrink and lose his vital parts, until nothing remained of his earth-encircling proportions except a wall.

In the year in which Galen bade farewell to the world, Origen was a pupil at the Catechetical School of Alexandria, the only academy of the time whose curriculum included Greek philosophy and the Scriptures. All his life Origen labored to reconcile the Grecian sages and the Christian apostles. Origen, a man of blameless character, was so much in earnest that he looked upon women as daughters of Satan, and to escape the call of the flesh, castrated himself. Origen's eloquent argumentation that the teachings of Aristotle and Plato were not incompatible with the teachings of Jesus Christ, acted as a bridge over which antiquity walked into medievalism. After many years at Alexandria, Origen continued his activities in Rome, Athens, Arabia, Cappadocia and Palestine. Origen's views on the preëxistence of the human soul of Christ before he became divine, aroused resentment among his brethren, and often coming into conflict with the Christian authorities, he was exiled and excommunicated. He was certainly as sincere, and often more orthodox than the orthodox who anathematized him—but from this time on, a new intolerance ruled the world: the ecclesiastical party which wielded political power was the only orthodox party, and in the name of God destroyed its opponents. Even the crimes of imperial Rome grow pale in comparison with the amount of human blood that was now to be shed over myths.

Persecution on a wholesale scale began in the fifth century, with the advent of St. Cyril, the assassin of Plato's last representative in Alexandria, the beautiful and learned Hypatia. No one could be more ascetic or orthodox than Nestorius of Constantinople, who cried, "Purge me, O Caesar, the earth of heretics, and I in return will give thee heaven." Between the patriarch of Alexandria, and the patriarch of Constantinople, the doctrinal differences were insignificant, but their personal animosity being considerable, they anathematized and counter-anathematized each other. At the Synod of Ephesus they met for a trial of strength: each was accompanied by many bishops and armed slaves. The proceedings would have disgraced rival gangs of bandits. Cyril was the more cunning politician, and by means of far-reaching bribery and criminal brutality, overthrew his antagonist. Nestorius, who had burned Arians and had hoped to exterminate all heretics, found himself proscribed as the arch-heretic of the age. It rarely happened that a heretic-hunter was not himself classed as a heretic by other heretic-hunters. Nestorius retired to his monastery at Antioch, until he was banished to Arabia and ultimately to the Great Oasis of Egypt, attempting to console himself by writing a book on the *Robber Synod of Ephesus*. The triumphant St. Cyril had placed a sword in the right hand of his church and a purse in its left, and militant Christianity embarked on its career of coercion.

Paganism was passing away, but the embattled Church needed enemies and victims. Men arose whose sole business was to destroy heresy, or to invent it if it did not exist. Thousands upon thousands were tortured in wars over words; multitudes perished in metaphysical quibbles which were as incomprehensible then as they are meaningless now.

The Nestorians, cut off from the prizes of power, were forced into fields of lesser rewards. It has happened more than once, that a race or sect, debarred from the politics of the day, found itself cultivating the healing art—with the result that the most pious of bishops and the most orthodox of rulers religiously swallowed their drugs from the spoons of heretics. The hunted Nestorians migrated to northwestern Mesopotamia, in the Babylonian-Assyrian-Israelitic town of Edessa—where the Hittites were ancient before the Hellenes came. Here, in the Christian era, we meet St. Ephraim, the Syrian hermit, who learned to speak Coptic and Greek, not by study, but through a miracle—according to his anonymous biographer. This saint had wandered far from his pagan fathers; small, bald and beardless, he never smiled; again quoting his first biographer: "water was his only drink, and his only food barley bread and sometimes pulse and vegetables. And his flesh was dried upon his bones, like a potter's sherd. His clothes were of many pieces patched together, the color of dirt." After him followed Rabbula, son of a heathen priest and a Christian mother. Rabbula did not adopt his mother's faith until converted by an example of miraculous healing; as a Christian, he sold all he owned, left his wife and family, and lived in solitude. His fame as a holy man caused him to be chosen bishop, and he who had been silent on the hill-slopes now preached incessantly against heretics, especially the Nestorians.

These men are of medical interest because Ephraim built the first large hospital in Edessa; and upon the ruins of pagan temples, Rabbula erected an infirmary exclusively for women. It is thus apparent that Christianity early promoted the hospital system, but to claim it as a Christian invention is to forget the asylums of the Egyptians at Heliopolis, the *iatreia* of the Greeks, the *valetudinaria* and military hospitals of the Romans, the numerous and fully-equipped hospitals of Buddhistic India. In the Pali narrative, known as the Mahavansa, the great chronicle of a thousand years of the history of Ceylon, it is related that Duttha Gamani, feeling his earthly journey ending (161 B.C.), asked the records of his reign be read to him, and among the last words the dying king heard were these: "I have daily maintained at eighteen different places, hospitals provided with suitable diet, and medicines prepared by physicians for the infirm."

When the Nestorians arrived at Edessa, its medical school and hospitals were active, and in time the heretics gained possession of the orthodox institutions. Under Nestorian influence, Edessa was regarded as a second Athens, or another Alexandria. This exaggeration at least is evidence of the reputation of the school. The Nestorians prospered at Edessa, until Bishop Cyrus whispered into the ear of Emperor Zeno; the lecture-halls were destroyed, and the bishop used the wreckage to build a church dedicated to Mary, Mother of God—a vindictive answer to the Nestorians, whose heresy consisted in the belief that Mary was the Mother of Christ, but not the Mother of God.

Expelled from Edessa, the Nestorians migrated to Persia, and in the medical school of Jundisapur they were destined to become the link between East and West. Admitted to Iran by

Cobades, they were welcomed by his son and successor, Chosroes, greatest of the Sassanid shahs. Chosroes—of whom it is difficult to say whether he burnt or built more cities—as the defender of Zoroaster, was severe with Persian heretics, but extended the hand of hospitality to foreign heretics. When Justinian closed the Academy of Athens, the seven exiled philosophers—"the last of the pagans"—found refuge with Chosroes, and when Rome purchased peace from Persia, Chosroes expressly stipulated, as one of the conditions, that these Greek Neoplatonists be permitted to live unmolested in the Roman empire.

As man and monarch, Persian Chosroes was superior to Roman Justinian. In 532, Chosroes, in concluding a treaty with this crowned thief, specified that Tribunus, Greek physician of Palestine, reside in his court for twelve months. At the end of that time, as Tribunus was preparing to leave Persia, Chosroes asked him what favor he desired. The physician pointed out some Roman captives, for whose freedom he pleaded, and Chosroes who was always despotic and generous on a large scale, liberated not only those named by Tribunus, but three thousand of their countrymen. Patron of Pahlawi literature, occupied with the army and administration, improving transportation and irrigation, encouraging trade and agriculture, erecting cities from their ashes and re-populating war-stricken provinces, Chosroes did not forget to send his physician Burzuya to India to investigate medical conditions. Burzuya returned with the lore of Susruta and Charaka—and the game of chess which ever since has been recommended as a method of treatment—and this visit of good-will paved the way for the coming of Hindu physicians to Persia.

Since the land that produced the *Vedas* in Sanskrit, and the land that wrote the *Zend-Avesta,* are geographic and ethnologic kindred, it may seem strange that their reciprocal relations should have been so vague—but rival religions formed a frontier that could not be crossed. The chief period of Indian medicine is coincident with the rise of Buddhism and corresponds with the classic age of Greece, and the parallelism between Hellenism and Hinduism is one of history's disputed problems. By the Code of Manu the physician was not permitted to attend funerals, and despite such thrusts as "The food of the physician is pus," and "The waggoner longs for wood, and the physician for diseases," Indian medicine produced these ethical and clinical observations:

To the sick man the doctor is a father: to the man in health a friend: the sickness passed and health restored, a preserver.

Without practical training and merely by hearing lectures and by the repetition of discourses, a pupil is like an ass with a burden of sandalwood, for he knows its weight but not its value.

He who knows only one branch of his art is like a bird with one wing. . . . He who is versed only in books will be alarmed and confused, like a coward on a battlefield, when confronted with active disease; he who rashly engages in practice without previous study of written science is entitled to no respect from the best of mankind, and merits punishment from the king; but he who combines reading with experience proceeds safely and surely like a chariot on two wheels.

The physician, the patient, the medicine and the nurse are the four feet of medicine upon which the cure depends. When three of these are as they should be, then by their aid the exertions of the fourth, the physician, are of effect, and he can cure a sore disease in a short time. But without the physician the other three are useless even when they are as they should be, just as the Brahmans who recite the Rig-Vedas and Sama-Vedas are useless at a sacrifice without the Brahman who recites the Yagur-Veda. But a good physician can cure a patient alone, just as a pilot can steer a boat to land without sailors.

The menstrual epoch is the most fruitful time for conception, for then the mouth of the womb is open, like the flower of the water-lily to the beams of the sun.

Susruta's instruction on the medical use of the five senses helps us to understand why the ancient Hindu physicians knew the sweetish taste of the urine of diabetes mellitus centuries before its recognition by European practitioners:

By the sense of *hearing* we can, for instance, determine whether the contents of an abscess are frothy and gaseous, for the emptying of such is attended with noise; by the sense of *feeling* we may know whether the skin is hot or cold, rough or smooth, thick or thin; by the sense of *sight* we can determine corpulence or emaciation, vital power, energy, and change of colour; by the sense of *taste* we can assure ourselves concerning the state of the urine in diabetes and other diseases of the urinary tract; and by the sense of *smell* we can recognise the peculiar perspiration of many diseases which has an important bearing on their identification.

Their surgical armamentarium—in which the hand figured as the first and most important of all surgical instruments—was extensive, including knives of steel that could divide a hair, reed-like catheters, fluid-removing trocars, bone-dividing nippers, polypus-forceps, cupping-glasses, and one hundred-and-one blunt instruments; when we remember that couching for cataract—they knew seventy-six eye-diseases—the surgical use of the lodestone, and plastic surgery, are Hindu discoveries, we can appreciate the pupils' request to Dhanvantari when he asked what branch of the healing art he should explain: "Teach us everything, but take surgery as the foundation of your discourse"; and the aphorism of Susruta, the Hindu Hippocrates: "Surgery is the first and highest division of the healing art, least liable to fallacy, pure in itself, perpetual in its applicability, the worthy produce of heaven, the sure source of fame on earth."

The Buddhist king, Asoka, was the first great builder of hospitals for man and beast; these animal-hospitals throw light on the Hindu injunction that the physician should refuse medical advice to criminals and to hunters who trap animals and ensnare birds. Buddhism is the gentlest and wisest, the most sceptical and scientific of religions—and the only one that does not worship the sword—and had it continued to prevail, Asiatic history would be different. But with the reëstablishment of Brahmanism, Buddhist hospitals and tolerance were destroyed. The modesty which Charaka advocated, "Even the most learned physician should never become puffed up because of his knowledge. Many recoil from the most skilful man if he is a boaster. And medicine is by no means easy to learn. Therefore let each one practise himself in it carefully and incessantly," did not appeal to the Brahman who claimed a monopoly of wisdom and superhuman privileges. The priestly class fastened upon India the immovable shackles of caste. No man dare differ from his father, none may aspire, but in the groove into which he is born he must live and die. Only the Brahmans are righteous, all others are unclean. Under Brahmanism, Indian science stagnated and disappeared, and India with its swarming millions became the land of the dead. The last words of the Buddha are indeed true: "We are but transient guests, and all things pass away"—but the memory of his graciousness lingers like the perfume of an eternal lotus-flower.

No story in medicine is more tender than Buddha's treatment of Kisagotami and her son. As is the Indian custom, Kisagotami was married in early girlhood; she was young when her son was born, young when he crept at her feet, and when he was able to run alone, she was still a child watching a younger child. The beautiful boy died, and the mother, crazed with grief, refused to part with him. She carried the body to friend and stranger, begging for a remedy to restore it to life. All pitied her, and one said, "I have no such medicine, but I know of one who has. Go to the Buddha." So Kisagotami sought out Buddha and rendered him homage. "O master," she said, "do you know any medicine that will be good for my child?" The Buddha shook his head. "Bring me mustard-seed"—and the girl was glad he named a drug she could obtain at once—"from a house in which no one has died." She went into the first house, and when the people heard her request, they said, "Here is mustard-seed, take it"; and when she asked if any had died in that house they answered, "Lady! what is this that you say? The living are few, but the dead are many." She went from house to house, and one said, "I have lost my son"; and another, "We have lost our parents"; and another, "I have lost my slave." She did not leave one house unvisited, and did not find one where death had not entered before her. At last she understood, and brought the body of her child to a forest, and left it there. Again she sought the Buddha and rendered him homage. "Have you the mustard-seed?" he asked. "O master," she said, "the living are few, but the dead are many."

Under Chosroes the Blessed (531-79), Greek, Hindu, Jewish, Nestorian, Syrian and Persian physicians mingled at Jundisapur, and Chosroes himself ordered Plato and Aristotle to be translated into Persian. The Nestorians became great polyglots, and Jundisapur developed into an international medical center that made it the *Civitas Hippocratica* of Asia. Chosroes passed from the scene, and in the following century the course of history was violently changed by an unexpected people. Savages rode out of the desert, and demanded the surrender of Byzantium and Persia. The Iranian monarch was amazed. "Who are you to attack an empire?" he asked. "You, of all peoples the poorest, most disunited, most ignorant." The messenger of the Saracens was unabashed: "All that you say was once true. The Arabians were clothed in the hair garments of beasts; their food was green lizards; they buried their infant daughters alive; they feasted on dead carcasses and drank warm blood; they slew their relatives and boasted of the property they stole; we knew not good from evil, nor could we tell what was lawful and what was unlawful. All this is true no longer. God in his mercy has sent us a holy prophet who has given us a sacred volume which teaches us the only true faith."

The man who accomplished this change—the swiftest in history—and within one generation gave his people a new religion and a national consciousness, was Mohammed. A more ignorant and unscrupulous adventurer never twisted destiny. Greedy, revengeful, murderous and lascivious—his harem increased with every victory—such was the founder of Islam and the Arabian Empire. Had he been otherwise, had he attempted to raise the status of woman or abolish slavery, had he hesitated in shedding human blood, had he ever felt the power of pity, the turbaned horsemen of the desert would not have overridden three continents in his name. The impulse for migration and invasion stirred the sands before the Prophet's time, but he unchained fanaticism as he preached: "The sword is the key of heaven. A drop of blood shed in the cause of God is of more avail than much fasting and prayer; whoso falls in battle, all his sins are forgiven; at the day of judgment his wounds shall be resplendent as vermillion and odiferous as musk"; instead of the Great Renunciation of Buddha, he was adroit enough to promise his followers a seventh heaven of many beds with a black-eyed houri in every bed—a paradise of eternal fornication.

After the death of Mohammed, his name on the lips of Moslems struck terror in Asia, Africa and Europe. All that Alexander had conquered fell into the hands of the Arabian, and where Caesar and Chosroes had ruled, a camel-breeder sat enthroned. The crescentade was invincible from the land of the Sphinx to the Gothic kingdom of Spain. The Mohammedan dominion then extended from the Mountains of Gold to the Atlantic Ocean; Memphis and Carthage were taken, and from the streets of Cordova to the banks of the Indus the mosques were alive with thanks to Allah. The victorious Saracen laughed at Rome, he wrested Jerusalem from the Christians, and in disdain he sold the Colossus, for old brass, to a Jew.

The Arabian Empire grew so unwieldy that, like the Roman Empire, it split in half: Bagdad on the Tigris, and Cordova in Spain, were not only the rival capitals of the eastern and western caliphates, but the most important cities of the time. After the lust of conquest was somewhat appeased and checked, the Arab became aware of the medical school at Jundisapur, and reacted as had the Roman to the superior culture of the captive Greek. From Jundisapur, Greek science spread throughout the Moslem world. When the intellect of Europe was so clouded by monkish fables that the monasteries were buying milk purporting to come from the breasts of the Blessed Virgin, barbarian brown-skinned tent-dwellers became the saviors of Greek philosophy. For the conquering Mohammedans were conquered by the Greek manuscripts. Their bigoted insularity disappeared in veneration of the Hippocratic aphorisms. No longer referring to all Europeans as unbelieving dogs, they pondered over the works of Dioscorides. As Athens and Rome now anathematized the pagan thinkers, Hippocrates and Aristotle and Galen left their homes, and far-stretching caravans of camels brought the parchments to Jundisapur and Bagdad. Aristotle, when his name was unknown in Paris and could not be pronounced at Oxford, was memorized at Nishapur and studied with awe at Samarcand.

Upon the stage of history many tragedies and comedies have been played, but never a world-drama stranger than this: persecuted Nestorians, excluded from church and state, devote themselves to the science of the Greeks condemned by Christendom, and driven by Byzantine intolerance from their school at Edessa in Mesopotamia, transmit Hellenic culture to Persian territory at Jundisapur, where the manuscripts are translated into Syriac and retranslated into Arabic, until the Arabic versions with their extensive commentary become so influential in the Occident that they are translated back into Latin, and Europe for centuries acknowledges the medical supremacy of Asia!

It came to pass that scholars in search of learning found it essential to acquire the Arabic tongue. Men who believed that Mohammed was able to put the moon within his sleeve, were at the same time men of science—a seeming inconsistency which is not altogether unknown among other people at the present day. From Hindu mathematics, the Arabians derived the system of numeration which we still use, and developed algebra, the word itself, like algorithm, dating from al-Khwarizmi's treatise, *al-jebr wal-muqābala*. The Caliph al-Mamun built a Hall of Science at Bagdad, whose pride was an observatory where his astronomers watched the skies and not only measured the height of the atmosphere and catalogued the stars, but spoke a language not heard on earth before: Aldebaran still shines brightly in the heavens, and the Arabic names of azimuth, zenith and nadir, are permanent parts of nomenclature. They established the first pharmacies; fostered the early steps of chemistry; discovered nitric acid, aqua regia, red precipitate, corrosive sublimate; either introduced or popularized such important drugs as camphor, rhubarb, senna, cassia fistula, nux vomica, nutmeg, tamarinds, musks and cloves; observed that colchicum is beneficial in gout; and gave us syrup, juleps, alkali, alembic and alcohol, which terms are as Arabic in origin as muslins from Mosul and damasks from Damascus.

The ninth century is the era of the Arabian Renaissance, and Hunain ibn Ishaq (809-77) was its herald. Hunain was born at Hira, the fertile land between the Euphrates and the Arabian desert, once known for its good air and collection of poets, but in his time already in physical and mental decay. Hunain, who was a Nestorian, journeyed to Bagdad to dispense drugs for Yuhanna ibn Masawaih (777-857), the leading Nestorian physician of his period. Yuhanna, son of the chemist to the Jundisapur Hospital, had come to Bagdad as medical attendant to Harun al-Rashid, remembered for the piety which caused him to prostrate himself a hundred times a day, for his patronage of the arts, for the elephant he sent to Charlemagne, and as the hero of the *Arabian Nights*. Dissection was practically unknown in Moslem lands, but it is said that Yuhanna dissected the species of ape that resembled man most closely. Of his numerous medical writings, his *Alteration of the Eye* is the earliest Arabic treatise on ophthalmology that has survived —though any day the dust may be blown from an older manuscript. The Arabians were acquainted with over one hundred diseases of the eye, and many ophthalmic operations. Yuhanna ibn Masawaih was known to the Latins as *Mesua Major,* and Hunain ibn Ishaq's Western name was *Johannitius*.

Many stories of Yuhanna's bad temper have come down to us, and his irascibility sometimes caused him to forget both his medical and religious creed. "I feel unwell in my stomach," complained a priest who consulted him. "Use the *Electuarium Susianum*," said Yuhanna. "I have already done so," responded the patient. "Use the *Electuarium Diacyminum*," said Yuhanna. "I have already taken some pounds of it," he replied. "Use the *Pentadicon*," said Yuhanna. "I have already drunk a whole vessel full," sighed the priest. "Use the *Confectio Ambrosia*," said Yuhanna. "I have already done so, and in large quantities." Yuhanna finally concluded the interview: "If you really want to get well, embrace Islamism, for that is good for the stomach."

Once Yuhanna was very ill, and some Nestorian priests approached his bed. He opened a sick eye and asked, "What are these rascals doing here?" Naturally enough, they answered, "We are praying that God will restore you to health." He drove them out with the retort, "A few pills will do more good than all your prayers, though they go on till the Resurrection." On another occasion, he remarked to a bore, "If the ignorance with which you are afflicted were converted into understanding, and then divided among a hundred beetles, each one of them would be more sagacious than Aristotle."

Yuhanna accepted Hunain as a pupil, but being annoyed by too many questions, wounded him with the words, "What have the people of Hira to do with medicine? Go and change money in the streets!" Evidently, Yuhanna had not forgotten that he came from Jundisapur, for al-Qifti explains: "These people of Jundisapur used to believe that only they were worthy of this science, and would not suffer it to go forth from themselves, their children and their kin."

Hunain wept in the streets, but through his tears vowed he would go to the lands of the West and learn Greek. He vanished, and Yuhanna believed he had followed his advice and turned tradesman. Long afterward, Hunain returned to Bagdad, bringing with him his translation of the *Aphorisms* of Hippocrates. Meeting the Caliph's astrologer, he asked him to show the version to Yuhanna, but not to mention his name. The quick-tempered Yuhanna was capable of enthusiasm, for after reading the translation he exclaimed, "This must have been written by the Holy Ghost." "Not at all," was the response, "it was written by the pupil whom you expelled."

Yuhanna, like a true scholar, begged to be reconciled to Hunain, and the two translators became co-workers. "I translated *De ossium dissectione* into Syriac for Yuhanna ibn Masawaih," says Hunain, "and I took pains to express the meaning as clearly as possible; for this man likes intelligible expression and urges constantly in this direction." In writing of Galen's *De simplicibus*, he states: "Later on Ayyub translated it better than Yusuf, but did not restore it as well as it should have been restored. After this I translated it into Syriac for Salmawaih and restored it as well as possible. The second section of this book had been translated by Sergius. Yuhanna ibn Masawaih asked me to collate and correct this section; I did so, although it would have been better to translate it afresh."

A sharp tongue is not incompatible with longevity, and Yuhanna reached the age of eighty. Upon his death, an Arabian poet was moved to satire:

Verily the physician with his physic and his drugs,
Cannot avert a summons that hath come.
What ails the physician that he dies of the disease
Which in times gone by he claimed to cure?
There died he who imported and sold the drug, and he who bought it,
And alike he who administered the drug, and he who took the drug.

As Hunain's medical reputation increased, it was inevitable that he should be presented at court. The caliph lost no time in telling him what he wanted—poison for one of his enemies: riches for Hunain if he complied, and prison if he refused. After a year in prison, Hunain was again led to the foot of the throne: on one side were heaped gems and gold, and on the other lay instruments of torture. The caliph pointed significantly to one pile and then to the other. "Which?" he asked. Hunain answered, "I have already told the Commander of the Faithful that I have skill only in what is beneficial, and have studied naught else." The caliph nodded for the sword of the executioner, and Hunain, feeling his last day had come, spoke: "I have a Lord who will give me my right tomorrow in the Supreme Uprising, so if the caliph would injure his own soul, let him do so." The tension was relieved by the caliph's smile; he had never intended to injure Hunain, and was simply testing his honesty. Such is the tale, and if any one can believe it, let him do so.

A preserved fragment of Hunain's autobiography complains that his fellow Nestorians accused him of being in the pay of the Byzantines—his intimate knowledge of Greek gave color to this accusation—and knowing he was an iconoclast they trapped him into insulting some sacred images, whereupon they imprisoned him, confiscated his property, and deprived him of the precious books he had accumulated during a lifetime of labor. But here too the legend-makers have been active with Hunain's alleged prison-dreams and his liberation by supernatural intercession. What we definitely know about Hunain is that he was the greatest of translators, and if ever this useful guild seeks a patron-saint, no one could be more appropriate than Hunain ibn Ishaq.

The Arabian passion for Greek manuscripts began before Hunain's time. The story of John the Grammarian who asked in vain for the Alexandrian Library, and the Caliph who destroyed it with the epigram, "If the books agree with the Koran they are superfluous; if they disagree they are pernicious," belongs rather to fiction than to history, since even Moslem fanaticism could not burn what Roman and Christian had already burned. The accusation is true to the extent that it indicated the early Mussulman's evaluation of the writings of infidels—an attitude which underwent such reversal that the Saracen confiscated a copy of Hippocrates or seized a codex of Dioscorides as the prize of victory; al-Mansur sent messengers to Constantinople for the works of Euclid; Harun al-Rashid, in dictating terms to the defeated emperor of the Byzantines, specified Greek manuscripts as his most coveted booty.

There were capable Greek translators into Syriac before Hunain—such as the sixth century medical priest, Sergius of Resaina—but Hunain's versions of Plato, Hippocrates, Aristotle, Euclid, Ptolemy, Dioscorides, Oribasius and Paulus Aegineta, set the standard; the little-known veterinary surgery of Theomnestus did not escape his zeal; he reviewed 129 books of

Galen, translating ninety-five into Syriac and thirty-nine into Arabic. He was the head and inspiration of a translation school, the most prominent members of which were his son Ishaq, his nephew Hubaish, and his disciple Isa; together they completed 106 Syriac and 108 Arabic versions of Galen alone, and much else. Hunain was not an easy master, as is obvious from this censure of his nephew: "Hubaish is a man of natural intelligence who wishes to follow my methods of translation; but I think that his diligence does not equal his talent." In time, despite his lame hand, Hubaish translated so accurately and industriously than even Hunain was satisfied.

In the dust of an oriental library a lost manuscript by Hunain has recently been found; it is an important document because it shows us how he worked:

I translated *De differentiis febrium* for Jibril when I was a youth, and this was the first of the books of Galen which I translated into Syriac. . . .

I translated Galen's *De facultatibus naturalibus* when I was a youth of about seventeen years of age, and I had translated previously only one book. . . .

I was a young man of about thirty years at the time when I translated Galen's *De constitutione artis medicae*, but I had already at my disposal a considerable amount of scientific material, some acquired by myself in the course of my private studies, and some contained in the books which I had accumulated. . . .

I sought earnestly for Galen's *De demonstratione,* and travelled in search of it in the lands of Mesopotamia, Syria, Palestine and Egypt, until I reached Alexandria, but I was not able to find anything except about half of it at Damascus.

I translated Galen's *De sectis* when I was a young man from a very defective Greek manuscript. Later on, when I was about forty years old, my pupil Hubaish asked me to correct it after having collected a certain number of Greek manuscripts. Thereon I collated these so as to produce one correct manuscript, and I compared this manuscript with the Syriac text and corrected it. I am in the habit of proceeding thus in all my translation work. Some years later I translated it into Arabic. . . .

Sergius had translated Galen's *Febrium,* but not in a creditable manner. I translated it first for Jibril when I was a youth; this was the first of Galen's books which I translated into Syriac. Later on, after having attained ripe manhood I revised the text and found a certain number of faults which I corrected with diligence, as I wished to have a copy for my son. I translated it moreover into Arabic for Abul-Hasan Ahmad.

It has been pointed out that these methods correspond with modern philological methods—but the rewards differ. When Hunain finished a treatise, he brought his work to the enlightened Caliph al-Mamun, in whose presence it was carefully weighed, and Hunain received for every manuscript-translation its weight in gold. It may strike us as curious that the Arabians who ransacked the globe for a Graeco-scientific manuscript, never translated a Greek poem or historical work, and it is likewise strange that the Latin authors simply did not exist for them. Hunain and his school were thus the executors through whom the legacy of Greek science passed to the Moslem world.

Among Hunain's contemporaries, Ali al-Tabari achieved distinction. Ali was the son of Sahl, the Persian Jewish scholar who combined in himself the professions of rabbi of Tabaristan, physician, mathematician, and astrologer-astronomer. The father was the first to translate into Arabic one of the crucial books in the realm of science—the *Almagest* of Ptolemy; and the son, who became a Mohammedan, wrote the first defense of Islam, entitled the *Book of Religion and Empire*. Ali's medical works consisted of treatises on cupping, amulets, preparation of food, hygiene, the correct use of drugs, and the manual known as the *Paradise of Wisdom*. Ali does not give case-reports, but quotes the ever-quoted Greeks, and the Nestorians Yuhanna and Hunain, and concludes with a summary of Hindu medicine, yet the *Paradise of Wisdom* acquires significance as one of the first Arabian textbooks for practitioners that is not a translation. The longest section—about two-fifths of the whole —is devoted to pathology, and in keeping with the custom, diseases are discussed in anatomical order from head to feet. Ali.

author of the aphorism, "An ignorant physician hastens death," insisted that whoever skimmed his *Paradise of Wisdom*, was similar to one who contemplated the gates of a garden, but whoever studied it attentively resembled one who wandered through its pleasant and fruitful paths.

Ali al-Tabari's manuscripts have only recently been discovered, and prior to these finds he was of interest as Rhazes' teacher. Rhazes, a Persian born in Rai near Teheran, turned his attention to medicine after he had reached middle-age—according to Ibn Khallikan, he was over forty before he began to devote himself to physic. When Rhazes was young, he played the lute and cultivated his voice, but according to Ibn Juljul, "on reaching the age of manhood, he renounced these occupations, saying that music proceeding from between mustachios and a beard had no charms to recommend it." A curious essay might be written on those men who undertook to study medicine late in life, and yet achieved success.

In those days traveling was a part of the medical curriculum, and Rhazes knew Jerusalem, and journeyed through Africa, and saw the lamps of Cordova—but he returned to the minarets of Bagdad, the magic city of the Arabian Nights. A hundred famous physicians contended for the directorship of the hospital of Bagdad, but the favor fell upon Rhazes. He developed into the chief clinician of the Arabian school, his material being so extensive that in recommending a mode of treatment for sciatica—sharp clysters until blood was drawn—he was able to say that he had seen this method successfully tried upon a thousand patients. It was the Golden Age of Arabian Medicine, and Rhazes was its effulgence. Pupils—Andalusian, Mozarab, Persian, Berbek, Hebrew, Egyptian—voyaged from afar to seek the teacher who had learned to say, "According to my own experience." What did they hear from the lips of Rhazes, over a thousand years ago, among the date-palms of Bagdad? Listen, as did those turbaned scholars, to a fragment of Rhazes' lecture, *On the Factors which Alienate the Public from the Physician:*

Among the circumstances which cause the hearts of the people to turn away from the reputable physician is the delusion that the medical man should know everything and should ask no questions. If he inspects the urine or feels the pulse he is supposed to know what the patient has eaten and what he has been doing. I myself, when I began to practise medicine, had resolved to ask no questions when the urine had been given me, and had been much honored. Later, when it was seen that I had made circumstantial inquiries, my reputation sank.

Another circumstance which brings physicians into contempt is that many diseases are too little removed from the border-line of health and are thus difficult to recognize and cure; others, malignant in themselves, externally appear trivial. When the layman sees that the physician is in doubt concerning his cure he draws it as a certain inference that the physician will understand still less of severer and more extensive illnesses. This is a false analogy. The symptoms of such diseases are less obvious because they are slighter deviations from the normal, and their cure is more difficult because no drastic remedies can be applied, but only those the effect of which is gradually brought about, such as diet, etc. An official of the hospital once complained of difficulty in moving some of his finger joints on account of a small but very hard sore which had for some time resisted the remedies he had applied. He openly reviled the physicians, saying: "If your art does not suffice to cure a small sore on the finger, how can you treat broken ribs and arms?" He then sought treatment from the women and the vulgar.

If it be argued that a malady should not be entrusted to one who may make a mistake, we rejoin: Matters must be entrusted to him who is furtherest from error, who errs most seldom. He who otherwise refuses to employ a physician would resemble him who would not ride a horse nor sleep in a canopied bed because horses stumble and the canopy might fall down—which are rare events.

A physician is sometimes undervalued who takes trouble over an incurable complaint; but the imperfection of the art should be considered, in this respect, unlike other arts, of which men know more than is necessary, while in medicine men have not yet attained to the indispensable and do not possess a remedy for every ill. The fault is therefore with the art, not with the physician.

The public demands that the physician should cure in a moment, like a magician, or that he should at least employ pleasant methods, which is not at all times and in all cases possible; to blame the physician on Nature's account is a great injustice. Thus it is that sorcerers make their fortune, even though they behave iniquitously, and their incompetent work brings them a good livelihood, while the physician must often endure poverty.

The heart of the public is further turned from the capable physician and towards fools because the ignorant sometimes succeed in curing complaints where this has not been done by the most famous physicians. The causes are manifold, luck, opportunity, etc. Sometimes the qualified physician effects an improvement which is not, however, yet visible; the patient is then placed under another doctor who rapidly brings about a cure and obtains the entire credit.

Many a quack is experienced in the treatment of a single complaint, or two, according to his practice, or because he has seen the treatment of an intelligent physician. Ignorant people, therefore, think that he has equal dexterity in everything and entrust themselves to him. It is a great mistake to think that, because he has a genuine remedy for one complaint, he has one for all. I have myself learnt remedies from women and herbalists who had no knowledge of medicine.

Remember that the well-trained physician is often in doubt and may take a long time to find the proper remedy. This occurred even to Galen.

Much of this sounds modern—and occidental. The voices of the past often speak in contemporary tones. We are all children of the same Mother Earth, and from the vocabulary of man the word "foreigner" should be erased.

Over two hundred treatises were written by Rhazes, including that vast undigested encyclopedic mass, the *Continent of Medicine*. Everything known to the medical art was put into these huge folios, but without method or arrangement, or any attention to style. Rhazes left this work in manuscript perhaps realizing that few could cross this unclassified *Continent*. But using the *Continent* as a basis, he prepared another work, dedicated to the Persian prince, al-Mansur, and thus known as the *Work to al-Mansur,* here the presentation being concise and elegant, and the topics so well arranged that it became one of the most popular of compendiums, and for centuries was used as a textbook in the colleges.

Physicians of the past have been aphorists, and the Rhazian adages will never lose their meaning: "Treat an incipient malady with remedies which will not prostrate the strength." "With a learned physician and an obedient patient, sickness soon disappears." "When you can cure by regimen, avoid having recourse to medicine; and when you can effect a cure by means of a simple medicine, avoid employing a compound one." "Truth and certainty in medicine is an unattainable goal; and the healing art, as it is described in books, is far inferior to the practical experience of a skillful and thoughtful physician."

The writings of Rhazes contain ingenious and acute observations on topics ranging all the way from hiccough and purgatives to spinal injury and embryotomy. He knew that the pupil contracts to light, and that the remedy for pediculosis of the eyelids is mercurial ointment. He urged the use of cold water in inflammatory fever, and insisted that fever be treated according to its causation. He taught that jaundice was caused by obstruction of the bile-passages, and was the first to describe the morbid deposit under a long bone's enveloping membrane (*spina ventosa*). European students of Arabian medicine credit Rhazes with having given a fuller account of curvature of the spine than any other author up to his time; he is further credited with being the first who wrote an entire book on pediatrics, the first who introduced chemical preparations into practice, and the first to maintain that disorders of the bladder are accompanied by blood in the urine (*hematuria*).

The Arabian school wrote much on gonorrhea, just as we do today, and Rhazes was so sagacious in this field that he may be considered a genito-urinary specialist. He gave a detailed description of strictures, and if they produced any degree of retention of urine (*ischuria*), he at once introduced the catheter, for he was a master of the principles of catheterism. To avoid obstruction from blood and pus, he bored numerous holes in the sides of the extremity which enters the bladder; not finding the classic bronze catheter sufficiently flexible, he invented one of lead. He was the first who consistently used urethral injections, and if his honeyed water or decoction of quince-seeds did not do much good, at least they did no harm—which cannot be said of many subsequent remedies. To abate the smarting pain during urination, he employed injections of tepid vinegar, or treated the bladder with injections of opium dissolved in rose water. He realized the need of relieving the inflammation and promoting healing of the urethra by local means and by internal medication. It seems that a gonorrheic was as safe in the hands of Rhazes as in our own.

No exposure of quackery is better known than Rhazes' spirited account:

There are so many little arts used by mountebanks and pretenders to physic, that an entire treatise, had I a mind to write one, would not contain them; but their impudence and daring boldness is equal to the guilt and inward conviction they have of tormenting and putting persons to pain in their last hours, for no reason at all.

Now some of them profess to cure the falling-sickness, and thereupon make an issue in the hinder part of the head, in form of a cross, and pretend to take something out of the opening, which they held all the while in their hands. Others give out, that they can draw snakes or lizards out of their patients' noses, which they seem to perform by putting up a pointed iron probe, with which they wound the nostril, until the blood comes: then they draw out the little artificial animal composed of liver, etc.

Some are confident they can take out the white specks in the eye. Before they apply the instrument to that part, they put in a piece of fine rag into the eye, and taking it out with the instrument, pretend it is drawn immediately from the eye. Some again undertake to suck water out of the ear, which they fill with a tube from their mouth, and hold the other end to the ear; and so spurting the water out of their mouths, pretend it came from the ear. Others pretend to get out worms, which grow in the ear, or roots of the teeth. Others can extract frogs from the under part of the tongue; and by lancing make an incision, into which they clap in the frog, and so take it out.

What shall I say of bones inserted into wounds and ulcers, which, after remaining there for some time, they take out again? Some, when they have taken out a stone from the bladder, persuade their patients, that still there's another left; they do this for this reason, to have it believed, that they have taken out another. Sometimes they probe the bladder, being altogether ignorant and uncertain, whether there be a stone or no. But if they don't find it, they pretend at least to take out one they have in readiness before, and show that to them.

Sometimes they make an incision in the anus for the piles, and by repeating the operation often bring it to a fistula or an ulcer, when there was neither before. Some say they take phlegm, or a substance like unto glass, out of the penis or other part of the body, by the conveyance of a pipe, which they hold with water in their mouths. Some pretend that they can contract and collect all the floating humors of the body to one place by rubbing it with winter cherries; which causes a burning or inflammation; and then they expect to be rewarded, as if they cure the distemper; and after they have suppled the place with oil, the pain presently goes off.

Some make their patients believe they have swallowed glass; so, taking a feather, which they force down the throat, they throw them into a vomiting, which brings up the stuff they themselves had put in with that very feather. Many things of this nature do they get out, which these impostors with great dexterity have put in, tending many times to the endangering the health of their patients, and often ending in the death of them.

Such counterfeits could not pass with discerning men, but that they did not dream of any fallacies, and made no doubt of the skill of those whom they employed; till at last when they suspect, or rather look more narrowly into their operations, the cheat is discovered. Therefore no wise men ought to trust their lives in their hands, nor take any more of their medicines, which have proved so fatal to many.

The textbooks of an age are much alike, and when Rhazes opened his *Division of Diseases* by first enumerating the maladies of the head, gradually descending to those of the feet, he was simply following the prevalent but unscientific fashion. But Rhazes wrote a slender *Treatise on Smallpox and Measles,* and here he followed no one. It is true he believed Galen was familiar with smallpox, and he quotes Aaron of Alexandria, the Arabian-Jewish physician Masarjawaih, and his teacher al-Tabari, but their references were indefinite; it was Rhazes who placed this disease on the medical map. His description stands out as unrivaled—the original and still surviving landmark in smallpox. For once, an Arabian touched hands with Hippocrates and Aretaeus. It is not his bulky *Continent*, but his tract on *Smallpox and Measles* which keeps alive the name of Rhazes.

Huge books, like unwieldy animals, have a tendency to become extinct. Haly Abbas, born in southwestern Persia of a Zoroastrian family, writing about half a century after Rhazes' death, said he knew of only two complete copies of the *Continent*—its size dismayed the calligraphist, and its cost alarmed the purchaser. Haly Abbas, who possessed a well-developed critical sense, remarked that Rhazes' *Continent* was too prolix, while his *Book to al-Mansur* was too condensed.

We need not be surprised that Haly judges his countryman, for not only Rhazes and Ibn Serapion, but Oribasius and Paulus Aegineta, and Galen and even the Father of Medicine pass in review before him: "Hippocrates who is the prince of the medical art and the first physician who ever wrote a book on this art, is the author of many treatises on all sorts of medical topics. But he writes in such a very concise manner that much of what he says is obscure, and as a consequence the reader, if he wishes to understand him, is obliged to seek the aid of a commentary."

Under these circumstances, there was nothing for Haly Abbas to do except to produce the right kind of textbook. He surveyed the entire subject, writing a complete system of medicine in 400,000 Arabic words. He dedicated it to his Emir, the founder of the Adudi Hospital of Bagdad, and the work is therefore known as the *Royal Book*. It is a well-arranged encyclopedia of the state of medical knowledge in the tenth century. Haly Abbas realized that book-learning did not suffice for a physician. "It is incumbent," he wrote, "that the student of this Art should constantly attend the hospitals and sick-houses; pay unremitting attention to the conditions and circumstances of their inmates, in company with the most acute professors of Medicine; and enquire frequently as to the state of the patients and the symptoms apparent in them, bearing in mind what he has read about these variations, and what they indicate of good or evil."

It is not to be expected that a textbook writer will differ materially from his predecessors, and when Haly writes that the womb is a wild beast, hungry for its food which is semen, he repeats what he has read and not what he has observed. Yet there were few pathologic conditions which he did not discuss with learning and judgment, and in dietetics and hygiene he discoursed on the value of sugar as food for infants; on the difference of the milk of cows, camels, sheep, goats and asses; on the influence of clothing upon health; on the action of mineral waters upon the system; on natural and artificial wines. His contributions to obstetrics include the observation, in opposition to older views, that in parturition the child does not actively emerge, but is expelled by the motion of the womb. It is doubtful, however, if Haly Abbas realized, as we moderns do, that the child's first thought in moving from the warm maternal nest into the cold and unfamiliar world, is the wish that it had never been born.

Haly Abbas perceived that both sexes are prone to depression at the approach of puberty, and he classified love under melancholia; he directed that lovesick youths undergo a moistening régime, since the black bile which afflicted them was equivalent, in the humoral pathology, to dryness. "They should take baths," said Haly Abbas, "moderate horse exercise, and anoint themselves with oil of violets. They should look upon gardens, fields, meadows and flowers, listen to sweet and low sounds as of the lute or lyre, and their minds should be occupied by stories, or pleasant and interesting news. But they must also have some work or business so as to keep them from idleness, and from thoughts of the loved ones; and it is good to excite them to quarrels and arguments, that their minds may be yet further distracted. Let them also cultivate the acquaintance of other young women."

In an age not characterized by fundamental discoveries, the salvaging of knowledge becomes important, and Haly's coördinated summary is a landmark in Arabian medicine. Rhazes' *Continent* was superseded by the *Royal Book* of Haly Abbas, until it was in its turn supplanted by Avicenna's *Canon*. Avicenna, the Ibn Sina of the Arabians, was a native of Bokhara, and thus the four outstanding physicians of the eastern caliphate —al-Tabari, Rhazes, Haly Abbas, Avicenna—were Persians.

Few tales in the Arabian Nights are stranger than the life of Avicenna. His amazing career began in his childhood, for at the age of ten he memorized the Koran; neither arithmetic nor Arabic poetry presented any difficulties; the *Isagoge* of Porphyry, the *Geometry* of Euclid, the *Almagest* of Ptolemy, were mastered with the aid of a green-grocer and a wandering tutor; philosophy and natural history followed; medicine was studied under a Nestorian, and Avicenna found it easy: "Medicine is no hard and thorny science, like mathematics and metaphysics, so I soon made great progress; I became an excellent doctor, and began to treat patients, using approved remedies. . . . At twelve years of age I disputed in law and logic. . . . When I found a difficulty, I referred to my notes and prayed to the Creator. At night, when weak or sleepy, I strengthened myself with a glass of wine."

He attended the sick without fees, and says he was rewarded by discovering new methods of treatment. When halted in the pursuit of higher philosophy, he put aside his books, and prayed in the mosque until the dark passages grew clear. The waking day and sleepless night were not sufficient, and even in dreams he solved problems. At sixteen he knew all subjects, but was sad because he could not comprehend the *Metaphysics* of Aristotle; he read it through forty times, and was able to repeat the words by heart, but could not fathom their meaning. One day on a bookstall he saw a commentary on Aristotle, written by the Turkish student of medicine and philosophy, al-Farabi. Avicenna knew that commentaries are often more mystifying than the text they seek to elucidate, but al-Farabi's little guide cost only three dirhems. He bought it and to his intense joy found he possessed the sesame that opened the door to the hidden treasures of Aristotle. He offered thanks to God, bestowed alms on the poor, and as his education was now complete, this youth of seventeen started upon his travels.

Adversity and glory were henceforth the inseparable companions of Avicenna. At eighteen he cured a king of a serious illness, and the fee enchanted him: he was permitted to use the royal archives with its manuscripts that had no duplicates. This irreplaceable library disappeared in fire, and before its ashes had cooled, the rumor was spread that Avicenna burned it to hide the sources of his knowledge—the echo of a calumny against a more ancient physician. After the extinction of the Samanid dynasty, Avicenna fled to escape capture by the sultan of Ghazna. He wandered to Khiva, through Nishapur and Merv, and at Jurjan sought the protection of Qabus, patron of learning. He came at the wrong time, for the army was in mutiny, and Qabus was starved to death. Avicenna reached Rai, the birthplace of Rhazes, and wrote many books, until the warfare between the royal mother and her second son drove him to Kazwin.

In the medieval East, fortune's wheel had no restraining axis: at Hamadan, Avicenna cured Shams Addaula of colic, and the grateful emir immediately raised the physician to the post of prime minister. Angry Kurds and Turks clamored for the Persian's head, and Shams Addaula saved the scholar's life only by stripping him of his honors and decreeing his banishment. Avicenna knew his patient's constitution, and instead of fleeing from Hamadan, secreted himself in the house of a friendly sheik, awaiting a summons that he felt was inevitable. After forty days, the emir sent for him, and offered his apologies in the Oriental manner: Shams Addaula again had colic, and Avicenna again became vizier.

His activity was extraordinary. The duties of statecraft ending at sundown, Avicenna spent the evening in study, dictating and lecturing, and expounding the *Canon*. To compose a treatise in twenty volumes was merely an incident in his career. Medicine, mathematics, astronomy, physics, chemistry, geology, philosophy, theology, poetry and music were enriched by his genius. The night was always young to Avicenna, and when manuscripts were put aside, the wine-jug was seldom empty, and he relaxed amid minstrels and dancing-girls. His sensualism was as famous as his scholarship, and all Islam asked: Which does Ibn Sina love the more—learning, or wine and women?

Adventure never deserted Avicenna. Concealment in an apothecary's house, imprisonment in a fortress, flight in the garb of a Sufite ascetic, escape from accumulating dangers, and chief citizen of Isphahan, are among the episodes of his latter years. Pouring out ceaseless productions in calamity and in prosperity, working, drinking, writing, laughing, pursuing wisdom and women to the end, the myriad-minded and merry-making Avicenna exhausted himself in his fifty-eighth year. Students of Persian literature believe that many verses of Omar Khayyam are unjustly attributed to others, but that at least one quatrain in the *Rubaiyat* was not written by the tent-maker who saw earth's sad destiny, but by Avicenna—the one beginning, "Up from Earth's Center through the Seventh Gate." Avicenna passed through this Seventh Gate before old age reached him.

The *Canon* of Avicenna, consisting of approximately a million words, is the most influential textbook ever written—for six centuries it dominated the medical schools of Asia and Europe. Upon every page we find something to admire and to condemn. His pharmacology was immense, but he thought he could deduce the therapeutic effects of drugs from their taste and smell and color. His study of symptoms is brilliant, but his division of pain into fifteen varieties is more subtle than scientific. His dual doctrine, "True according to faith; false according to reason," was wholly baneful in its effects. In treating gonorrhea, Avicenna was probably the first to use catheters made of the skin of various animals, and he mentions intravesical injections by means of a silver syringe. That he advised a louse to be inserted in the meatus of persons suffering from retention of urine, is simply additional evidence of the easy capacity of the Arabians to mix absurdities with their rational procedures. It is almost unbelievable how frequently Avicenna's louse, modified at times to a bug or a flea, reappears in the venereal literature.

He proves himself an indulgent physician when he says, "All our study, all our care, should be directed to forming and molding the character of the child. Care must be taken that he does not blaze out with anger, nor be overwhelmed with fear, nor cast down by sadness, nor harassed by wakefulness. So we must always notice what he wants, what he is eager for, and this should be provided for him and given to him, but what he dislikes should be taken out of his way. For hence comes a two-fold advantage, one to the mind, the other to the body." But when he directed, "If the child does not sleep properly, mix some poppy with his food," he became the mischievous father of soothing-syrups.

The *Canon* is both the epitome and the summation of Graeco-Arabian medicine. What Galen did for the Romans, Avicenna accomplished for the Moslems. It established itself as law, and criticism was regarded as sacrilege. "The Lord saith, Every kind of game is comprehended in the Wild Ass," wrote Nizami of Samarcand, "and all this and even more is in the *Canon;* from him who hath mastered the first volume thereof, nothing will be hidden concerning the general theory and principles of Medicine, so that could Hippocrates and Galen return to life, it would be proper that they should do reverence to this book. Yet have I heard a wonderful thing; one hath taken exception to Ibn Sina in respect to this work, and hath embodied his criticisms in a book which he hath entitled the *Rectification of the Canon*. It is as though I looked upon both, and saw how foolish is the author and how detestable his work. For what right hath any one to find fault with so great a man, when the very first question in a book of his is difficult of comprehension? . . . May God by his grace and favor keep us from such stumblings and vain imaginings!" Pilgrims who visit his brickwork tomb in Hamadan, swear that Avicenna cured them, and native doctors study his books word for word, and prescribe according to his precepts. Avicenna has been sleeping since the year 1037, but he still treats all the invalids of Persia.

After Avicenna, the star of Islam set in the East to rise in the West. Spain, which in its Roman days gave birth to the Senecas, Lucan, Quintilian and Martial, produced Albucasis, Avenzoar, Averroes and Maimonides in its Moslem period. Glamorous Bagdad on the Tigris found its counterpart in Cordova on the Guadalquivir. Europe was darkened at sunset, Cordova shone with public lamps; Europe was dirty, Cordova built a thousand baths; Europe was covered with vermin, Cordova changed its undergarments daily; Europe lay in mud, Cordova's streets were paved; Europe's palaces had smoke-holes in the ceiling, Cordova's arabesques were exquisite; Europe's nobility could not sign its name, Cordova's children went to school; Europe's monks could not read the baptismal service, Cordova's teachers created a library of Alexandrian dimensions. Throughout its long history, Spain has been an evil and intolerant nation, spreading its piety over two hemispheres at the point of the sword; out of its blood-stained past, only its Moorish hour emerges resplendent, and in its turn succumbed to Mohammedan fanaticism.

Albucasis is a solitary figure, standing apart as the only Arabian who wrote a separate treatise on surgery. Christian historians have asserted that from the manner in which he describes the rite of circumcision, there can be no doubt he was a Jew, but Jews have not claimed him. His practice does not divulge his religion, for he relates, with impartiality, that he extracted a large arrow which lodged below the eye of a Jew, and took out a barbed arrow which was sticking in the throat of a Christian, and in each case the patient recovered. Albucasis described and pictured about two hundred surgical instruments, and it was long believed these were the first surgical drawings extant, but earlier ones have recently been found in manuscripts.

His *Surgery* is largely an abstract of the compilation of

Paulus Aegineta, but he amplifies his author. Albucasis appears to have been the inventor of the sponge-tipped probang for dislodging foreign particles from the gullet, of the grooved probe for urethral investigation, and of an ear-syringe which he thus describes: "You may also introduce into the cannula a specially adapted copper piston or a stylet, the end of which is armed with cotton. Then fill the cannula with oil or some other suitable fluid, introduce into one end the stylet armed with cotton, and push it onward until the liquid enters the ear."

The well-known obstetrical position, in which the parturient woman lies supine, with her hips at the edge and her legs hanging over the table, was first described by Albucasis. The Arabians indulged in strange perversions, but Moslem modesty did not permit men to examine women, and even in so serious an operation as cutting for stone (*lithotomy*), Albucasis directs the midwives to undertake the task: "The finger should be introduced into the rectum of virgins, into the vagina of married women; then an incision should be made, in virgins to the left and below into the labium, in married women between the urethra and os pubis, so that in both cases the wound is oblique." In fracture of the pubic arch he recommended a tube to be attached to a sheep's bladder, and the latter to be inserted in the vagina; by blowing forcibly into the tube the sheep's bladder would be distended until the vaginal cavity was filled sufficiently to restore the injured pelvis. His illustrations of obstetrical instruments include forceps with crossed blades, and dilators with screw action. With such tools, we would expect results, but prejudice stood in the way of progress. For example, Albucasis did not love wine like Avicenna, yet prescribed it medicinally: a Moslem who copied his codex added the pious warning, "Allah has forbidden wine. If it be granted to the sick to recover, they will do so without wine." It was this attitude which was responsible for the ultimate sterilization of Arabian medicine.

It is difficult to explain the magnificent specimens of Etruscan bridgework, for all things Etrurian are as mysterious as its unreadable language. In the post-Roman era, to the great calamity of the human race, dental knowledge decayed. If Albucasis is not the restorer, at least he is the conservator of dentistry in the Arabian period. Histories of dentistry are always embellished with illustrations of his instruments for shaking, loosening and removing teeth, the earliest type of turn key for extraction, dental saw and file, set of fifteen dental scrapers, small axe for resection of irregular teeth, elevators and forceps for extraction of roots, vulsella for removal of portions of the jaw, and the gold and silver wire with which he bound a loose tooth to a sound one. He realized that irregular or projecting teeth are particularly displeasing in women, and described the operation for their correction.

In the absence of a dental chair, his method of holding a patient during extraction, was sensible: "The head of the patient should be taken between the knees of the operator, in order to keep it steady." He was a pioneer in discussing oral deformities, dental arches, formation of tartar, replanting teeth, and artificial teeth: "The space left by missing teeth can be filled up with artificial ones made of ox-bone; such teeth can be anchored with a suitable gold wire to the firm teeth; they will be found of esthetic and functional value."

Albucasis thumbed his Paulus in vain if he expected to find a reference to those individuals whose blood will not clot and thus face death at every pin-prick or at the pulling of a tooth. So Albucasis wrote the first account of bleeder's disease (*hemophilia*), the peculiar condition which females transmit to their male offspring alone: "I found men in a certain village who told me that whenever they suffered a severe wound, it bled until they were dead, and they added that when a child rubbed his gums they began to bleed, and went on bleeding till he died. Another also having had a vein opened by a phlebotomist bled to death; and they said that, in general, most of them died thus. I have never seen such a thing save in this village; nor do I find it noticed in ancient writers. I know not the cause of it, but as for the cure, I suppose a cautery should be applied at once; but I have never tried it, and the whole thing is marvelous to me."

It is almost as marvelous to us today, for we know little more about it than Albucasis did. But in his paragraph there is an ominous word which we have long discarded—the cautery. The Arabs have been described as blood-shy and knife-shy, but it was Albucasis who made the actual cautery their national instrument. He who pictured all the instruments of surgery, preferred the branding iron. He who knew that the hemorrhage of wounded arteries could be stopped by styptics, ligature, and complete division, favored cauterization. Where Antyllus would have incised, Albucasis burned. He mentions more than fifty diseases which he himself treated with fire. How low was the state of surgery in his time is obvious from his lamentation, "The operative Art has disappeared from among us almost without leaving any trace behind. Only in the writings of the ancients do we find some references to it but these, by bad translations, by errors and alterations, have become nearly unintelligible and useless." Such was the surgical confession of the greatest of Arabian surgeons.

Avenzoar, sage of Seville, also practised surgery, but is remembered as the foremost clinician of the Western Caliphate. It has been frequently asserted, and as frequently denied, that he was a Jew. His ancestors were distinguished statesmen and jurists in Spain, and his grandfather and father were eminent physicians. The family was one of unusual independence; the father had such slight respect for Avicenna's Canon that he wrote his own prescriptions on the blank space of the margins; however, when Avenzoar was puzzled over a case and asked his father's advice, the old man bade him read Galen.

Avenzoar is responsible for a superstition which prevailed for centuries; not satisfied with claiming that he cured his dysentery by wearing an Emerald upon his belly, he wrote the first account of the Bezoar Stone: "That is the best which is found in the east, near the eyes of stags. Great stags, in those countries, eat serpents to make them strong; and, before they have received any hurt from them, run to the streams of water, and go into it so far till it comes up to their heads; this custom they have from natural instinct; and there they continue without tasting the water (for, if they should drink it they would die immediately), till their eyes begin to trickle: this liquor, which there oozes out under the eyelids, thickens and coagulates; and continues running, till it increases to the bigness of a chestnut or a nut. When these stags find the force of the poison spent, they come out of the water, and return to their usual haunts; and this substance, by degrees growing as hard as a stone, at last, by their frequent rubbing it, falls off. This is the most useful Bezoar of all."

As an antidote for poison, the bezoars were much in demand, though their location was transferred to the stomach instead of the canthus, and other animals than the stag were deemed capable of producing these medicinal stones. Druggists sold bezoars in such quantities that an indignant surgeon protested these specimens had never been inside any wild goat, antelope, or ape. Their reputation rose with time, and physicians prescribed them for all fevers, and for skin diseases including leprosy. Men carried them, in gold and silver cases, as amulets; during plague, those who could not afford to buy, rented one by the day. False bezoars were burnt by the authorities, but if declared genuine they were sold at great price and treasured as heirlooms. According to Abdalanarack, a castle in Cordova was given in exchange for one of these stones. Most remarkable of all, the Bezoar Stone as an official remedy was admitted into the London Pharmacopeias until the mid-eighteenth century.

Avenzoar's faith in emeralds and bezoars did not interfere with his clinical insight; delusion and discernment may dwell within the same convolutions, and Avenzoar's folly is wiped out by Avenzoar's wisdom. The itch mite (*Acarus scabiei*) has caused the human race to scratch itself throughout the ages, but it was first described by Avenzoar: "Sometimes there arises on the body, under the external skin, little swellings which the vulgar call *soab*, and if the skin be removed, there issues from various parts a very small beast, so small that he is hardly visible."

The Hippocratic school looked at a growing malignant tumor, and was reminded of a moving crab (*karkinos, karkinoma,* cancer). Galen explains, "Just as a crab's feet extend from every part of its body, so in this disease the veins (he did not know the lymphatics) are distended, forming a similar figure." Paulus repeats the comparison, and adds: "But some say that cancer is so called because it adheres to any parts which it seizes upon in an obstinate manner like the crab." The masterly description of Celsus ends with the melancholy reflection that nothing can be expected from medicines or corrosive applications or burning irons or the scalpel. The Arabians received their knowledge of malignancy from the Greeks; like their teachers, they sanctioned operation in cancer of the breast and extremities, and realized it may be extirpated only in its initial stage—and what more do we know of this frightful malady today?

Clinical examinations enabled Avenzoar to diagnose cancer of the stomach: "One of Ali's courtiers long had an obscure disease, with indigestion, loss of flesh, and occasional fever. I found him much prostrated with a slow, irregular serrate pulse. In the epigastric region I felt a round hard mass like an apple, painful on deep pressure." Equally graphic is his account of cancer of the gullet, "commencing with mild pain and difficulty in swallowing, and gradually increasing to complete occlusion."

Here Galen did not serve as guide, and without written authority Avenzoar faced the problem of the slow but ever-tightening stricture that was closing his patient's gullet. He answered it by inserting down the throat a silver pipe through which he poured fresh milk or gruel. Vomiting or obstruction at times made this impossible, and when the invading tumor rendered its victim incapable of swallowing food, how was he to be fed? Should the doomed man be placed in a bath of warm milk in the hope that the pores of the skin would be able to absorb nourishment? Avenzoar mentions this procedure, but on the whole rejects it as frivolous. He favored a plan of his own, although it contradicted Galen who had said that by means of the nutrient clyster no particles can reach the stomach for digestion.

Avenzoar agreed that on normal occasions an intestinal injection, "introduced by violence, will never ascend so high as the stomach, for the contractile force of the intestines themselves resists and endeavors to throw it back; the case is quite different when the body is in great want of nourishment and the intestines are empty: then there is an attractive power in the stomach and guts, which gradually draws upward any nourishment which lies in the way, from one intestine to another." This remarkable passage foreshadows knowledge of reverse peristalsis, and Avenzoar continues: "Why may we not suppose that milk or broth may be by this force of attraction carried through the intestines up as far as the stomach, since seeds put in a pot, or any other earthen vessel, manifestly attract and imbibe nourishment and moisture beyond the extent of the vessel itself?"

His practice in these cases was to wash out the lower bowel, then with a goat's bladder into which a tube was fastened, he injected milk, eggs and gruel into the gut. Contemporaries, and successors for centuries, ridiculed the nutrient enema, but modern medicine utilizes the rectum, not only for the introduction of pre-digested food, but for the administration of drugs. To Avenzoar belongs the credit of being the first advocate of nutrition *per rectum*.

All printed editions of Avenzoar's *Theisir* are bound with the *Colliget* of Averroes, and never was a bibliographic union more appropriate, for Averroes was Avenzoar's pupil and friend. Averroes admired his teacher so much that he was ready to stand against Galen if only Avenzoar were on his side. For example, Galen recommended that the new-born be salted, but Avenzoar thought it more useful to rub them with oil of nuts, and Averroes agreed with his countryman. Descended from a line of jurists, Averroes was bred to the law, which he followed until science claimed his attention. His social position, combined with his rectitude and talents, brought him such positions as cadi of Seville, chief magistrate of Cordova, governor of Morocco. Even the pleasure of appointing judges and modifying his country's laws could not seduce him from study; it is said that the night of his father's death and the night of his wedding-day were the only nights which Averroes did not devote to intellectual labor.

He wrote much on the healing art, but a great philosopher has never been a great physician, and Averroes' observation that smallpox does not attack the same person twice—an adumbration of immunology—constitutes his sole original contribution to medicine. His lifework was the interpretation of Aristotle, in which he was so successful that he was entitled The Commentator. After knowing Aristotle, Averroes could not be confined by the Koran, and realizing that the Mohammedan creed, no more than the Jewish and Christian sects, sought scientific truth, he evolved into pantheist and freethinker, the great Moslem heretic of the twelfth century. Despite his scepticism, he was credulous at least once: he believed a woman who assured him she had conceived in water, whereupon the unsuspecting inquirer promulgated the doctrine that a female may become pregnant by entering a bath in which a male has had a seminal emission.

Both Avenzoar and Averroes suffered much from Moslem piety. Avenzoar's father was persecuted by the Almoravides, and died in prison. Avenzoar also was kept in Ali ibn Jussuf's dungeons, from which he was taken, from time to time, to treat the court. As the hands of Ali were raised in supplication to Allah, the Almoravides were swept from power by another sect of Islam, the relentless Almohades. An obscure lamplighter in a mosque produced a deformed son; crooked in mind and body, Mohammed ibn Tumart was hated for his harshness and ugliness; many towns spurned this undersized misshapen beggar, little thinking he was a destined conqueror. He appointed himself censor of Islam, and preached the sinfulness of laughter and song, of poetry and painting; gathering crowds of fanatics around him, he wrecked wine-shops and music-halls in Morocco; growing in insolence and power, he attacked Ali's sister, because she walked the streets of Fez unveiled; with the sword of intolerance he was invincible, and after his death in a monastery, his followers ruled Northern Africa and Moslem Spain.

The enemies of Averroes now had their opportunity. His

character was unimpeachable, but they invoked the graver charge of heresy—his deeds did not count if he believed a forbidden creed. Averroes, declared guilty of freethought, was exiled from Cordova to a town inhabited only by Jews. There was public clamor for his death, but according to Leo Africanus, another punishment was reserved for the aged philosopher: bareheaded and in rags, Averroes stood by the door of a mosque, and all the orthodox were permitted to vent their indignation by spitting in his face. It is reported, though on insufficient evidence, that when Averroes was informed the Saracens and Christians had combined to burn his books and to condemn his soul to eternal fire, he answered: "Let my soul be with the philosophers."

The dark days of Spain, begun by the Almoravides, and continued by the Almohades, were the prelude of darker days to come. Under the magnificent Abdurraham and his son Hakam, the Hebrew, Christian and Moslem of Spain spoke the same tongue, read the same literary and scientific masterpieces, and applauded the same dancing-girls. Under the Almohades, the order went forth that all Christians and Jews must choose between conversion to Islam or perpetual banishment. From the grave where he had lain for twenty years, the fleshless hand of Mohammed ibn Tumart destroyed every Church and Synagogue in Andalusia. Writers, not consulting their chronology, say that when Averroes was degraded amid the Jews, he was protected by his pupil, Moses Maimonides. The family of Maimonides was expelled from Cordova in 1148, and Averroes did not fall from office until 1195, at which time Maimonides had long been living in another continent. Averroes found a patron in the third emir of the Almohades, who restored him to his rank and library, but the sorrows and wanderings of Maimonides—which began in his thirteenth year—were of long duration. His father Maimon, exegete and moralist, had placed him under distinguished Moslem teachers, and personally instructed him in rabbinical lore. The philosophical works of both Maimon and Maimonides were usually composed, not in Hebrew, but in Arabic.

Adrift from their accustomed surroundings, these scholars

carried on the Jewish Tradition; nomads and outcasts, there was no place in Spain they dared call home. Danger increased with the years, and in 1160 Maimon took his daughter, his sons Moses and David, and sailed to deep-valleyed Fez, the university town of Morocco, the pride of Moorish Africa. In secret they consorted with Jews, and outwardly wore the mask of Islam. Discovery of this dual life meant death; thus was the leader of the community, Judah ibn Shoshan, detected and executed. Maimonides was saved by the influence of an Arabic poet, but Fez had grown too perilous. Like thieves in the night, the family of Maimon stole out of Morocco in 1165, and set forth for Palestine. They survived a storm and a threatened shipwreck, and in a month reached Acre, the little town fertilized by countless fallen warriors of conflicting faiths. Eighty miles to the south lay Jerusalem, where Maimonides wept at the Wailing Wall, but could not remain.

The emotional appeals of Peter the Hermit, which caused multitudes of peasants to follow the hoof-prints of his mule; the preaching of Pope Urban that Christ's Sepulchre must be recovered from the infidel; the assurance of Bernard of Clairvaux that whoever slays an unbeliever is certain of Paradise; the interference of the Turks with Christian pilgrims; the desire of Penitents to wash out their sins in the blood of heretics; the chivalry of knights which made it necessary for them to kill; the demand of nobles for new territory; the ambition of merchants for the rich markets of Asia; the lure of adventure, and the migration instinct; pestilence coming down from Flanders, and famine in Lorraine—these were among the factors, religious, commercial, personal, political—which again launched the West against the East.

Across Europe, through Germany and Hungary, beyond Bulgaria and Thrace, marched the army of the First Crusade, torturing and destroying unoffending populations, pillaging and ravishing, whitening its track with bones and reddening it with blood. At Antioch a priest hid and found a Saracen spear, announcing the discovery of the Holy Lance which pierced the side of the Saviour: superstition accomplished the rest, and despite obstacles and dissensions, the soldiers of the Cross moved on to the winepress of the Lord. Blunder and disharmony could not stay them, and history will not forget the afternoon when Godfrey of Bouillon stood with unsheathed sword on the walls of Jerusalem. The orgy that followed is one of the worst in human annals. Water never flowed through the parched Holy Land as did blood through days and nights; men who were rumored to have swallowed gold, were ripped open; few women in that City of God escaped rape; the soldiers picked up infant Arabs and battered out their brains against the stones; children were tossed in the air and flung from the parapets; only after the third day did the Crusaders begin to weary of stabbing 70,000 Moslems; no graves could hold the unburied dead, from whose putrefying bodies arose pestilence; the unresisting Jews were herded in their synagogues and burnt, the smell of the roasting flesh of blasphemers being incense to pious nostrils. Modern historians, after relating these events, interpret them as beneficial to mankind, because the Crusades introduced to Europe the knowledge of sugar and lemons, the use of glass mirrors and the rosary, and the Arabic terms of tariff and corvette; but the memory of the massacre was too vivid in the days of Maimonides, and unaware that the Crusades had brought such musical instruments as the lute and the naker to Frank and Norman, he departed for Egypt. The second Moses came to the home of the first Moses, and in Fostat, the old section of Cairo, he achieved such renown that his contemporaries said: "From Moses unto Moses there arose not one like Moses."

Misfortune did not desert Maimonides during his early years in Egypt. Informers who had known him in Morocco, denounced him for apostasy to Islam; his life hung on a legal thread, until a remarkable decision came out of Egypt: a forced conversion is not a conversion, and since he had never been converted, he could not be accused of relapsing from conversion. His father died, and his brother, a dealer in precious stones and the financial support of the family, was drowned with his fortune in the Indian Ocean. It was more than he could endure, and eight years later he wrote to one of his friends at Acre: "It is the heaviest evil that has befallen me. His little daughter and his widow were left with me. For a full year I lay on my couch, stricken with fever and despair. Many years have now gone over me, yet still I mourn, for there is no consolation possible. He grew up on my knees, he was my brother, my pupil; he went abroad to trade that I might remain at home and continue my studies; he was well versed in Talmud and Bible, and an accomplished grammarian. My one joy was to see him. He has gone to his eternal home, and has left me confounded in a strange land. Whenever I come across his handwriting or one of his books, my heart turns within me, and my grief reawakes. I should have died in my affliction but for the Law, which is my delight, and but for philosophy, which makes me forget to moan."

Maimonides had never earned a living, and with old Hebraic wrath he flays those who trade their holy knowledge for gain. Now that David was gone, the elder brother could not continue the jewelry business alone, and he turned to medicine. He had first studied the principles under Moslem teachers as a part of general culture, and it was now necessary to practise for bread. After a long period of obscurity and struggle, he was appointed physician to the court of Saladin. The most fortunate event in the troubled life of Maimonides, the one saving circumstance, was Saladin. To have been his contemporary, his subject, and physician to his family, gave Maimonides the opportunity to develop into the most famous Jew of medievalism. In an age when sectarian hatred was the chief of virtues, when toleration was heresy and crime, when even a Maimonides insisted a Jew should not save from death an idolater who falls into the water, Saladin stands out as the pattern of courtesy and graciousness. A Kurd by race, a student of the Koran, and the most devout of Mohammedans, he was nevertheless the champion of international justice, and it is characteristic of him that his medical staff comprised Jews, Christians and Moslems.

In his time the crusaders were brigands, the few who honestly sought salvation being overwhelmed by the many who frankly sought plunder; the Knights Templars and Hospitallers took the vow of poverty and accumulated wealth beyond all computation; the adventurous Reginald of Chatillon terrorized the desert with his raids on caravans and his insults to Mohammed. The protests of Saladin were met by coarse defiance and additional violence. Saladin could not lay aside the Koran, but he read it on horseback as he advanced toward the Holy City. His was the gentlest hand that ever slit a Christian throat, or wiped out an army. His kindness to women and his love for children were known to all. In October 1187, he entered Jerusalem as conqueror, purifying the city by prayer and rose-water, and by pulling down the golden cross—the work of Godfrey of Bouillon was undone. The cries of ravished Moslem women, and the blood of children beaten to death by the first crusaders, called for revenge. Had this loose-sleeved, green-turbaned man drawn his scimitar, massacre would have been answered by massacre. Saladin looked at his helpless captives, at the widows and orphans, and his eyes grew moist with pity. His power was absolute, and he used it by opening his purse to the poor, by protecting the needy, and by guarding the sick. In the meantime Europe heard a different version: the news spread that the Holy Sepulchre was profaned by the sultan's horses, and peasants from Ireland to the Levant were horrified to hear that Saladin ate Christian children for breakfast. This propaganda was the signal for the Third Crusade, and whoever did not take the cross was burdened with the tax known as Saladin's tithe. Richard the Lion-Hearted appeared on the scene, blustering and barbarous, running many Moslems through with his terrible lance. The climate disagreed with the English warrior, and as he tossed in his sun-baked tent he received a rare gift from the hospitable Saladin—a caravan of camels carrying snow to soothe his fever.

The troubadours sang a thousand lies about the valiant Richard, and perhaps an Arabian historian added another when he maintained that the Plantagenet offered Maimonides the post of medical attendant to the English court. Since King Richard suggested a marriage between his own sister and Saladin's brother, he may also have asked for the Sultan's physician, but we doubt this often-told tale. If Maimonides actually received such an invitation, he must have reflected that Cairo was less turbulent than London, and that it was unwise to exchange a Moslem saint for a Christian savage. How busy he eventually became as a practitioner is apparent from a letter which he wrote in September 1199 to ward off the impending visit of his disciple Samuel ibn Tibbon:

Now God knows that in order to write this to you I have escaped to a secluded spot, where people would not think to find me, sometimes leaning for support against the wall, sometimes lying down on account of my excessive weakness, for I have grown old and feeble.

But with respect to your wish to come here to me, I cannot but say how greatly your visit would delight me, for I truly long to commune with you, and would anticipate our meeting with even greater joy than you. Yet I must advise you not to expose yourself to the perils of the voyage, for beyond seeing me, and my doing all I could to honour you, you would not derive any advantage from your visit. Do not expect to be able to confer with me on any scientific subject for even one hour either by day or by night, for the following is my daily occupation:

I dwell at Fostat and the Sultan resides at Cairo; these two places are two Sabbath days' journey (about one mile and a half) distant from each other. My duties to the Sultan are very heavy. I am obliged to visit him every day, early in the morning; and when he or any of his children, or any of the inmates of his harem, are indisposed, I dare not quit Cairo, but must stay during the greater part of the day in the palace. It also frequently happens that one or two of the royal officers fall sick, and I must attend to their healing. Hence, as a rule, I repair to Cairo, very early in the day, and even if nothing unusual happens, I do not return to Fostat until the afternoon. Then I am almost dying with hunger. I find the antechambers filled with people, both Jews and Moslems, nobles and common people, judges and bailiffs, friends and foes—a mixed multitude, who await the time of my return.

I dismount from my animal, wash my hands, go forth to my patients, and entreat them to bear with me while I partake of some slight refreshment, the only meal I take in the twenty-four hours. Then I attend to my patients, write prescriptions and directions for their various ailments. Patients go in and out until nightfall, and sometimes even, I solemnly assure you, until two hours and more in the night. I converse with and prescribe for them while lying down from sheer fatigue, and when night falls I am so exhausted that I can scarcely speak.

In consequence of this, no Israelite can have any private interview with me except on the Sabbath. On that day the whole congregation, or at least the majority of the members, come to me after the morning service, when I instruct them as to their proceedings during the whole week; we study together a little until noon, when they depart. Some of them return, and read with me after the afternoon service until evening prayers. In this manner I spend that day. I have here related to you only a part of what you would see if you were to visit me.

Now, when you have completed for our brethren the translation you have commenced, I beg that you will come to me, but not with the hope of deriving any advantage from your visit as regards your studies; for my time is, as I have shown you, excessively occupied.

Correspondence in the Middle Ages was far more important than it has since become, and a letter from Maimonides was an epoch-making event to a Jewish community. He was the official head of his people in Cairo, but the Jews of the world consulted him on all possible subjects, and his response was practically law. Yemenites and the Provençal Jews asked him questions, his decisions settled debates in the island of Sicily, and a Jew who traveled from England to India would find that Jews all along the route abided by his dicta. The *Responsa* of Maimonides were oracular: whoever disagreed with him either did not understand him, or was an ignorant fool or worse—this being the medieval method of discussion.

His main work—*Commentary on the Mishnah* (1168), *Re-*

ligious *Code* (1180) and *Guide of the Perplexed* (1190)—was the complete codification and interpretation of Biblical, Talmudical and Rabbinical literature. It is one of the monuments of medieval scholarship, and caused a eulogist to say, "He made of Israel again one people, and brought one to the other, so that they became one flesh." In a certain sense this is true, yet it is equally true that Maimonides cleft Israel in twain. The unadulterated Jews held it sinful to know of the existence of the writings of non-Jews; Maimonides was stigmatized because he read Aristotle, with the aid of the commentaries of al-Farabi and Avicenna—three blaspheming dogs. Maimonides undertook the impossible task of harmonizing Aristotle and Moses, and although this attempted syncretism of Hebraism and Hellenism was foredoomed to failure, at least he showed his people that science and philosophy did not begin and end in the Talmud. He was regarded as the liberalizer of Judaism, and as its destroyer. His adherents greeted his books as the new sacred canon, and his opponents pronounced them heretical. The two views were expressed on his tomb. An adoring Jew wrote: "Here lies a man, and still no man; if thou wert a man, the shadows of angels must have sheltered thy mother." Another Jew spat as he read this inscription, and erasing it, wrote: "Here lies Moses Maimonides, the excommunicated heretic." A generation after his death he was the storm center of a Holy War; the Bagdad Goanate quoted even Moslem philosophers against their coreligionist, and the rabbis of northern and southern France hurled curses at each other. So furious did the dispute become, so deep was the hatred of the opposing Jews, that the anti-Maimonidists brought the matter to the attention of the Christian authorities. The Inquisition answered by burning the books of Maimonides, and when his followers accused their opponents of delation, the Inquisition cut out their tongues. Fanaticism is indeed the incurable cancer of the human soul.

The admiration of Maimonides for Aristotle was profound, and he exalted the Stagirite at the expense of Plato: "The words of Plato, Aristotle's teacher, are obscure and figurative; they are superfluous to the man of intelligence, inasmuch as Aristotle supplanted all his predecessors. The thorough understanding of Aristotle is the highest achievement to which man can attain, with the sole exception of the understanding of the Prophets." This praise was largely responsible for the growth of the Jewish legend of Aristotle, although its germ is to be found as far back as 200 B.C., in the assertion of the Jewish philosopher, Aristobulus of Paneas, that Biblical revelation and Aristotelian reasoning are identical. Flavius Josephus bolstered up the legend by quoting passages indicating that Aristotle discoursed with a Jew and was impressed by his erudition, dietary laws, and the difficulty of pronouncing Jerusalem.

The legend languished until Maimonides raised Aristotle to the pinnacle of pagan glory. Pious Jews felt sad that one who was not of their race should receive so much credit. Thereupon they remembered that when Alexander conquered Jerusalem, he gave the writings of King Solomon to Aristotle who plagiarized their wisdom. Then it was said Aristotle, arguing with Simon about the ascertainment of truth, was convinced the reasoning faculty is less important than divine revelation. As the legend grew, the son of Shem-Tob saw it written in an old book that Aristotle was converted to Judaism on his death-bed. Later Gedaliah ibn Yahyah also found an old book (so he said) in which Aristotle accepted the Mosaic account of creation, acknowledged the Torah, and recanted his errors. Even this did not suffice, and the learned Abraham Bibago triumphantly announced that Aristotle was born in Jerusalem, a Jew of the tribe of Benjamin. Thus may a full-fledged legend arise out of nothing, but in this connection we must remember that if a legend permitted itself to be embarrassed by a fact, there would be no legends.

There is another legend, enveloping Maimonides himself, which requires examination. His compatriots have repeated so often that he was a great scientist and physician that their estimate is generally accepted. Some will be shocked to hear that he does not merit the name of scientist, and did not possess the scientific attitude. Averroes studied Aristotle, believing he was going back to the Greeks, but since he was unhampered by prejudice, he was really advancing toward Nature. Maimonides studied Aristotle through the spectacles of Moses. As long as he could induce an amalgam between them he was content, but when even the subtlest dialectics could not force them to unite, he invariably deserted Aristotle. For example, the keen mind of the Greek realized the eternity of matter, and hence the impossibility of a special act of creation. As this view could not be reconciled with the Mosaic account of creation, Maimonides clung to the *creatio ex nihilo* of Genesis. Aristotle saw the universe governed by immutable law, nature unchangeable, and nothing supernatural: Maimonides admonished his pupil, Joseph ibn Aknin, to reject this cosmic conception because it leaves no room for miracles, for prayer, for prophecy, and for revelation. Maimonides could not follow Aristotle very far along the paths of science, because the Old Testament blocked his way.

Maimonides was indeed a learned physician. He knew what the authorities had written, and his aphorisms were extracted from Galen. He was perfectly willing to be guided by Galen until Galen came in conflict with Moses. However, when Galen said Moses was unscientific—"I do not agree with Moses that anything is possible with God, and that God can suddenly turn a stone into a man or make a horse or cow from ashes. . . . In this matter our opinion and that of Plato and of others among the Greeks who have written correctly concerning natural science differs from the view of Moses"—Maimonides threw Galen overboard with Aristotle.

Maimonides' medical compositions include treatises on asthma and hygiene, written for Saladin's ailing son; on coitus, dedicated to Saladin's nephew, the sultan of Hamat; on poisons and antidotes; on hemorrhoids; and imitations of the aphorisms of Hippocrates and Galen. These writings do not deserve their high reputation. "A physician," said Maimonides, "should begin with simple treatment, trying to cure by diet before he administers drugs"—all of which is eminently true, but the Greeks had said it a hundred times. "Unripe fruit is harmful": this too is true, but any housewife could have told him as much.

In fact, most of his health rules—"Do not continue eating until the belly is distended; avoid poisonous foodstuffs; bathe every seven days; live in moderation"—were platitudes before the twelfth century. We find more medical wisdom in Seneca's letters to his friend Lucilius than in all the hygienic tracts of Maimonides. To few topics did Maimonides devote so much attention as to toxicology, yet he reached the conclusion that a fasting man's bite is the most dangerous poison, and that the most valuable remedy is the powder of precious stone. It is said he materially improved the method of performing circumcision, but his interest in the operation was rabbinical rather than surgical. Maimonides' *Prayer for Physicians* is beautiful, and deserves to rank with the Oath of Hippocrates, but as this Prayer was composed six centuries after the time of Maimonides, he knew nothing about it.

Maimonides was an authority on, and advocate of, sexual intercourse, writing two treatises on its hygienic aspects. "When erection," he said, "occurs in a natural and unconscious manner, and when after directing one's thoughts towards other subjects one feels the erection persist, and if there is a sluggish sensation in the regions of the kidneys, and the cords of the testicles are tightened and the flesh is warm, then one needs to have sexual intercourse and it is hygienic to perform the act." He asserts, "Copulation is life: strength to the body, and light to the eyes," and yet knew so little about it that he asserts coitus will not be fruitful if performed in the sitting posture or standing.

Extraneous arguments are not needed to demonstrate the status of Maimonides as a physician, for he reveals it in a letter to Jonathan of Lunel: "Although from my boyhood the Torah was betrothed to me, and continues to hold my heart as the wife of my youth, in whose love I find a constant delight, strange women whom I first took into my house as her handmaids become her rivals, and absorb a portion of my time." Maimonides' strange woman was Medicine, and the result was inevitable: for Medicine is a jealous and absorbing wife, demanding wholehearted fidelity, permitting a little straying only that the wanderer may return with more eagerness to the legitimate consort, not granting her rewards to mortals who seek her for pastime or for bread, but whispering her secrets to those who slave with joy for her sake alone. Maimonides was not one of these.

Maimonides acquired an extensive reputation throughout Europe, many of his works being put into Latin for the Schoolmen. Such theologians as Alexander of Hales, William of Auvergne, Albertus Magnus, Thomas Aquinas, Vincent of Beauvais, and Duns Scotus frequently quoted their precursor, for they attempted to fit Aristotle into Christianity, just as Maimonides had attempted to reconcile him with Judaism. Adopting the method of Maimonides, these Franciscans and Dominicans simply stretched Aristotle from the Old Testament to the New. It is a sober statement that Maimonides is entitled to a place among the Fathers of the Church much more than he is entitled to a place among the scientists. He grappled with Aristotle less in the interests of truth than in the interests of the Torah.

The achievements of the Jewish physicians of the Middle Ages have often been exaggerated. It must be remembered that they never dissected, and without anatomical and physiological knowledge they could be no more than servile imitators of the Greeks. If they shine, it is because of the surrounding darkness of monastic medicine. What discoveries of fundamental importance did they make in science? Not one can be named. The Semitic races gave man his theology—Judaism, Christianity, Islamism—and not his science. The great Jewish investigators date from the mid-nineteenth century, and not from medievalism, and they derive from Hippocrates and not from Maimonides. Not Jerusalem, not Mecca, but Hellas is our holy land.

Nestorians and Syrians were the midwives of Arabian medicine; Persians brought it to maturity; and Jews nursed it through all its stages. It is thus apparent that although we use the term Arabian medicine, the term is a misnomer—Mohammedan culture, racially and geographically, penetrated far beyond Arabia and its inhabitants. True indeed, Arabic was the prevailing language, but we do not consider Roger Bacon a Roman because his works were written in Latin. Appropriately enough, the biographical history of Arabian medicine closes with the name of Bar Hebraeus, the tireless compiler of the thirteenth century. The son and pupil of the Jewish physician Aaron, who was converted to Christianity, Bar Hebraeus bore no trace of his origin except his name. His works were composed in Syriac and Arabic, and there is no evidence that he even knew Hebrew. His Jewish descent was so thoroughly forgotten that he was appointed bishop of Aleppo and catholicus of the Jacobites. Physician, poet, philosopher, theologian, grammarian, and historian above all, his *Syriac Chronicle* places him among the foremost of Syrian scholars.

Medical attendant to the Tatar King of Kings, Bar Hebraeus edited Dioscorides and Hunain in Syriac, and translated Hippocrates and Galen into Arabic. Bar Hebraeus, the last of the great Syrian physicians, has left us, in his *Chronicle*, a picture of Jundisapur, the cradle of Arabian medicine: "And Sapur built for himself a city which was like unto Constantinople, and its name was Jundisapur and he settled his Greek wife therein. And there came with her skillful men from among the Greek physicians, and they sowed Hippocratic medicine in the East. And there were also excellent Syrian physicians, such as Sergius of Rishaina, who was the first to translate the philosophical and medical works of the Greeks into Syriac, and Atanus of Amid, and Philagrius, and Simon the monk, who belonged to Taibuthah, and Gregory the Bishop, and Theodosius the Patriarch, and Hunain, the excellent man, the son of Isaac, and many others after them until this day. These were all Syrians, but Aaron the Elder was not a Syrian. Gosyos, an Alexandrian, translated his book from Greek into Syriac."

Medical licensure originated at Bagdad in 931. In that year, a case of fatal professional ignorance was brought to the attention of al-Muqtadir, and the Caliph determined to wipe out the evil at once: exempting the leading physicians of the city, he forbade the others to continue their practice unless they proved their competence. According to al-Qifti, eight hundred and sixty trembling candidates appeared before Sinan ibn Thabit, the first official medical examiner.

One day, among these practitioners, stood a man of such scholarly and venerable mien, that Sinan did not question him, but rather sought his corroboration in the problems presented. The old man remained grave and silent, and when the others had gone, Sinan remarked, "I should like to hear from the professor something which I may learn from him, and also to know who was his teacher in the profession." To Sinan's surprise, the old man placed before him a purse of gold which he pulled from his sleeve, saying, "I cannot read or write well, nor have I read anything systematically, but I have a family whom I maintain by my professional labors, which therefore I beg you not to interrupt." The examiner laughed and answered, "You may have your license provided you do not prescribe phlebotomy, or any purgative drugs except for simple ailments." The old practitioner replied, "That has been my practice all my life, nor have I ever ventured beyond oxymel and jalap."

The following day a comely youth arrived. "With whom did you study?" asked Sinan. "With my father," said the young man. "And who is your father?" asked the examiner. "The old gentleman who was with you yesterday," said the young man. "A fine old gentleman!" commented Sinan, "and do you follow his methods? Yes? Then see that you do not go beyond them." Sinan ibn Thabit was distinguished as physician, mathematician, astronomer, statesman and humanitarian, and he did not become pompous even on this historic occasion.

Sinan is especially noteworthy for his efforts on behalf of prisoners and sick criminals, and for his administration of the hospitals of Bagdad. Moslem hospitals constitute one of the brightest phases of Arabian medicine, and as early as 707 the Caliph Welid established infirmaries at Damascus for the blind and for lepers. As the Nestorian hospital at Jundisapur declined,

Islam founded hospitals throughout its dominions. Aside from the numerous ones at Bagdad, Damascus, Cairo and Cordova, others were maintained at Antioch, Jerusalem, Mecca, Medina, Mosul, Hamar, Aleppo, Rai, Isphahan, Shiraz, Fez, Algericas, and of course in Alexandria and elsewhere.

The tale is told that when Rhazes was invited to choose a hospital site, he exposed meat in various sections of Bagdad, and selected the location where there was the most resistance to putrefaction. Equally interesting is al-Warraq's reminiscence that he encountered an aged inhabitant of Rai who informed him of Rhazes' method of instruction in hospitals: Rhazes held his clinic surrounded by his pupils, who themselves were surrounded by their disciples, and these in turn had other pupils about them. The patient who came for consultation, addressed himself first to the last, and if these knew what to say, they displayed their knowledge; if not, it was the turn of the next to speak; and if these could not give the correct answer, then Rhazes himself solved the difficulty.

Harun al-Rashid, in ordering the Jewish physician Shammakh to poison an inconvenient Iman, was carrying on an old tradition, but he established a tradition of his own by attaching a college and a hospital to every mosque. He opened an asylum for the insane—Arabian lunatics were treated much better than their European brothers—and in the twelfth century, the Jewish world-traveler, Benjamin of Tudela, passing through Bagdad, found sixty hospitals, "All well provided from the king's stores with spices and other necessaries, and every patient who claims assistance is fed at the king's expense until his cure is completed."

Nureddin, most honest of monarchs, had no jewel to give to his favorite sultana, but he possessed a scimitar which destroyed the crusaders led by three kings. In gratitude to God, he dedicated a great hospital which was strictly a charitable institution. "I am rich enough," protested Ibn al-Athir, "to pay for my drugs." The superintendent replied, "No doubt you can do without our medicines, but here no one despises Nureddin's benefits.

In the name of God, I assure you that Sultan Saladin's sons and their whole families send here for medicines, and never pay." Long afterward, Khalil Daheri exclaimed, "It has never had its like in the world," and he writes that even the healthy feigned illness to gain admittance: "While making the pilgrimage to Mecca, I stayed at Damascus, and had with me a certain Persian, a man of wit and intelligence, who followed the rites of the four orthodox sects, performing them all at the same time. When he went over the hospital and saw the patients' diet, and all their comforts and advantages, which are without number, he pretended to be ill and stayed three days there. The physician having felt his pulse recognized his case and prescribed any diet he liked, so he was fed upon young chickens, cakes, and sherbet, and all manner of fruits. But after two days the doctor wrote a prescription implying that a guest should not stay beyond the third day. They say the fire has never been put out at this hospital since it was built."

Nureddin's Hospital was surpassed only by its offspring, the Mansurian Hospital of Cairo. Mansur Gilafan, during a political campaign was stopped at Damascus, not by an onslaught of the enemy, but by an attack of colic. The physicians treated him with medicaments from the Nureddin Hospital, which he visited upon his recovery, and marveling at what he saw, the emir swore to build a hospital if God made him sultan. After seven years, in the summer of 1283, he was in a position to keep his vow. The house and grounds of the high-born Cotbia appealed to him, and as the Arabian historian relates: "When the Sultan chose the Cotbian House for his hospital, he called the Eunuch Hasam to carry on the negotiations for its purchase, knowing that through his wisdom the matter could soon be settled, and that Cotbia would not hesitate to give her consent." These are the words of al-Macrizi, who wrote the best account of Moslem hospitals, but neglected to add what would happen if Cotbia had been unwilling. She received a sum of money and the Emerald Castle in exchange, and likewise consented to move without delay, for she overlooked some things—8000 female slaves, and costly treasures including a remarkable ruby, while from her courtyard they dug up a sealed pitcher filled with gold, and a casket containing a pearl that astonished all. The Arabian historian is too tactful to suggest that she was kicked out, but he admits, "The value of what she left behind her was quite as much as the cost of the hospital." There are so many Mansurs—the name means the Victorious—in Arabian annals that only oriental scholars can differentiate them, but this one is memorable for showing hospital executives how to erect a great hospital without expense.

Mansur Gilafan was as arbitrary with the builders as he had been with Cotbia. He brought three hundred prisoners to the spot, and took all the workers from Cohere and Misi, with the result that these two cities were at a standstill; whoever passed and looked at the projected hospital, was forced to help; proud soldiers and high officials were dismounted and compelled to pick up a stone and carry it to its destination; the sultan himself rode every day to the rapidly-rising walls, and his people saw him polishing stones. In less than a year the Mansurian Hospital was ready, supplemented by an academy, library and mosque.

For Mansur did not forget the spiritual needs of his subjects. Fifty alternating lecturers read the Koran day and night; a professor and two adjuncts taught the tradition of the Prophet to students; the muezzins, from the most beautiful tower in all Egypt, called the faithful to prayer. Yet the orthodox did not come. They remembered the expulsion of Cotbia and the enforced carrying of stones; they whispered the hospital was founded on injustice, and preferred to worship Allah elsewhere.

The sick could not afford to be so scrupulous. They heard of the comfortable beds and their coverings, of the kitchens where food and syrups were prepared, and balms and eye-salves provided. Neither the number of patients nor their length of stay was limited; male and female attendants ministered to their wants; there were drugs and physicians for all possible diseases, and separate wards for cases of fever, ophthalmic patients, for the wounded, and those suffering from dysentery. The section for convalescents was divided for men and for women; a long tent permitted them to walk in the shade. Water flowed from the springs into the courtyard, and each hall had its fountain. Even an out-patient department was not lacking, and invalids confined at home were supplied with every necessity. Managers and overseers kept written records, and so well endowed was this Mansurian Hospital that the poorest were readily admitted, and on their departure received funds which made it unnecessary for them to seek work until they were restored to health and strength.

Medicine has reached a high stage of development when the doctors know the time to throw away their drugs. The Arabians are fond of telling this tale: A young woman suffered from paralysis of the arms, and her physician asked her to stand in the presence of the assembled court; without warning, he removed her veil, causing her to blush deeply, and he added to the indignity by suddenly raising her clothes over her head; the young lady instinctively lifted her arms to pull down her garments, and was cured.

An emir was rheumatic, and could not walk; his physicians were unable to help him, and Rhazes was summoned. Rhazes refused to cross the swollen Oxus in the frail boat provided for him, so the royal messengers carried him across as prisoner. Even Rhazes' treatment was unsuccessful, and eventually he said, "Tomorrow I shall try a new treatment, but it will cost you the best horse and mule in your stable"; too ill to argue, the joint-stiffened emir assented. Outside the city was a bath where Rhazes took his royal patient, they entered the hot room, and Rhazes carefully administered douches of hot water. Then he excused himself, and the emir was left sitting alone. When Rhazes returned he was fully dressed, and he menaced his naked patient with a knife, crying, "Thou didst order me to be bound and cast into the boat, and didst conspire against my life. If I do not destroy thee for this, my name is not Mohammed ibn Zakariyya." The effect of these insults and threats may be imagined, and consumed with fear and rage the crippled emir sprang to his feet.

He called his guards in vain, for the physician and his servant had escaped on the horse and mule that he had unwittingly provided. On the seventh day, the servant returned with the animals and this letter from Rhazes: "May the life of the King be prolonged in health and authority! Agreeably to my undertaking I treated you to the best of my ability. There was however a deficiency in the natural caloric, and this treatment would have been unduly protracted, so I abandoned it in favor of *psychotherapeusis,* and when the peccant humors had undergone sufficient coction in the bath, I deliberately provoked you in order to increase the natural caloric, which thus gained sufficient strength to dissolve the already softened humors. But henceforth it is inexpedient that we should meet." The grateful emir, rid of his rheumatism through psychotherapy, begged Rhazes to return for his fee, and despite his refusal, "rewarded him with a robe of honor, a cloak, a turban, arms, a male and female slave, and a horse fully caparisoned, and further assigned to him a yearly pension of 2000 gold *dinars* and 200 ass-loads of corn."

A member of the House of Buwayh suffered from the fixed idea that he was a cow. Nothing could dispel this delusion, and the melancholy prince refused to eat, crying each day, "Kill me, so that a good stew may be prepared from my flesh." The physicians were so helpless, and the situation grew so critical, that Avicenna, already overwhelmed with work as prime minister, was compelled to take charge of the case. He directed an assistant to shout that the butcher was on his way, and then Avicenna came with a cleaver, asking, "Where is this cow, that I may kill it?" Satisfied at last, the sick prince began to moo, and the physician ordered him thrown to the ground and bound with ropes; Avicenna felt him all over in the manner of a butcher, and announced, "This cow is too lean, and not ready for the slaughter; it must be fattened." The patient therefore ate readily, and with the return of strength, his mind was entirely cured.

The foregoing anecdotes are from the *Four Discourses* of the Persian Nizami, the court-poet of Samarcand; and Nizami of Ganja, the poet from the hills of Kum, in his *Treasury of Mysteries,* describes a frightened physician who was commanded to smell a rose upon which an incantation had been breathed, and died from fear of the rose; these tales may not be literally true, but they are remarkable for twelfth-century recognition of suggestion and psychotherapy.

The more familiar the Occidental student becomes with the Arabian physicians of medievalism, the more is he impressed with their mental resources; and for this reason, the more is he inclined to ask: Why did the Medicine which produced the chemical discoveries of Geber, the hospital administration of Sinan ibn Thabit at Bagdad, the educational activities of Hasdai ibn Shaprut at Cordova, the observations of Rhazes on smallpox and measles, the textbook of Haly Abbas, the system of Avicenna, the dietetics of Isaac Israeli, the surgery of Albucasis, the ophthalmology of Ali ibn Isa, the speculations on contagion of Ibn el-Chatib, the clinical acumen of Avenzoar, the immunologic suggestion of Averroes, the botanical investigations of el-Beithar, the medico-historical researches of Useibia, and scholars extending over five centuries from Yuhanna and Hunain to Maimonides and Bar Hebraeus—why should this Medicine, having reached a certain fruition, become sterile and leave no seed for posterity?

The answer seems difficult, yet a minor incident throws much light on the problem. Abdallatif of Bagdad, traveling physician and naturalist of the twelfth century, after living at Mosul and Damascus, visited Cairo for the purpose of conversing with Maimonides, the "Eagle of the Doctors." During his sojourn in Egypt, where he remained long enough to become the graphic annalist of a famine and plague he witnessed, Abdallatif took part in a discussion on the advantages of personal inspection over reading. A chance remark about a mound of unburied bodies induced him to visit the spot, and Abdallatif stood on a hill in the midst of twenty thousand skeletons. He picked up a mandible, and could not believe his eyes: the infallible Galen had written it was composed of several pieces, but Abdallatif could see only one. He looked at two hundred of these lower jaws, he sent them to other physicians for examination, and all agreed it consisted of one bone. His experience was similar with the sacrum: Galen said it was multiple, but Abdallatif found it was usually single. Holding these bones in his hand, Abdallatif was the first who saw that Galen could be wrong, and his simple observations are the sole Arabian contributions to anatomy.

Unburdened by tradition, fresh from nature observation, ancient Greece erected the structure of scientific medicine. Much of that structure stands today, but with the passing of time a new foundation was needed—the foundation of Anatomy and Physiology. Medievalism could not build this foundation, because the materials were lacking. The alleged differences between the three great Semitic religions stained continents with blood and strewed the earth with corpses, but all shrank with equal horror from the anatomist's knife. All united in the belief that whoever touches a cadaver is guilty of sin, and Medicine remained without a true basis for centuries. Hence Arabian medicine could not endure, and under accumulating knowledge it collapsed completely. Had the Koran not prohibited dissection, the gifted Arabians would not have been mere copyists of the Greeks. Had Rhazes, the most original member of the Arabian school, been permitted to explore the secrets of the human body, he would not have said: "If Galen and Aristotle are of one mind on a subject, then of course their opinion is the right one. When they differ, however, it is extremely difficult to know the truth." This is the tragedy of Arabian medicine.

VII

EUROPEAN MEDICINE IN THE MIDDLE AGES

WITH the passing of Galen at the end of the second century, the thread of rational medicine snaps; in the coming centuries an Oribasius and a Paulus Aegineta gather up the broken strands, but no new patterns are woven, for the science of antiquity has run its course. Medicine now spins at a ghostly loom, producing charms and amulets, and the distaff of the age is the Abracadabra. The book of *De medicina praecepta* which wound out to fifteen hundred hexameters, entangled the profession and public alike; whether written by Serenus Sammonicus who was murdered at a banquet by Caracalla, or by his son who bore the same name, is undetermined, but the superstition inculcated —adoration of odd numbers, and dirt and dung from wagon-ruts to cure colic—brings us to the Dark Ages. Classics which should have been immortal have perished, while the rubbish of Serenus Sammonicus has survived, for its formulas were repeated in countless incantations, and the sick wore the magic word—

```
ABRACADABRA    abracadabra
 ABRACADABR     abracadabr
  ABRACADAB      abracadab
   ABRACADA       abracada
    ABRACAD        abracad
     ABRACA         abraca     ABRACADABRA
      ABRAC          abrac      BRACADABR
       ABRA           abra       RACADAB
        ABR            abr        ACADA
         AB             ab         CAD
          A              a          A
```

Serenus Sammonicus explained that the entire word must be written out on the first line, and a letter dropped with each succeeding line, thus forcing the demon of the disease gradually to release its grip upon its victim:

> Thou shalt on paper write the spell divine,
> *Abracadabra* called, in many a line;
> Each under each in even order place,
> But the last letter in each line efface.
> As by degrees the elements grow few
> Still take away, but fix the residue,
> Till at the last one letter stands alone
> And the whole dwindles to a tapering cone.
> Tie this about the neck with flaxen string;
> Mighty the good 'twill to the patient bring.
> Its wondrous potency shall guard his head,
> And drive disease and death far from his bed.

Sextus Placitus treats fever by cutting a splinter from a door through which a eunuch has passed, and Marcellus Empiricus removes an abscess of the right eye by touching it with three fingers of the left hand, expectorating, and repeating thrice: "The mule brings into the world no young, nor does the stone produce wool; so may this disease come to no head, or if it comes to a head, may it wither away." Another ophthalmological prescription from his *De medicamentis empiricis* is characteristic of his book: "A very long-legged white spider rubbed up with oil removes white spots from the eye if assiduously used; therefore mind and rub up a good many with sufficient oil lest the medicine be exhausted before the cure is complete."

An envious Druid gives Saint Patrick a cup of poisoned ale; the snake-banisher makes the sign of the cross, and recites the incantation: "Tuba fis fri ibu, fis ibu anfis; Fis bru uatha, ibu lithu," and adds the name of the Savior. At these words, the poison freezes and falls to the ground as he inverts the cup. The good ale remains, and the saint now quaffs it without harm.

The *Leech Book of Bald* contains a musical charm against fever:

A man shall write this upon the sacramental paten, and wash it off into the drink with holy water—

+ + + Λ + + + + + C D + + + + + + + + +

and sing over it, *In principio erat verbum,* &c. (John i, 1). Then wash the writing with holy water off the dish into the drink, then sing the Credo, and the Pater Noster, and this lay:—*Beati Immaculati,* the psalm (Ps. cxix) with the twelve prayer psalms.

From this Anglo-Saxon *Leech Book of Bald* we learn that a medicine is more effective if drunk out of church bells:

A drink for a fiend-sick man, when a devil possesses the man, or affects him from within with disease, to be drunk out of a church bell:

Take githrife, yarrow, betony, and also other worts; work up the drink with clear ale, sing seven masses over the worts, add garlic and holy water, and drip the drink into every drink that he shall hereafter drink; and then let him drink it out of a church bell, and let the mass priest sing this over him after he has drunk it: *Domine sancte pater omnipotens,* &c.

A strange mysticism has come over men, and even their senses cannot be trusted. Saint Augustine, most influential of theologians, writes in his famous *De civitate Dei:* "When I was Bishop of Hippo, I came with some Christian slaves to teach them Christ's Evangelium. There we saw many men and women who had no heads, and whose eyes were fastened in the breast, but otherwise their limbs were like ours." These words have a familiar ring, nor do we have to search far for their source. They occur in Pliny by way of Ctesias, and evidently Augustine read the old pagan author and imagines that what he had read he has actually seen. Pliny, with his inexhaustible credulity, becomes the favorite naturalist of the middle ages, and tales which Aulus Gellius disdained—"I was seized with disgust for such worthless writings, which contribute nothing to the enrichment or profit of life"—are precisely suited to an age which believes all things without evidence.

Wherever we turn, the era of magic is upon us. Greek medicine, which in its classic days had been free from superstition, has ceased to function. Experiments are not performed, but miracles are expected. Nature is overwhelmed by supernaturalism, and a fact is not believed unless it is supported by a fable. The shadows deepen, and it is sacrilege to know more mathematics than is necessary to compute the date of Easter. Hippocrates and Aristotle and Galen are in exile, and their legacy is claimed by the Arabians. Europe is satisfied with the biological knowledge of the *Physiologus* or *Bestiaries,* where it reads the wonder-tales of pelicans that revive their dead by sprinkling them with blood, of crocodiles that weep because they have eaten a man, of salamanders that quench flames and phoenixes that arise from ashes, of ichneumons that cover themselves with mud to kill dragons, and of unicorns that can be caught only by virgins.

The minds of men have grown childish; they cannot reach the adult conceptions of old; if they ask questions at all, they are foolish ones, mainly about astrology, for the *zodiac man* is everywhere in the ascendant. Aristarchus of Samos, of the third century B.C., was the first to realize the immensity of the universe and to teach that the earth moves round the sun. Eratosthenes of Cyrene—both Aristarchus and Eratosthenes were astronomers of the Alexandrian school—had measured the earth in a manner that we consider modern, but medieval astronomy is molded according to the views of Joshua. Archimedes' treatise *On Method* is erased to make room for a prayerbook; lost in a library at Constantinople, this palimpsest sleeps in dust until our own day; to the joy of scholars, the original writing is decipherable and Archimedes is rescued, but many scientific classics of antiquity, despoiled in medievalism, can never be recovered.

It is a tragic day for Europe when it exchanges the myths of the Greeks for the myths of the Jews. Jupiter smiles in Homer and laughs aloud in Hesiod, but Jehovah of the Jews is a chronic dyspeptic, belching fire and brimstone, threatening and cursing, hating and slaughtering the human race. Intolerance is his keynote, and destruction is the passion of the Lord of eternal vengeance. The gloom of the Scriptures descends upon medievalism; this world is dross, and only the world to come is of value; the body is not worth knowing and saving—it is vile clay imprisoning the immortal soul. The Greek had gloried in his nude and beautiful flesh; the hammer of the monk smashes many an ancient statue in protest. A weariness of life overtakes medieval Pagan and Christian. Porphyry tells us that his master Plotinus, the coryphaeus of Neoplatonism, is ashamed his "soul is in body." The violent Saint Jerome asks: "Does your skin roughen without baths? Who is once washed in the blood of Christ needs not wash again."

The pleasures of the flesh are the lures of the devil; the body must be scorned in the upward climb to salvation. Life is a transient journey in a world of sin, but Death releases the soul at the crossroads of Heaven and Hell. All earthly learning is vain; Tertullian says, "Investigation is unnecessary since the Gospel." Behold, the day of the Lord cometh with wrath; his terrible lips are ready to blow the trumpet for the Last Judgment—and what then shall avail the science of the Greeks? Thus is closed, throughout the Dark Ages, the road of inquiry leading to knowledge of the human body.

We hear the voice of Gregory of Tours pronouncing it blasphemy for the sick to consult earthly physicians instead of the shrine of St. Martin. Since disease is an expression of God's wrath, is not an appeal to the saints more effective than the drugs of the apothecary? Believers are exhorted to heed the Epistle of James: "Is any sick among you? let him call for the elders of the church; and let them pray over him, anointing him with oil in the name of the Lord: And the prayer of faith shall save the sick, and the Lord shall raise him up."

Many tales are related of the demons exorcised by holy men and women; the annals and chronicles of the times speak of expelled devils which can be seen, sometimes in droves, leaving the bodies of their victims. Against these visitations of Satan, mundane remedies cannot suffice, but the evil spirits are vanquished by invoking the saints. The sufferer from toothache appeals to St. Appolonia; with consecrated water, Hugo the Holy draws a serpent from a woman's body; a friar choking over a fishbone is saved by St. Agnes; a man, mute from birth, attends vespers at the shrine of St. Anthony, and speaks; a journey to the altar of St. Gall is the true remedy for gout; a blind person, groping for the blood-stains on the chapel of St. Magnus, is blessed with vision; a hunchback kneels at the tomb of St. Andreas, and arises straight; a child suffocated by the Devil is restored by St. Melanus; a hundred slain infants awake at the intercession of St. Coleta, and whoever drinks from her cup recovers from catalepsy; an idiot regains his reason by touching the relics of St. Anastasius; a dying king is restored to vigor by a fragment of the true cross.

Long after the Arabians scan the West for Greek manuscripts, the monasteries search the East for sacred relics. The abbey of Saint Gall is fortunate enough to receive a box containing souvenirs of Abraham, Isaac and Jacob—and sickness disappears from the neighborhood. A Cistercian monk secures part of the body of Saint George and the bones of John the Baptist; substantial pieces of the true cross are distributed throughout Germany, and yet the cross itself remains intact; Venice too possesses the genuine cross, and the head of John the Baptist.

Constantinople falls in the Fourth Crusade, and the rage of Christian against Christian is almost unparalleled in the annals of the human race: the library is burned, and homes and palaces wantonly reduced to ashes; horses and mules stumble beneath the weight of stolen plunder; a prostitute dances in the seat of the patriarch; soldiers of the cross get drunk from the chalices of the church; pilgrims gamble on church-tables bearing the picture of Christ; in the deluge of the blood of their fellow-believers, in the midst of violation of mother and matron, of virgin and nun, they gather booty greater than that of many kingdoms: the stone on which the head of Jacob rested, the magic staff which Moses transformed into a serpent, the complete skeletons of Saint Luke and the Prophet Simeon, the garments of the Holy Virgin and droplets of her milk, the cradle in which Jesus slept, one of his teeth, a hair of his beard, a crumb of bread from the Last Supper, and a small bottle of the Savior's blood. Wherever these talismans are deposited in Western Europe, a healing-shrine springs up, and the sick and the lame seek it in pilgrimage, with hope in their hearts.

After Galen's time, the Greek tongue begins to disappear from the Western Empire, and in the fourth century Rome is again a Latin City. Europe's inability to read the Greek language means the loss of continuity of Greek learning; only in the "heel and toe and shin of Italy" a corrupt Greek lingers, yet even this drying seed is later to bear important fruit. The Ostrogothic statesman-historian of Syrian descent, Cassiodorus (*c.* 490-585), retires from the world's turmoil to establish upon his estates on the Calabrian gulf a monastic academy and library, where he teaches his monks to preserve, copy and translate Greek manuscripts into Latin, thus inaugurating the period of Monastic Medicine. The idea spreads to other monasteries, and monks copying manuscripts form one of the familiar pictures of medievalism; it is more a matter of calligraphy than of scholarship, and often a monk spends a lifetime in illuminating a single manuscript. They are as undiscriminating as a catalogue, and among the manuscripts found in a monastic library is a version of Soranus on childbirth.

Throughout ages of disorder, the monastery is often inn and hospital, school-room and shelter. Physic-gardens are sometimes attached to the monasteries, and we see the squinting monk, Walafrid Strabo, celebrating in hexameters the medicinal virtues of the twenty-three herbs that grow in his monastery-garden. The verse is gentle and the picture pleasing, but nothing moves. Greek medicine is immured in the monasteries, awaiting its resurrection. The periods which produce a Rhazes and an Avicenna in the East, bring forth only drug-lists and antidotaria in the West.

It is confusing that the many centuries which intervene between Galen and the Renaissance should be spoken of collectively as the Middle Ages, for an event of great importance divides the earlier middle ages from the latter. Paradoxically enough, when Moslem culture is already on the point of decline, it is discovered by Europe. The stream of learning from the West which had fructified the East, now turns and flows from East to West. Greek science which for centuries had sojourned in the lands of Islam, returns to Europe in Graeco-Arabic guise. This is the daybreak of the Dark Ages, and the man who accomplished the epochal task of linking East and West is Constantinus Africanus. By his work, Latinity is able, through the far-winding Arabic roads, to find the highway to Hellenism.

The life of Constantinus, in spite of Peter the Deacon, remains legendary, or at least uncertain. According to Peter the Deacon, he was born at Carthage and studied at Babylon, but attention has been called to the fact that neither Carthage nor Babylon existed in the eleventh century. It has been said he was the most important professor at the School of Salerno which owes to him its greatest literary activity, and it has also been said he never taught at Salerno. He has been decried as an ignorant and dishonest worker, because his Latin was barbarous and he palmed off his translations from the Arabic, especially the writings of Haly Abbas and Isaac Israeli, as his original work, and others hail him as Magister orientis et occidentis, and maintain his acknowledgments to the Arabian authors were complete and generous; some say that Constantinus, during his career as monk of Monte Cassino, hid all traces of the origin of his books in order that he alone might receive the glory, and others say he was obliged to suppress the Arabian sources in order to facilitate their acceptance by Christian Europe. Strange to say, it so happens that not one of these points is important, and even if it should be proven that Constantinus was guilty of all the accusations which Stephen of Pisa levelled at him, he still remains a pivotal figure in the history of medicine. For this much is undeniable: Constantinus Africanus, after long years in the Orient, imported Arabic manuscripts to Italy, and when he translated them into Latin, the intellectual ferment that resulted was the first step in the lifting of the Dark Ages.

Europe suddenly realized that the wisdom of the past must

be read from right to left. Whoever understood the tongue of Islam was at a premium. The Arabic-speaking Jews of Spain were fêted and caressed. If the evidence were not extant, it would be difficult to believe that for two centuries the chief occupation of Christian scholars was the translation of Greek-inspired Arabic works into Latin. Their mutual enthusiasm for Greek manuscripts once joined Nestorians and Arabians in the East, and the same cause now united Christian, Jew and Spanish Moslem in the West.

John the Saracen, disciple of Constantinus, completed his master's translation of Haly Abbas; Stephen of Antioch also translated Haly Abbas; the western nations learned mathematics and astronomy from the Latinized versions of Arabic editions of Euclid and Ptolemy; Aristotle had been expatriated so long that he was almost as Oriental as Avicenna: in Latin garb both reigned as the intellectual monarchs of medieval Europe; Galen too returned, looking swarthy and wearing a turban—in fact, seven of his anatomical books, forever lost in the original Greek, survived only in Arabic. Hermann the German employed and encouraged Saracen translators.

In the early thirteenth century, the Guide of Maimonides was Latinized, and later, Blasius at Barcelona translated Maimonides' treatise on Poisons for Pope Clement V. The scholarly Jewish physician of Italy, Faraj ben Salim, had sufficient courage to transform Rhazes' Continens into Latin! Faraj worked under the patronage of Charles of Anjou, who esteemed his work so highly that he ordered the chief illuminator of the time, Friar Giovanni of Monte Cassino, to draw portraits of himself and Faraj on the manuscript. Thus, in the middle ages, a king felt it added to his glory to be pictured with a translator, and there is an even more interesting thirteenth-century manuscript showing Jewish translators receiving an Arabic medical book from an Eastern ruler, and returning it in Latin to a Western king.

The list of the twelfth and thirteenth century translators is long and impressive, but special mention is due to Raymond, archbishop of Toledo, who established in this city a school of translators in association with the archdeacon Domingo Gundisalvo and the Hebrew John Avendeut. Here, to the Moslem schools of Spain, came Gerard of Cremona, in search of Ptolemy whom he could not find in Christian Europe. What Hunain was to the East in the ninth century, Gerard became to the West in the twelfth. He translated Ptolemy from the Arabic —a version which overshadowed the anonymous Sicilian translation from the Greek; he translated Menelaus of Alexandria, whose works had perished in Greek and existed only in Arabic and Hebrew; Messahala, whose mathematical knowledge aided the building of Bagdad, was now given to the Latin world by Gerard of Cremona; he translated al-Kindi, the myriad-minded philosopher and scientist of the Arabs; al-Khwarizmi, whose name looms so large in the annals of mathematics; numerous other mathematicians and astronomers, including al-Farghani, Ahmad ibn Yusuf, al-Nairizi, and al-Zarqali; the treatise on twilight by the great Alhazen who boasted he could control the Nile, and whose epoch-making Optics contains the first scientific investigation of the *camera obscura*. Gerard's medical translations from the Arabic include the writings of Serapion the Elder, the surgery of Albucasis, the Canon of Avicenna, and Ali ibn Ridwan's commentary on the Ars parva of Galen. It is not strange that Gerard of Cremona has long been considered the greatest of translators.

The introduction of Arabic science to England in the twelfth century is an interesting cultural chapter. Adelard of Bath, who played the cithara before an unknown queen, traveled in many lands and brought Arabic learning to England. Walcher, prior of Malvern, studied the skies through an Arabian astrolabe. Robert of Ketene spoke with the tongue of the East, and translated the Algebra of al-Khwarizmi. Various Jews from Spain, converted ones like Petrus Alphonsi, and unconverted ones like Abraham ibn Ezra, visited England, and their presence meant an increased interest in astronomy and mathematics; the latter once summed up his life of a wandering scholar in the words, "There I resided as a stranger, wrote books, and revealed the secrets of knowledge." Daniel of Morley was another Englishman whose quest of philosophy led him across the Pyrenees, and the Christian scholar carried back to his native land the manuscripts of Moslems. In England, as elsewhere in Europe, the Middle Ages ceased to be static under the Arabian touch.

Early in the next century the mysterious figure of Michael Scot, of somewhere on the Scottish Borders, begins to haunt the scene. Master of the Black Arts, he called spirits by their proper names, and they answered; he knew how to confine a demon in a bottle; from a sneeze he could foretell the future; a hair of the head or a drop of menstrual fluid revealed much to him; and in a footprint of the dust he read grave portents. If we wonder what connection can exist between this necromancer and the transmission of scientific knowledge, we must remember we are in the thirteenth century, and that Michael Scot, familiar with Hebrew and Arabic—the angels neglected to teach him Greek—was the first to give Aristotle's biology, including the Aristotelian commentaries of Avicenna and Averroes, to medieval Europe.

His severest critic, Roger Bacon, who claimed Michael Scot was ignorant of sciences and linguistics, and that most of the work was done by Andrew the Jew, admits the Wizard of the North raised the banner of Aristotle in the Latin world. It may appear strange that this credulous sorcerer, with his head buried in shadows, imagined himself an opponent of magic, but inconsistency reaches its limit when we find him in the South, the central figure in the most sceptical court of Europe. Frederick II, essentially a freethinking rationalist of modern mold, the clearest, keenest mind of the Middle Ages, retained Michael Scot as his astrologer and scientific adviser.

Among the medieval Roman emperors, not even a Charlemagne approaches Frederick in versatility and intellect. Both of his grandfathers, Roger II and Barbarossa, were among the most remarkable men of their time, and were surpassed only by their unequaled grandson. Frederick's career upset and remade history. He led the Sixth Crusade and placed the iron crown of Jerusalem on his head—a deed which medievalism was never to witness again. Europe trembled at the spectacle of an unbelieving and excommunicated Crusader winning the Holy Land as the enemy of the Pope and ally of the Moslem—Europe could much easier understand Saint Louis of France, who said the best argument with a Mohammedan was to see how far your sword could sink into his bowels. In an age when the interdict put even an emperor outside the human pale, it was inevitable that Frederick should eventually be defeated by the Vatican, but the Vatican never recovered from the blows inflicted by Frederick.

This monarch spoke six languages at a time when kings did not speak any. His curiosity opened his Sicilian court to Jewish scholars: he knew about Maimonides, and encouraged Jacob Anatoli and Jehuda ben Solomon Cohen; he ordered lectures in Hebrew to be delivered at the university of Naples, which he founded in opposition to papal Bologna; Jewish translations of Averroes were dedicated to his attendant, Michael Scot, and hopes were entertained that the Messiah might come in his reign. His international interests proved him a true descendant of the Roger who embellished his Norman-Byzantine church at Palermo with Arabic arches and scripts; in the chronicle of the English monk, Matthew Paris, we read that Frederick would rather be surrounded by Moslems than by Christians—which however did not prevent him, on occasion, from persecuting heretics.

To his contemporaries he was always the World's Wonder (*stupor mundi*), whether they contemplated his battles or legislation, his extensive learning or oriental luxuriance, his scholars or eunuchs, the magnificence of his menagerie or the variety of his harem. Pietro da Eboli dedicated to him his poem on the healing springs of Pozzuoli, and for him Adam of Cremona wrote on military hygiene; in his court Pier della Vigna wrote the first Italian sonnet, and Leonard of Pisa popularized Arabic arithmetic; Frederick arrived at Ravenna with many animals never before seen in Italy, and gave Europe its first sight of a giraffe. In the thirteenth century, only Frederick had the audacity to transport camels across the Alps, and take a bath on Sunday, and address a scientific questionnaire to Mohammedan scholars in Persia, Asia Minor, Syria, Yemen, Egypt and Morocco, asking them, amid a whole course of penetrating questions, "Why do objects partly covered by water appear bent?" and "What is the cause of the illusion of spots before the eyes?" and "Why does Canopus appear bigger when near the horizon, whereas the absence of moisture in the southern deserts precludes moisture as an explanation?"

It is doubtful if any of the professional savants whom Frederick attracted or enticed to his court, rivaled him as an observer or investigator. The stories told of him—that he sent the diver Nicholas, known as The Fish, to explore the waters of Scylla and Charybdis; isolated newborn infants from the sound of the human voice to determine whether the first words they uttered would be in Hebrew or a more modern tongue; cut open the abdomen of men to note the effect of rest and exertion on digestion—are evidence of his ruthless, restless, experimenting mind. His book on falconry (*De arte venandi cum avibus*) is largely independent of current scholasticism: gathering first-hand information, based on international research, making comparative records of all things that fly, studying feathers and molting, observing the nests and habits of cuckoos, testing whether the eggs of ostriches can be hatched by the sun's heat, sealing the eyes of vultures to learn if they obtain food by sight or smell, disproving the legend of barnacle geese hatched from barnacles, Frederick accepts no statement without investigation. He refers several times to Aristotle, but rather in the spirit of a teacher pointing out the errors of a pupil who lacks experience in the subject. This amazing Hohenstaufen undertook to compose a treatise on a cruel sport, and concluded as the author of an important contribution to zoölogy.

It would have been better for Roger Bacon, if instead of finding fault with the translations of Michael Scot, he had followed his countryman to Frederick's court. The generally accepted statements are that Roger Bacon was born about 1214 near Ilchester in Somerset, studied in Oxford, became a Franciscan friar in Paris, returned to Oxford as teacher, was sent to France for ten years of silence and discipline, was forbidden by his superiors to write anything, received a papal decree to the contrary, was in a quandary how to obtain the necessary parchment, finally completed three large treatises (*Opus majus, opus minus, opus tertium*) for the friendly pope, returned to Oxford, devoted himself to experimental science and attacking the corruption of the church of which he remained an orthodox member, was condemned by an antagonistic pope, was imprisoned for fourteen years on account of certain suspicious novelties (*propter novitates suspectas*), was released shortly before his death, after which his books were nailed on a door, exposed to wind and weather. Some of these data are now being seriously questioned.

The old legend that Roger Bacon constructed a Brazen Head and asked the Devil to make it speak—naturally the Devil obliged him and the Head uttered oracles—has been replaced by the newer legend that Roger Bacon was an unadulterated scientist with a modern outlook on nature. Neglected in the centuries following his death—there are no Baconian incunabula—he is overrated today, being regarded as a phenomenon, an independent thinker of the thirteenth century, free from Greek and Arabic influences. Yet in the best of his medical essays, a brief tract on the faults of physicians (*Erroribus medicorum*), occupying less than twenty pages in print, he quotes Hippocrates, Euclid and Pliny, refers twice to Ptolemy, six times to Galen, appeals twenty-five times to the authority of Aristotle, and among the Arabians quotes Serapion, Isaac Israeli, Alhazen, al-Kindi, Rhazes thrice, Haly Abbas six times, Avicenna seventeen times, and among the later workers quotes Constantinus, Michael Scot and Platearius. Evidently he was more erudite than independent. In this tract he regards Aristotle as an astrologer, relies on the pseudo-Aristotelian *Secretum Secretorum*, and complains "A fourth defect is that physicians do not study the heavenly bodies upon which all alteration of bodies in the lower world depends, while purgations, venesections and other evacuations and constrictions, and the whole of medical practice are based on the study of atmospheric changes due to the influence of the spheres and stars. Wherefore a physician who knows not how to take into account the positions and aspects of the planets can effect nothing in the healing arts except by chance and good fortune." On several other occasions he declares that a knowledge of the astrological aspects of critical days is the essence of medicine.

He condemned magic and wrote on the "nullity of magic," without once realizing that he believed as firmly in magic as any of his contemporaries. His work on the preservation of youth and the cure of old age—a subject which interested him greatly —is of the same caliber as most rejuvenistic literature. He tells us of "a case attested by the evidence of a papal letter, that Almanicus, when a captive among the Saracens, took a medicine through the effect of which he prolonged his life five hundred years," and that "Artephius, who wisely studied the forces of animals and stones for the purpose of learning the secrets of nature, especially the secret of the length of life, gloried in living for one thousand and twenty-five years." After such case-reports, we are not surprised that Bacon believes a circle drawn around venomous animals prevents them from moving, and that Ethiopian sages ride dragons through the air at top speed and consume their flesh, "for no education which man can give will bestow such wisdom as does the eating of the flesh of dragons."

Out of this circle of superstition there emerges another Bacon, the Bacon who was a pioneer of comparative philology, the Bacon who followed the mathematical method, the Bacon who stood forth as an apostle of experiment (*scientia experimentalis*), the Bacon who visualized the Machine Age. Roger Bacon's popular fame today is largely based on a passage in his *De secretis operibus:*

Machines for navigation can be made without rowers so that the largest ships on rivers or seas will be moved by a single man in charge with greater velocity than if they were full of men. Also cars can be made so that without animals they will move with unbelievable rapidity; such we opine were the scythe-bearing chariots with which the men of old fought. Also flying machines can be constructed so that a man sits in the midst of the machine revolving some engine by which artificial wings are made to beat the air like a flying bird. Also a machine small in size for raising or lowering enormous weights, than which nothing is more useful in emergencies. For by a machine three fingers high and wide and of less size a man could free himself and his friends from all danger of prison and rise and descend. Also a machine can easily be made by which one man can draw a thousand to himself by violence against their wills, and attract other things in like manner. Also machines can be made for walking in the sea and rivers, even to the bottom without danger. For Alexander the Great employed such, that he might see the secrets of the deep, as Ethicus the astronomer tells. These machines were made in antiquity and they have certainly been made in our times, except possibly a flying machine which I have not seen nor do I know any one who has, but I know an expert who has thought out the way to make one. And such things can be made almost without limit, for instance, bridges across rivers without piers or other supports, and mechanisms, and unheard of engines.

An even more prophetic passage—though marred by the lynx's eye, against which Alexander Neckam had already expressed doubts—occurs in *De multiplicatione specierum;* his generation must have thought the *Doctor mirabilis* was indulging in more magic when Roger Bacon thus anticipated radiology:

No substance is so dense as altogether to prevent rays from passing. Matter is common to all things, and thus there is no substance on which the action involved in the passage of a ray may not produce a change. Thus it is that rays of heat and sound penetrate through the walls of a vessel of gold or brass. It is said by Boethius that a lynx's eye will pierce through thick walls. In this case the wall would be permeable to visual rays. In any case there are many dense bodies which altogether interfere with the visual and other senses of man, so that rays cannot pass with such energy as to produce an effect on human sense, and yet nevertheless rays do really pass, though without our being aware of it.

The *Compendium Medicinae* of Gilbertus Anglicus—his name indicates his European reputation—is the first complete treatise on general medicine by an Englishman. Since Gilbertus was one of the foremost physicians of his time, no other evidence is needed to illustrate the degraded status of medicine in the thirteenth century. For the Compendium is a collection of disgraceful superstitions, an epitome of scholasticism, polypharmacy, amuletic and astrologic medicine. Nor can the Compendium be dismissed as the opinion of an individual practitioner, for it is plainly an "abstract and brief chronicle of the time." Here is his method of treating sexual impotence:

Let a man, twenty years of age or more, before the third hour of the vigil of St. John the Baptist, pull up by the roots a specimen of comfrey (*consolida major*) and another of heal all (*consolida minor*), repeating thrice the Lord's prayer. Let him speak to none while going or returning, not even one word, but in deep silence let him extract the juice from the herbs, and with it write on parchment this charm: The Lord said increase x Utiboth x and multiply x thabechay x and replenish the earth x amath x. If a man wears around his neck a card inscribed with these identical words written in this juice, he will beget a male; conversely, if a woman, she will conceive a female.

Gilbertus has such faith in the potency of this charm that he immediately informs the wearer what to do if it produces satyriasis. In other fields he is not more sensible: he mentions asses' hoofs attached to the patient's leg as treatment for gout, the water in which a murderer has rinsed his hands as an aid in childbirth, and a grunting sow tied to the bed as the cure for lethargy—perhaps an effective empiric remedy.

But we cannot leave the Compendium on this note, for we must learn that in the medieval writings strange passages are readily blended with valuable ones. For example, John of Arderne gave the profession this charm for cramps: "Take a sheet of parchment and write on it the first sign Thebal, Suthe, Gnthenay. In the name of the Father and the Son and of the Holy Ghost, Amen. Jesus of Nazareth, Mary, John, Michael, Gabriel, Raphael. The Word was made Flesh—after every word make a cross within a square. The sheet is afterwards closed like a letter so that it cannot be readily opened. And he who carries that charm upon him in good faith and in the name of the Omnipotent God and firmly believes in it will without doubt never be troubled with the cramp." Yet John of Arderne, revelling in amulets, began to think surgically as soon as he held an instrument in his hands—he called himself a surgeon among physicians (*chirurgus inter medicos*). He virtually created the operation for *fistula in ano,* and was probably correct in claiming to be the only man of his time, in England or beyond the Sea, who could terminate this tragedy.

Gilbertus indicates that he himself is not favorably disposed toward some of the remedies he describes, but he hesitates to omit what others have included; in places he intimates he would willingly discard the popular complicated formulae of his time for the simple expectant treatment of Hippocrates, but he does not wish his contemporaries to regard him as peculiar—which reminds us of Daniel of Morley's fear of being "the only Greek among the Romans." Gilbertus Anglicus was not the first to know the contagiousness of smallpox, since Avicenna had already spoken of smallpox and measles as "of all diseases the most contagious," but Gilbertus appears to have been the earliest to mention the use of red colors in its therapy. How John of Gaddesden—the first Englishman employed at Court as a physician—later treated the son of Edward II by this method, is well known: "When the son of the illustrious king of England had the smallpox, I took care that everything about his couch should be red, and his cure was perfectly effected, for he was restored to health without a trace of the disease." The reasons behind this could not be given until recent times. Gilbertus' belief that impure coitus is the cause of leprosy may not have been as far-fetched as it seems, for it is possible that medieval syphilis was hidden under the label of leprosy.

Among those who frequently quoted the Compendium of Gilbertus was the Portuguese physician known as Petrus Hispanus, himself the author of many medical treatises, including the famous Treasury of the Poor (*Thesaurus pauperum*), book on eye-diseases (*Liber de oculis*), and extensive commentaries on the dietetics and urology of Isaac Israeli. Numerous other works —notably a letter to Frederick II on the rules of health—are attributed to him. Ptolemy of Lucca expressed contemporary opinion when he described Petrus Hispanus as "in all things, a scholar; and in medicine, a specialist." If then we read Petrus Hispanus, we know we are following the approved methods of medical practice in the thirteenth century. That Peter could not be easily fooled is evident from his prescription for hysterical women: "I can say from experience that if a large cupping glass (a common jar will do) be applied to the lower part of the patient's abdomen, with free use of the red-hot iron, it will most thoroughly cure this disease. In hysterical fainting blow pepper and salt up the patient's nose. She will soon come round."

He knew that scabies could be cured in a day by sulphur, and many of his medico-philosophical speculations are brilliant. We must not, however, praise him too soon, for like the rest of his contemporaries, he believed in witchcraft and demons, advised epileptics to carry a parchment bearing the names of the three wise men of the East, and declared that "wearing the heart of a vulture makes one popular with all men and very wealthy, and that by vivisecting the bird hoopoe and eating its palpitating heart one may learn the future and all secrets concealed in men's minds." Even in an age when remedies were valued according to their nastiness, Peter managed to distinguish himself as the champion of the therapeutics of dung.

Peter's parallel careers in medicine and theology were so successful that in the same year (1276) he was physician to Pope Gregory X and cardinal-bishop of Frascati. Christendom was then in a state of confusion, for three popes had died within seven months; the Church naturally grew shy of decrepit cardinals, and felt the first requisites of the Supreme Pontiff should be youth and health. Peter was not old, and two other factors were in his favor: his knowledge of hygiene and his prediction that he would live long. Peter of Spain thereupon became Saint Peter's successor as Pope John XXI; despite his prophecy, within seven months the roof of the palace fell upon him, and the Colmar Chronicle thus wrote his obituary: "John the Pope, a magician skilled in all the sciences, an enemy to men of religion, a despiser of the decrees of the General Council, died this year 1277." Peter's gross superstition and keen intelligence, his reputed friendship with both the skeptical Frederick II and the orthodox Gregory X; his own elevation to the papacy, and the charges constantly brought against him that he was a heretic and hostile to God and Church; his fame as a physician at a time when a priest was not supposed to be a physician—all this makes us realize that the Middle Ages are not easy to understand.

Bernard Gordon, who taught at Montpellier, was probably a Frenchman of Scotch descent. He has been hailed as Gordonius the Divine because of his Lily of Medicine (*Lilium Medicinae*), which bred John of Gaddesden's Angelic Rose of Medicine (*Rosa Anglica*)—it is a sidelight on the times that physicians, in entitling their books, competed with ballad-mongers; works dealing largely with the therapeutics of excrements bore the poetic names of Flowers of Medicine or Laurels of Practice. Gordon names the eight diseases which at that time (1305) were considered contagious: acute fever, phthisis, scabies, epilepsy, erysipelas, anthrax, conjunctivitis, leprosy (*febris acuta, ptisis, scabies, pedicon, sacer ignis, anthrax, lippa, lepra, nobis contagia praestant*). To understand these conditions at all, it may be admitted that by acute fever he meant bubonic plague, that scabies may have been confused with syphilis, that in conjunctivitis he probably included trachoma, and that leprosy may have covered syphilis. Even then the list is most confusing, but it is important as an early epidemiologic note.

Gordon's book contains the first reference in medical literature to eye-glasses, which were first made from the stone beryllus, and hence Gordon calls them *oculus berellinus,* but he spoils it by adding that whoever uses his eye-salve—the best that God has revealed—will find spectacles unnecessary. He is thus in the same class with John of Arderne, for when this surgeon realized that not enough people were afflicted with *fistula in ano* to enable him to get rich, he announced that all the world must take an enema at least twice a year, but to be effective the enema must be performed under his instructions with the new syringes he invented for the purpose—and according to the appended scale of fees.

Gordon's views on venereal disease needed clarification, for while he knew that gonorrhea was due to sexual contact, he also thought it could be caused by undue lust or sitting on a cold stone. For retention, he introduces the inevitable bug of Avicenna. He said that strangury did not permit a man to study, nor to sleep nor to digest his meat. His treatment was interesting because it was directed primarily toward the relief of constipation, and considerable attention is paid to diet, though blood-letting is the cardinal remedy.

The middle ages which were successful in quarantining leprosy, failed in their efforts against prostitution. The oldest of problems has been present in every age, and every age has treated it without understanding. Saint Augustine's words have gone unheeded through the centuries: "Suppress prostitution, and capricious lust will overthrow society." Theodora, the crowned whore, thought of a way of reforming other prostitutes; she transferred five hundred from the brothels of Constantinople to a peaceful retreat on the Asiatic shore of the Bosphorus; it was a beautiful home, half prison, half convent, entirely safe from male invasion: many of the inmates threw themselves in the sea, and others died from unbearable boredom. A German emperor decreed that prostitutes be plunged naked in cold streams, and ordered all who observed them to laugh and jeer—but even more barbarous laws did not avail. Saint Louis of

France, badly defeated in his crusades against the Saracens, returned to his kingdom to wage an equally ineffective warfare against the harlots of his realm: he deprived them of their dwellings and tunics, and the troubadours tell us that "disconsolate maidens might be seen everywhere, followed by excellent citizens, victims of their amatory charms."

The unnatural conditions of the middle ages favored the prevalence of prostitution. The armies of the crusaders were followed by armies of women, and in one year the Knights Templars paid for thirteen thousand prostitutes. The number of occupations in which women could engage was extremely limited, and the situation was aggravated by constant wars, especially the vast butchery of the crusades, which left about seven females for every male. The medical profession was not invited to solve the problem, and at best could have done nothing. Such was the reputation of medical students, that any woman living in their quarters or found in their society, was by that fact alone regarded as wanton—it was believed that the mental concentration of scholars made them unable to resist physical fascination.

But no class was exempt: emperor and noble, cleric and tradesman, all knew the Frauenhaus. The old Parliamentary suggestions to brothel-keepers—"No host shall receive a female from ecclesiastical institutions, nor shall he receive a married woman," and "No host shall keep a maiden who has the dangerous burning disease"—are revelatory. Sexual laxity was the rule, and amiability the fashion. Iron drawers, which could not be removed except with the husband's key, were made for women, and were not always worn voluntarily. Prudent men, before departing on a journey, guarded the honor of the home and the virtue of the wife by thus padlocking the genitalia. These girdles of chastity were sometimes manufactured from old armor, but at other times were exquisite samples of the goldsmith's art —velvet-covered hoops fitting snugly around the waist, from which projected a sheet of gold anatomically covering the parts to be protected, with ingenious openings allowing for the performance of the natural functions, the entire apparatus kept in place by a lock responding only to a special key. Of course, stories were current of the lady's locksmith outwitting the husband's goldsmith, and the duplicate key took its place in the social satire of the time.

If Hildebrand had emasculated his clergy instead of merely forbidding them to marry, he would have deprived the middle ages of their choicest scandals. The celibacy of priests became a grim jest, and their housekeepers (*focariae*) were judged at their true worth. People who did not know Latin knew enough to protest against the expulsion of women from the monasteries, since these concubines in some measure protected the wives and daughters of the peasantry from monkish lust. More than one abbess was proprietress of a brothel, the erudite archbishop of Mayence kept as many prostitutes as books, and an English cardinal purchased a *lupanar* as an investment. Repentant females who entered nunneries were often not permitted by the father-confessors to carry out vows of future chastity. The pursuit of licentiousness filtered down from St. Peter's chair to the lowest vagrant monks. The infatuation of monastic lovers diverted to concubines sacred vessels of gold and silver belonging to the church; the anchorite of St. Gall who deserted his cloister for the embrace of a Jewess, is proof that the middle ages were human. The subterranean passages connecting monasteries and nunneries, and the numerous skeletons of infants unearthed in their vicinities, were the inevitable results of an unnatural prohibition.

Diverse estimates of the middle ages are inevitable, for so many contradictory things are true. Attempts at rigid classification are upset by exceptions and inconsistencies, which of course may be said of any period. Did they believe the earth was round or flat? In the patristic writings of Isidore of Seville we find passages indicating a belief in both the sphericity and the flatness of the earth. Were lepers invariably excluded from all human contact? We know that acquaintances and strangers came from afar to enjoy the discourse of the learned leprous Abbot of St. Albans, Richard Wallingford.

What was the ecclesiastical attitude toward the knowledge of the time? Many devout churchmen were enemies of science, and many devout churchmen were friends of science. The differential diagnosis between the occult and the actual did not then exist, and often the same individual was a devotee of both. We must read the books of those days to realize the anomalous situation that an astrologer forecasting the future from the stars, could also be a truth-seeker, a scholar and a discoverer.

The University of Paris was the medical headquarters of the middle ages, and it was precisely the University of Paris which ruined medicine by outlawing surgical operations and bedside examinations. There were times in the middle ages when the Jews were the only practitioners, and there were times when the Jews were forbidden to practise at all. Some regarded Satan as the inventor of the healing art, and some regarded Christ as the supreme physician. Against Saint Bernard and Saint Agatha, who recoiled at the mention of medicine, may be placed Cosmas and Damian, the patron saints of medicine. If an author produced a work of philosophical speculations, there was no way of knowing beforehand whether he would be persecuted as a heretic, or rewarded with a bishopric.

When we come across the statement of Albert Bollstädt that with his own eyes he saw a beautiful emerald crack to pieces because a toad gazed fixedly at it, the explanation being that the emerald was of weak virtue, as otherwise the gem would have burst the toad, we may be puzzled why his contemporaries called this man Albertus Magnus, but when we read his botanical writings his title of *Doctor universalis* becomes clearer.

We learn that medievalism was so lacking in the experimental method that when the question arose of the number of teeth in the horse, no one thought of opening the horse's mouth, but consulted the authorities of antiquity for an answer. Yet a medieval astrologer, Oliver of Malmesbury, was sufficiently experimental to equip his hands and feet with wings and fly with the wind from a tower: after falling and breaking his legs, his experiment taught him he needed a tail. It is true that Petrus

Lombardus asked "Do the bowels move in Paradise?" but it is equally true that Petrus Hispanus wished to know "Can natural death be retarded?" If the thirteenth century was so unobservant as to believe magic could alter the laws of nature, this same century must have made many experiments before it was able to read through spectacles.

The pictures of anemic saints and bleeding martyrs are offset by the gross carousals of lusty men and willing wenches. The opening clause of charters, "In view of the approaching end of the world. . . ." would convince us the middle ages were melancholy, if at the same time we did not hear the joyous strains of troubadour and minnesinger.

Perhaps nothing brings us so close to medievalism as its university life. Their *trivium* and *quadrivium*—grammar, logic, rhetoric; and arithmetic, geometry, music, astronomy—may not correspond to our conception of the seven liberal arts, but the student is an eternal figure. When we read the cunning and piteous money-begging letters addressed by the medieval scholar to *paterfamilias*, we are reminded of the modern student who writes to father for an additional allowance to purchase a caeliac axis. Many tavern-songs of European students of today are echoes of those of the twelfth and thirteenth centuries. The Middle Ages could not have been too ascetic, since they produced the rollicking rhymes of the Goliards, in praise of women, wine and riotous living. A popular song of the medieval *vagantes* ran as follows:

> We in our wandering,
> Blithesome and squandering,
>   Tara, tantara, teino!
>
> Laugh till our sides we split,
> Rags on our hides we fit;
>   Tara, tantara, teino!
>
> Jesting eternally,
> Quaffing infernally:
>   Tara, tantara, teino!

The surviving manuscripts are indisputable testimony that the mental activity of the middle ages was enormous, though often misdirected. An age could not advance far which substituted the syllogism for science, and we feel that many a recondite treatise requires the antidote of the old Greek laughter. Upon the whole, the positive contributions of European medievalism to scientific thought are meager, for the visions of Hildegard of Bingen and the illumination of Raymond Lull, the credulity of Thomas of Cantimpré and William of Auvergne's worry whether Hell will remain vast enough to contain all the damned, are its characteristic features.

Although tons of medieval literature may safely be exchanged for one of Socrates' harangues on the street-corners of Athens, or for a page of Hippocrates, volumes have been and will continue to be written on medieval contributions to science and civilization: depending upon what angle we focus, the middle ages appear correspondingly dark or bright. If a general scrutiny conveys the impression that between the peaks of Hellas and the Renaissance there intervenes the marsh of medievalism, at least among its moss-grown superstitions we find the seeds of truth and beauty.

Grandfather Roger, probably as the result of his Arabian contacts, issued (1140) the first European law of medical licensure: "Whoever will henceforth practise medicine, let him present himself to our officials and judges to be examined by them; but if he presume of his own temerity, let him be imprisoned and all his goods sold by auction. The object of this is to prevent the subjects of our kingdom incurring peril through the ignorance of physicians."

A century later, Frederick II followed in the family footsteps, but characteristically went far ahead; in the law he promulgated (1240) for the regulation of the practice of medicine in the Two Sicilies, under the jurisdiction of the School of Salerno, he recognizes that the physician must be an educated man, and requires a general preliminary course of three years before beginning the medical curriculum of five years; after the academic degree has been earned, he must obtain by examination a license from Government officials; even then he is not permitted to practise until he has served as assistant to an established practitioner for a full year; he must visit his patients twice a day, and once in the night if necessary; the fees in the daytime are regulated according to the distance; the poor are to be treated gratis; the licensed physician must not enter into business relations with apothecaries, and is not permitted to own an apothecary shop; inspectors are appointed to see that remedies are prepared conscientiously, and whenever possible, prescriptions should be compounded in their presence; if these inspectors are so faithless to the duties entrusted to them that they countenance frauds, they shall be punished by death; a physician who decides to practise surgery, must obtain from his teachers a certificate testifying to his proficiency in human anatomy. Such a man was Frederick, that only the most recent medical legislation has caught up with some of his provisions.

Salubrious Salerno, on the Tyrrhenian Sea about thirty miles from Naples, was a health resort since the days of Horace; imperceptibly, by the merging of Greek, Latin, Hebrew and Arabic influences, the Hippocratic City developed the first medical school of Christian Europe. The origin of the School of Salerno is as yet undetermined, just as we still wonder whether to regard Trotula as the first woman professor of gynecology at Salerno, or to transfer her, chair and all, to the nursery as Dame Trot. Although Salernitan literature is abundant, the earliest official document of Salerno—the charter granted by the enlightened Frederick (1231)—belongs to its period of decline. We know of Frederick's interest in anatomy, but the statement that he ordered a human body to be dissected at least once every five years in the presence of the physicians and surgeons, is evidently another legend of Salerno. At any rate, Salernitan anatomy is didactic and porcine—that is, the professors read anatomical texts on the pig, and if swine were dissected, the object of the dissection was to illustrate the text, not to dispute it.

As time went on, other schools arose to share the glory that had once been Salerno's alone; Alexander Neckam believed a snake-bitten weasel seeks medicinal plants, for "educated by nature, it knows the virtues of herbs, although it has neither studied medicine at Salerno nor been drilled in the schools at Montpellier." Aegidius of Corbeil laments that where once masters had taught, prematurely-sprouting seedlings who should still be under the teacher's cane, mount professorial chairs in pompous procession. "Far from the heights of thy fame art thou sunk, O Salerno!" he cries. Later Petrarch writes: "The story goes that medicine took its rise in Salerno, but all falls alike a prey to withering age." As Salerno grew old, looking back with pride upon the work of its early teachers—the *Passionarius* of Gariopontus, the *Antidotarium* of Nicolaus Salernitanus, the *Circa instans* of Matthaeus Platearius, the *Anatomia porci* of Copho—medical leadership passed to its rival in the north, Bologna.

At first, the lawyers dominated the University of Bologna, and curiously enough, without any design on their part, the legal faculty proved of greater service to anatomy than their medical colleagues, who were still content to read to their students the Latin translations of Arabian translations from the Greek. In cases of suspicious death, the Bolognese jurists directed the physicians to open the body and report their findings; inadequately performed, and under the auspices of jurisprudence rather than natural science, nevertheless these early medico-legal post-mortems brought the knife to the cadaver.

Then Taddeo Alderotti of Florence came to Bologna. Born in poverty, he was not able to study medicine until he reached maturity; his fees increased with his celebrity, and in the pursuit of gold he overcharged nobles and argued with the pope; he became so rich that his avarice did not detract from his popularity, and the Bolognese exempted him from the payment of taxes. Enthusiastic contemporaries called him "the greatest physician in Christendom," and his activity raised the medical department of Bologna into prominence. Taddeo proclaimed himself an Hippocratist, but he combined philosophy and medicine which Hippocrates had separated. The legal spirit of Bologna was reflected in the teachings of Taddeo, whose Hippocratic glossaries were further embellished with *quaestiones, disputationes, recollectiones, quodlibetationes*. According to Taddeo, medical education consists of, and medical problems are solved by, "assertion, evidence, objection, counter-objection, solution"—a lawyer in a physician's gown. Taddeo carried scholasticism to such a pitch, that he is really the father of medical dialectics; hence his influence has been largely mischievous, but in his favor it is believed he stimulated his pupils to study anatomy, for several of them mention autopsies and dissections.

The most important of these pupils, from the standpoint of anatomical progress, is Mondino de' Luzzi, called Mundinus, the son of a Bolognese apothecary. In January and March 1315, when Mundinus was about forty years old, he obtained the bodies of two females, and dissected them for his students. Preservatives were unknown, and haste was essential: first he opened the belly, in order to be able to cast aside, as soon as possible, the corruptible abdominal organs; next he demonstrated the thorax; at the third lecture he dissected the head; the fourth and last session was devoted to examination of the extremities.

Soon afterwards (1316), Mundinus wrote a practical handbook of anatomy, which for the next two hundred years was the favorite *Anatomia* of all the medical schools. This compendium therefore reveals to us the anatomical knowledge of the fourteenth and fifteenth centuries. Since Mundinus had the advantage of actual dissection, we may expect his manual to be based on first-hand information. If, in his brief introduction, we are surprised to find the familiar names of Plato and Galen, and later on to encounter Haly Abbas, Serapion and Rhazes, and to meet the omnipresent Hippocrates and Aristotle again, we must remember that two cadavers do not make an anatomical revolution.

Mundinus dissected, not as a rebel against ancient authority, but to confirm their authority. He tells us, "as Avicenna doth state," and "whoever desires to learn these parts, let him read Avicenna." Galen is quoted on almost every page, and often several times on a page. Mundinus is saturated with the old Galenic teleology: he says the Creator purposely made the abdominal walls lax to allow them to stretch in case we suffer from flatulence and dropsy. He does not correct a single ancient error, but he repeats many. On the first day of his memorable dissection he saw the woman's caecum, but not her vermiform appendix; he still describes the third mythical ventricle of the heart; and he echoes Michael Scot by giving us a uterus of seven chambers—"three to right and three to left and one in the midst at the top"—the purpose of these cells being to facilitate seminal and menstrual coagulation.

What then did Mundinus discover, since he neither added to nor took anything away from the Galenic-Arabic anatomy? Aside from an incidental mention of the pancreatic duct, he discovered nothing, for it was not an independent Mundinus who dissected. He looked at the cadaver through the eyes of Galen, and "as Avicenna doth saith," guided his scalpel. Yet Mundinus is a landmark in anatomy, and its acknowledged restorer. He taught on the cadaver, and was thus the first inheritor of the Alexandrians, and the forerunner of the anatomists who were to dissect and to see what they dissected.

The times were not propitious for anatomical inquiry, or for breaking with the past. Emperor Frederick's decree that surgeons must be familiar with human anatomy, is not to be interpreted as meaning demonstrative anatomy. It must again be emphasized that in those days men thought they were studying anatomy if they read anatomical texts. In the early middle ages anatomical investigation hardly existed, and in the age of Mundinus an accident prevented its development. Humble crusaders who died in the East, mingled their lime with Moslem soil; but if the crusader was a man of influence, his bones were boiled and transported home for burial. Thus the skeletons of nobles and kings went traveling and rattling over Asia, back to Europe; it was not the pleasantest of customs, and in 1300, Pope Boni-

EUROPEAN MEDICINE IN THE MIDDLE AGES

face VIII stopped it with the following Decretal (*De sepulturis*):

> Persons cutting up the bodies of the dead, barbarously boiling them, in order that the bones, being separated from the flesh, may be carried for burial into their own countries, are by the very act excommunicated.
>
> As there exists a certain abuse, which is characterized by the most abominable savagery, but which nevertheless some of the faithful have stupidly adopted, We, prompted by motives of humanity, have decreed that all further mangling of the human body, the very mention of which fills the soul with horror, should be henceforth abolished.
>
> The custom referred to is observed with regard to those who happen to be in any way distinguished by birth or position, who, when dying in foreign lands, have expressed a desire to be buried in their own country. The custom consists of disemboweling and dismembering the corpse, or chopping it into pieces, and then boiling it, so as to remove the flesh before sending the bones home to be buried —all from a distorted respect for the dead.
>
> Now, this is not only abominable in the sight of God, but extremely revolting under every human respect. Wishing, therefore as the duty of our office demands, to provide a remedy for this abuse, by which the custom, which is such an abomination, so inhuman and so impious, may be eradicated and no longer be practised by others, We, by our apostolic authority, decree and ordain that no matter what position or family or dignity they may be, no matter in what cities or lands or places in which the worship of the Catholic faith flourishes, the practice of this *or any similar abuse with regard to the bodies of the dead should cease forever.* (Italics ours.)

On the face of it, there is no direct reference to anatomists in this document; in fact, there were not enough dissecting anatomists to make a Bull worth while. Yet the effect of the Bull was disastrous to anatomy. The few who desired to investigate the cadaver were deterred by the pope's unfortunate expression, "or any similar abuse." This could easily be construed as including anatomy, and that was precisely what occurred. The reaction of contemporary anatomists to the Bull is well illustrated by Mundinus himself. In his description of the ear, he says, "The bones which are below the os basilare cannot be well seen unless they are well removed and boiled, but owing to the sin involved in this I am accustomed to pass them by." A generation later, Guido de Vigevano began his own anatomical treatise with the admission, "It is prohibited by the Church to make an anatomy on the human body." The Pope's intentions were good, but he should have been more careful about his phraseology.

However, history is a record of contradictions: before the Bull of Boniface, there was no public dissection, but immediately afterwards sporadic dissection began in various places. Is it possible that the prohibition of dissection, actual or alleged, served as a stimulus? Before the fourteenth century had run its course, dissection ceased to be a novelty: in 1399, the famous Florentine, Coluccio Salutati, weighing the relative merits of law and medicine, decided that law is the pleasanter profession, because its practitioners are not obliged to demonstrate viscera:

> Doctors of the laws, when they teach and dispute, do not depart from the examination of reason. But yours so teach by reason and disputations that unless many things are present before the eyes of the doctor they cannot fulfill their function. Whence it is that the human frame ought to be shown by dissection and that you are accustomed to display whatever is especially deserving of knowledge. Yet it is repulsive to inspect and demonstrate by the hands of the one performing that service the viscera of man through veins, arteries, cartilages, bones, medullas, muscles and joints, and the very human intestines, heart, liver, lungs, stomach, ilia, and colon and bladder and whatever diligent nature has no less curiously concealed than constructed,—all which so far departs from humanity that one cannot even hear of it without a certain horror, and I do not see how the caverns of the human body can be viewed without effusion of tears. Why need I mention the impurities, disagreeable to smell, foul to the sight, and unsettling to the stomach, through which your consideration of the human body wends its way, or the examination of urine proceeds, or the judging of corrupted blood, and the inspection you must make of the very excrement.

It is difficult to estimate the frequency of dissection during the fourteenth and fifteenth centuries, because the dissection itself was entirely barren of results. Anatomical illustration remained absolutely traditional and stationary: the human body as depicted on fifteenth century manuscripts is precisely the same human body as found on thirteenth century manuscripts—incredibly crude and without a trace of anatomical observation. To realize their worthlessness, these pictures must be seen. It is obvious that not one of them was drawn from the dissected cadaver, but all are derived from older manuscripts or codices. Irrespective then of the century, whether of oriental or occidental origin, whether representing the external structure, the viscera, the generative organs, the pregnant woman, or the osseous, muscular, nervous or vascular system, these anatomical illustrations remain as an eternal indictment and exposure of medievalism.

Ecclesiastical opposition, popular prejudice, and the degradation of surgery were among the factors prohibiting progress. The edict of the Council of Tours in 1163, "The Church shrinks from blood" (*Ecclesia abhorret a sanguine*), was a powerful deterrent. But medicine was not guiltless. Medicine drew her scholastic robes about her, and separated from surgery—and both suffered. The conceits of the pedants and faculties reached such a pass that they refused to hold a knife, or perform a venesection themselves, or make a physical examination; when the hand was banished from the realm of science, much of reason went with it.

Surgery was regarded an unfit occupation for a gentleman and scholar, and was largely relegated to barbers. The contemporary attitude toward surgeons is apparent from this notandum: "If possible, the surgeon should avoid a bad reputation, because the people, since ancient times, consider all surgeons to be thieves, man-killers, and the worst kind of frauds." This description certainly fitted many surgeons of that time and since, yet the main interest of medieval medicine lies in its surgery: in achievement, the scalpel surpassed the urine-flask.

Roger of Palermo, who introduced the seton in Europe—it is credited to Rhazes in the East—was the first to describe hernia pulmonis, and suturing the intestines over a hollow cylinder: "Insert into the intestinal canal a small tubular piece of elderwort and then stitch the raw edges of the bowel over it." Had he stopped there, his fame would be brighter today, but he was an advocate of the healing of wounds by second intention, with all the attending horrors of granulating surfaces and laudable pus. Roland of Parma walked in his footsteps, and the work of both is preserved in the commentary of the Four Masters of Salerno, which may be considered the earliest medieval textbook of surgery.

These teachings were opposed by Hugo of Lucca and his son Theodoric of Cervia. Hugo did not write, but Theodoric was author, surgeon and bishop. To Theodoric's pen we owe the most luminous passage in medieval surgery: "For it is not necessary, as Roger and Roland have written, as many of their disciples teach, and as all modern surgeons profess, that pus should be generated in wounds. No error can be greater than this. Such a practice is indeed to hinder nature, to prolong the disease, and to prevent the conglutination and consolidation of the wound."

Taking a suggestion from the *Antidotarium* of Nicolaus Salernitanus, Hugh and Theodoric taught the use of the sleeping sponge (*spongia somnifera*) to produce stupefaction—a sponge saturated with the mixed juices of opium, hyoscyamus, mandragora, conium and other narcotic plants, dried in the sun, dipped in warm water when required and applied to the patient's nostrils. Hugh and Theodoric thus stand out as medieval pioneers of antisepsis and anesthesia. If a recent experimenter has found that these medieval narcotics "do not make even a guinea pig nod," at least Hugh and Theodoric realized the need of the conquest of pain. It is difficult to determine how much Theodoric owes to the Calabrian surgeon, Bruno of Longoburgo, in whose writings occur the remarkable expressions, "healing by first intention," and "healing by second intention." Various similarities in the books of Bruno and Theodoric are undoubtedly due to their common Graeco-Arabian sources.

William of Saliceto, professor at Bologna and afterwards official physician at Verona, was the chief surgeon of his time. He is notable as the author of the first treatise on surgical anatomy, as the champion of the knife against the Arabic cautery, as one of the earliest to emphasize the relationship of coitus to venereal disease, and for his good advice to physicians: "Do not hold any conversation with the lady of the house upon confidential matters." Saliceto, in his attempt to reunite medical and surgical thinking, was encouraged by his eminent pupil, Lanfranchi of Milan. In fact, Lanfranchi indulged in a wholesome, much-needed outburst of wrath: "Good God! why this abandoning of operations to lay persons, disdaining surgery, as I perceive, because they do not know how to operate—an abuse which has reached such a point that the vulgar begin to think the same man cannot know medicine and surgery. . . . I say however that no man can be a good physician who has no knowledge of operative surgery; a knowledge of both branches is essential."

In Lanfranchi's day, it was almost impossible to avoid involvement in the quarrels of the Guelphs and Ghibellines, and like many other Italians, he fled to France, just as many Frenchmen fled to Italy. He remained long enough at Lyons to compose a book on surgery, and the exile then proceeded to Paris. He lost no time in calling the French surgeons *idiotae*, but decided, that in spite of them, Paris was the earthly paradise. The university stood temptingly before him, and his ability was recognized by the chancellor: but within its portals only celibates were permitted to teach, and Lanfranchi could not deny he was a married man. He became a member of Jean Pitard's Collège de St. Côme, and his lectures brought Italian surgery to French soil. He is credited with being the first to describe concussion of the brain, and his work on injuries of the head is still regarded as one of the classics of medieval surgery; nevertheless, in fractures of the skull he felt the safest treatment was the "invocation of the Holy Ghost," which carried on the tradition of Theodoric of Cervia, who wrote, "when the brain is involved, the patient will have the best chance of recovery if the surgeon applies a simple ointment, and sprinkles thereupon the *pulvis mirabilis* of Hugh of Lucca in the form of a cross, at the same time calling upon the holy and undivided Trinity for help."

Saliceto and Lanfranchi may be regarded as the fathers of venereal prophylaxis, since they advised that after every suspicious connection, the parts be washed with water and vinegar, or with one's own urine. In this simple manner they initiated a problem which is still mooted, for there are physicians practising today who believe illicit coitus is as bad as burglary or murder, and claim the sinner should not be protected. In the treatment of gonorrhea, Lanfranchi brought forward formula after formula, each one of which he boosted in the most enthusiastic style. When it was suggested that if his remedies were really so wonderful, fewer should suffice, he responded: "I answer by referring to Avicenna, who, when one remedy was not effective, selected another. For a remedy may be good for Peter but not for John, and a remedy may be good at one time and not at another." This was the same clever Lanfranchi who said, "Do all you can for the poor, but get all you can from the rich."

Lanfranchi paved the way for Henri de Mondeville and for French leadership in surgery. At Montpellier, and later in Paris, there must have been much laughter when Henri de Mondeville stood in the professorial chair, denouncing the follies of the female sex or uttering epigrams: "Never dine with a patient who is in your debt, but get your dinner at an inn, otherwise he will deduct his hospitality from your fee." "If you have operated conscientiously on the rich for a proper fee, and on the poor for charity, you need not play the monk, nor make pilgrimages for your soul."

Henri shows his insight into human nature (of all times) by his suggestion: "Keep up your patient's spirits by music of viols and ten-stringed psaltery, or by forged letters describing the death of his enemies; if he is a canon, inform him that his bishop has just died and he has been elected in his place." His cutting remark, "God did not exhaust all His creative power in making Galen," was evidence that the middle ages were growing restless under the weight of ancient authority. There is nothing new in Henri's anatomy, but his plea for surgical cleanliness is valiant—and hundreds of years in advance of its time:

> Many more surgeons know how to cause suppuration than how to heal a wound.
>
> Wash the wound scrupulously from all foreign matter; use no probes, no tents—except under special circumstances; apply no oily or irritant matters; avoid the formation of pus, which is not a stage of healing but a complication. Wounds dry much better before suppuration than after it.
>
> Do not follow Galen and allow the wound to bleed, with the notion of preventing inflammation; for you will only reduce the patient's strength, give him two diseases instead of one, and favor secondary hemorrhage.
>
> When your dressings have been carefully made, do not interfere with them for some days; keep the air out, for a wound left in contact with the air will suppurate; however, should pain and heat arise, open and wash out again, or even a poultice may be necessary; but do not pull your dressings about, nature works better alone.
>
> Always put your needles and thread in order before you begin to operate and the thread not in a tangle, or you will have to wait and rethread it; now blood will not wait.
>
> Needles are to be of various sizes, triangular and sharp, and clean, or they will *infect* the wound.
>
> If treated on Theodoric's and my instructions, every simple wound will heal without any notable quantity of pus.

The dominant surgical figure of the fourteenth century was Guy de Chauliac, whose *Chirurgia magna* (1363) brought medieval surgery to a focus. His three thousand quotations, from a hundred authors, disclose how heavily the middle ages leaned upon authority, and his two hundred references to Albucasis alone, demonstrate the supremacy of the Arabians. Like many others, before his time and after, Guy de Chauliac denounced his contemporaries, but venerated his predecessors.

Guy was a careful surgeon if he kept his scalpels as sharp as his pen; here are a few samples of his criticism: "Then came Theodoric, who compiled a book by stealing everything Bruno had said, with some fables of his master, Hugh of Lucca." "There is a sect composed of military men, German chevaliers and others following the army, who with conjurations and potions, oil, wool, and cabbage leaves, dress all wounds, basing their practice on the maxim that God has given his virtue to herbs and to stones." "Another sect consists of women and of many fools who treat all diseases by referring them to the saints." After receiving John of Gaddesden's *Angelic Rose of Medicine*, Guy thus reviewed it: "They have sent me this insipid rose; I thought I might find some fragrance in it, but discovered only vapidness." In spite of this judgment, we need not be surprised that Guy extracts from John's book, without any acknowledgment, his idea of the suspensory or truss, for John had taken it in the same manner from another.

Guy de Chauliac was educated in the foremost schools of Italy and France; his learning enabled him to erect a literary monument of much historical value, but scholarship is not the essence of surgery. The presence of Galen in Guy's private library made it impossible to contradict the omniscient Greek. Guy de Chauliac had eighteen Arabian authors on his shelves, and overquoted them. For example, a venereal patient can teach his physician more than books, but too often Guy writes: "Now the method of bringing on micturition is according to Haly Abbas, Avicenna and Albucasis, etc." He endeavors to promote urination by prescribing cantharides, because Rhazes had prescribed it; and he inserts an insect in the meatus, because Avicenna had inserted it.

Guy deserves little admiration for his popularization of scorpion oil as a diuretic in venereal disease. Long afterwards, a medical traveler, the very man who translated Guy's work into French, tells of meeting a convoy of ten mules, all heavily laden with living scorpions—a significant sidelight on the prevalence of gonorrhea. Guy appears to have understood the cause and nature of chordee, which he treated by means of camphor, Galen's wax salve, and the application of a sheet of lead. Guy de Chauliac has been considered the greatest surgeon of the middle ages, but he was too devoted to the Graeco-Arabians to challenge his idols.

As the result of his experience in Bologna, he emphasized the importance of anatomical knowledge for the operator; nevertheless, he himself was too busy studying, correcting, criticizing and systematizing, to be an innovator. Unfortunately for the human race, Guy de Chauliac did not agree that nature works best without interference; he thought nature needed the authority of Guy de Chauliac and his salves. By his energetic probing and plugging of wounds, by his everlasting plasters and irritants, he promulgated the doctrine of pus. Thus medieval surgery—like the surgery of the next five hundred years—ends on the note of suppuration.

Guy de Chauliac had so high a conception of the duties of a physician that he did not desert his post during the Black Death of 1348, though he realized, only too well, that the best remedy was flight. Even his reason for remaining among the plague-stricken is not to his discredit: "As for me, to avoid infamy, I did not dare absent myself, but still I was in continual fear." What living thing on earth was free from fear in 1348 and after? When Clement VI asked for the number of the dead, there were whispers that half the world's population had died; others said not quite so many; the statistics which the Pope finally received accounted for 42,836,486 corpses; in Europe alone, 25,000,000 perished—the total mortality of the Black Death was over sixty millions. Guy de Chauliac, because of his eminence, was asked to explain the origin of the plague, and he answered, "The grand conjunction of the three superior planets, Saturn, Jupiter and Mars, in the sign of Aquarius, produced the Black Death." Not until recent times was there a physician who knew that plagues were caused, not by the grand conjunction of planets, but by the more ominous conjunction of rats and fleas.

Terrible stories were told of the plagues: of parents deserting their children; infants sucking the poisoned breasts of dead mothers; the boy who returned to his native village and met an old man who said, "I am the only survivor"; the goose-girl who dressed herself in gowns and jewels and went walking through the empty manor like a princess—there was none to stop her, for she was the sole inhabitant left in the town; ghost-ships that drifted through the seas with lifeless crews; wolves living in houses in which all the people had died; entire Jewish communities burned to death in the belief that they caused the plague through malice—rabble, princes and clergy wallowing in their blood and gold; galley-slaves appointed gravediggers at high salaries; beggars in possession of untold wealth—for a day; hysterical merriment in the midst of universal destruction; women running naked through the streets; unbridled debauchery until the last moment of life; violation of dying women, and of their bodies after death; every variety of sexual perversion; dancing on the corpses of relatives; physicians and popes fleeing from the pestilence; the crazy songs of the flagellants; the end of law, since there were no officials to enforce the law.

The Black Death of 1348 can never be forgotten, for its chroniclers include Petrarch and Boccaccio; the latter's *Decameron*, though not exclusively for its epidemiological data, remains one of the most widely-read books in the world. In one of his famous letters, Petrarch exclaims: "Oh happy posterity, who will not experience such abysmal woe and will look upon our testimony as a fable." It was an embittered Petrarch who survived the Black Death, for in the early morning of April 6, 1348, the body of Petrarch's Laura lay among the plague-victims at Avignon.

The unbroken friendship between Petrarch and Boccaccio ranks as one of the noblest in literature. Their united efforts did much for the revival of learning, and even their ignorance of Greek did not dampen their enthusiasm for classicism. It was due primarily to Boccaccio that Leontius Pilatus was appointed the first professor of Greek in Italy, and both Boccaccio and Petrarch sat at the feet of this unworthy adventurer, whose sole merit was his excellent command of the tongue of Homer.

Boccaccio, entering the library of the monastery of Monte Cassino, found a doorless room, the window covered with grass, the manuscripts in dust, the bindings fallen apart, pages torn from the codices and sold by the monks as amulets. Boccaccio's purse rescued some manuscripts, and the number he copied with his own hand has astonished posterity. One of Petrarch's most precious possessions was a manuscript of the Iliad in the original, which he reverenced but could not read. Such was the plight of the leading humanists in the fourteenth century.

Petrarch's love of the Ancients combined itself with hatred of the Arabians, and since the medicine of his time was largely Arabic, Petrarch became its chief satirist. Not a desire to make others laugh, but genuine animosity drives his pen in his antimedical crusade. He robs even the doctor's graduation ceremony of its moment of solemnity and dignity: "Now the young man appears, puts on an air of importance, and murmurs unintelligibly while the people stare at him with astonishment, and his friends congratulate and applaud him. The bells are rung, trumpets sounded, rings and kisses exchanged, and the round cap of the Magister is placed on his head. Whereupon he, who had mounted the ceremonial chair a blockhead, descends from it a wise man. This is a metamorphosis of which Ovid knew nothing."

The physician had been taught he must dress well if he wished to succeed, and perhaps the medieval invalid preferred his attendant to visit him in a hat of velour, with gloved hands, in a fur-trimmed cloak falling from the shoulders; but luxurious clothes on a medical back stirred Petrarch's wrath, and he wrote to Boccaccio: "Add to this the indecent finery of usurped garments, of purple mixed with other colors, sparkling rings, gilded spurs, and tell me where is there an eye, healthy as it may be, which can defend itself against such dazzling magnificence?"

While it is difficult to blame Petrarch for this outburst against dandyism, we must remember the tyranny of costume in the middle ages: the long robe and other evidences of professional status were as much a part of the scenery as the cowled monk and the armored knight, the laced boot of the peasant and the cloth of gold of the prince.

That Petrarch, the divine sonneteer, could readily indulge in biting remarks, is obvious from the following: "Within a few years you were given up three times to the Heavenly Physician, who finally made you well." The Hippocratic aphorism (Life is short, and the Art long: *vita brevis, longa ars*) which the whole Latin world quoted with approval, received this additional commentary from Petrarch: "Life in itself is short enough, but the physicians with their art, know to their amusement, how to make it still shorter."

Such epigrams, however, were only preludes of the coming storm, which burst in full force in Petrarch's letter to Clement VI. This document is of intense psychological interest, for in writing to the sick pope, Petrarch forgets his rôle as the founder of humanism; this Greekophile, who even when gray hairs were entwined with his laurel-wreath, still hoped to learn Greek and cited Cato—"Nor do I yet despair; and the example of Cato suggests some comfort and hope, since it was in the last period of age that he attained the knowledge of the Greek letters"— now quotes the same Cato and Pliny because of their bias against all things Greek.

From his letter to Clement, we could never imagine it was penned by the same hand which wrote, on receiving a copy of the Iliad and Odyssey, "I have seated Homer by the side of Plato, the prince of poets near the prince of philosophers; and I glory in the sight of my illustrious guests. Of their immortal writings, whatever had been translated into the Latin idiom, I had already acquired; but, if there be no profit, at least there is pleasure, in beholding these venerable Greeks in their proper and national habit." It was a different Petrarch who on March 13, 1352, enrolled under Pliny's pro-Roman banner, and aroused the sick-chamber of the pope with this declaration of war against Graeco-Arabia:

> I was much alarmed, gentle Father, to hear of your sickness, and this news sent a frosty shiver over my limbs. I know that your bedside is beleagued by doctors, and naturally this fills me with fear. Their opinions are always conflicting, and he who has nothing new to say, suffers the shame of limping behind the others. As Pliny said, in order to make a name for themselves through some novelty, they traffic with our lives. With them—not as with other trades—it is sufficient to be called a physician to be believed to the last word, and yet a physician's lie harbors more danger than any other. Only sweet hope causes us not to think of the situation. They learn their art at our expense, and even our death brings them experience: the physician alone has the right to kill with impunity.
>
> Oh, Most Gentle Father, look upon their band as an army of enemies. Remember the warning epitaph which that unfortunate man had inscribed on his tombstone: "I died of too many physicians." Entirely appropriate to our time is the prophecy of the ancient Cato: "When the Greeks have flooded us with their literature, and especially their physicians, they will ruin everything for us."
>
> As we fear to live without physicians, although countless nations have lived, better perhaps and healthier, without them—Pliny says the Romans themselves lived so for more than 600 years at the time of their greatest epoch—then find yourself a single one of their band who is worthy, not on account of the grace of his expressions, but because of his knowledge and his integrity. For in the act of forgetting their profession, they are eager to step out of their sphere; they set their feet upon the blooming acres of poesy and the wide fields of rhetoric, as though it were not their province to heal but to convince. Thus they discuss with much vocal effort at the bedside of the unfortunate, and while their patients are dying, they spin their Hippocratic theories with Ciceronian eloquence, and even when the result is fatal, they find means of being proud of the elegance of their oratory.
>
> That physicians may not believe I have any personal motive in making these accusations, I advance the name of Pliny, who said more about medicine and medical men than any one else—if he were alive today he would say still more. He is my guide in this letter,

and you may now hear his words: "The physician who distinguishes himself by his beautiful talk, becomes the arbiter of our life and death." When a physician excels, not through wisdom, but through facility of speech, avoid him as you would an assassin who is ready to throw a noose around your body. To him are suited the words which the old man in Plautus' *Aulularia* addressed to the garrulous cook: "Go to—you are paid to cook, and not to talk." Take care of yourself, and be of good hope and cheer: this works a true miracle in healing. Your health is ours and that of the Church, which now is ill with you, and will again be well with you. And God keep you.

Clement VI may be considered—if we overlook his addiction to nepotism and taxation—one of the good popes, but he was human enough to relish a quarrel. He did not hide this document in his archives, neither did he adopt the poet's suggestion to dismiss his physicians; he retained his medical advisers, but showed them Petrarch's letter—perhaps to put them on their mettle. He smiled at their rage and unchristian cries of revenge, until the physicians in their turn showed him another letter from Petrarch—in which the poet criticizes the pope for remaining at Avignon instead of reigning at Rome.

The Supreme Pontiff's displeasure added fresh fuel to Petrarch's fury. The myrtle slips from his brow to his spleen, as the lyrist of love descends to vituperation and sarcasm; he is careful however not to mention any physician by name: "That would suit you indeed, that through me, the celebrated poet, you should become immortal. . . . How does it happen that the entire medical camp is thrown into commotion because I scolded some bad physicians? Do Homer and Cicero feel themselves injured when clumsy versemakers or incompetent orators are rebuked?" In this strain, one epistle of invective followed another.

Petrarch's reference to medicine as a low trade which neglects the soul and cares only for the body, belongs with his Cato-Pliny revival among the follies of poets; yet the unfortunate aspect of his battles with the physicians is the essential truth of many of his complaints. Above the *Invectivae*, arise his denunciation of medico-scholastic Arabism, his scorn of syllogisms whose excessive verbiage conceals faulty knowledge, his repudiation of astrology and alchemy, of uroscopy and coproscopy; as we listen to his appeal to follow Nature instead of Galen, to shake off the trammels of authority for independent observation, we hear a voice that transcends medievalism. When that voice ceases to be solitary, and becomes the language of a group, the Middle Ages have ended, and awakened Europe enters the Renaissance.

VIII

MEDICINE IN THE RENAISSANCE

THE generation which lived with one foot in the Middle Ages and the other in the Renaissance, did not realize it was straddling two epochs. The children of the Middle Ages who became the fathers of the Renaissance were not conscious of any abrupt break with the past. Only when the Renaissance was in maturity, could it be seen that the new art of movable type and paper-making, the discovery of America and the rounding of Africa, the decline of scholasticism and the rise of humanism, the impairment of ecclesiasticism and the spread of the Reformation, the emancipation from authority and the reawakening of the experimental method, had changed man's outlook on the world.

It must not be imagined that the coming of the Renaissance at once meant a brighter and better world. The spirit of Spain in the Renaissance was well expressed by Isabella: "In the name of Christ and his maidmother," said the Queen, "I have caused great misery, and have depopulated towns and districts and provinces and kingdoms." The Inquisition was indeed established in the Middle Ages, but it flared into greatest activity in the Renaissance. The innocent blood now shed was always at high tide: countless victims accused of heresy to enable the Church to confiscate their property; rapacious cardinals attending the tortures and executions with troops of merry-making prostitutes; master of unbelievable orgies, Pope Alexander VI, poisoner and plunderer of Europe, again and again assassinating rich prelates and nobles to obtain their ducats for his illegitimate children; permitting his favorite son, Cesar Borgia, to murder his brothers and terrify all Italy with his unspeakable monstrosities; the characteristic remark attributed to the worldly Pope Leo X, "And all these privileges have been secured to us by the fable of Jesus Christ"—this is a part of the picture of the Renaissance, and belongs to the terrible history of humanity.

The new theology was as credulous as the old, and equally hostile to science which contradicted the scriptures. When Copernicus published his book on the orbits of celestial bodies, the Protestant joined with the Catholic in a chorus of denunciation, and Martin Luther declared, "The fool wants to upset the whole science of astronomy, but as Holy Scriptures show, Joshua commanded the sun to stand still, and not the earth." Modern alienists who examine his celebrated *Table Talk*, become convinced that the sixteenth was the darkest of centuries. There is nothing in the annals of demonology more appalling than Luther's tales of the devil's changelings: he believed the devil begets children in the image of man and substitutes them for the real children which disappear from the world, while the changelings are brought up by the unsuspecting parents; it was thus inevitable that he should suspect certain children of being changelings and not human children, and of course he suggested they be drowned.

Luther suffered from labyrinthine disease, and the constant noises in his head made him hear the roaring of the devil. "Is that thou, devil?" was his earnest cry. It has been charged against him that he transformed the medieval devil from a prankish Robin Goodfellow into the malignant man-hating archfiend of the sixteenth century. In Luther's day there must have been sincere men who sighed for the good old times of medievalism, when witches were fewer, and Satan himself less active. Destiny may choose a victim of superstition to liberate us from superstition: on December 10th, 1520, when Martin Luther burned the papal bull *Exurge Domine* in public—and the heavens did not fall—mankind took a long step forward.

Of the cultural factors which brought about the Renaissance, the most important was the recovery of the original texts of the classics. Medievalism had abundant versions, but an author is obscured, rather than clarified, by too many translators, commentators and glossators. Aristotle, for example, was studied in the schools of Europe from a "Latin translation of a Hebrew translation of an Arab commentary upon an Arab translation of a Syriac translation of the Greek text." In this tumult of tongues, Aristotle had scant opportunity to speak for himself. Such compilations had sufficed for the scholastics, but the enthusiasts of humanism refused to drink any longer from these transmitted sources—they thirsted for the fountain-head of knowledge, for the original manuscripts of Greece and Rome.

A crucial date is therefore 1443, in which year Tomaso da Sarzana found Celsus in a church at Milan. The Middle Ages knew little of Celsus, but the Renaissance received from this manuscript an epitome of Hippocratic medicine in flawless Latin —much different from the dog-Latin so long in vogue. Celsus was one of the first medical classics to be put into print, and *De re medicina* became a favorite book of the new era. The Graeco-Latino-Arabic nomenclature of Avicenna-Mondino began to be replaced by the vocabulary of Celsus; such words as occiput, vertebra, scapula, humerus, radius and ulna, patella, abdomen, uterus and anus, have descended to us from Celsus.

In 1453, Christendom was in mourning. Constantinople, the gate to Europe and Asia, for over a thousand years the capital of the Byzantine Roman Empire, was conquered by the Turk. The scimitar and the seraglio of a cruel and lustful sultan emptied the City of the Golden Horn of its inexhaustible treasures and despoiled its maidens and young men. Nicholas V, hearing of the catastrophe, and of the manuscripts consigned to the flames, wept for the double death of Jesus and Homer. This learned Pope who founded the Vatican Library—and was no other than the Tomaso da Sarzana who ten years previously had discovered the Celsus manuscript in the church of Ambrosius—was not entirely correct. The fall of the Roman empire in the east caused a scattering of Greek scholars throughout the west; these exiles may have been in rags, but through their tattered coats could be seen manuscripts which they saved from the holocaust of Constantinople. In the same way, after the sack of Mainz (1462) by Archbishop Adolph of Nassau, the fugitive German printers spread the knowledge of Gutenberg's invention to other lands.

In its earliest phase, the Renaissance was a rebellion against Arabism. This furnishes us an admirable example of the relativity of truth: in the twelfth century, Arabism was a stimulus which aroused Europe from its torpor; before the fourteenth century had run its course, Arabism had become a narcotic which lulled Europe to sleep. When Avicenna arrived in Europe, he was a keen-witted savant who knew medicine from *Alif* to *Ya*, and his ideas were advanced and novel; within two hundred years he had grown into a heavy, verbose professor, who talked more and more as he had less to say. There was Jacques Despars of Turnai, who for twenty years in Paris continuously expounded Avicenna's *Canon of Medicine*, without reaching the end of the book—some students were beginning to find this a bore. The first battle of the Renaissance was between the conservatives who clung to Avicenna, and the radicals who fought for the new texts of Galen—the original Galen instead of the oriental Galen.

A new spirit of criticism overwhelmed the Arabs. Niccolo Leoniceno of Vicenza put his finger on the mistakes of Avicenna and Serapion; his pupil Giovanni Manardi aided him; the Silesian Johannes Lange said Hippocrates and Galen must be studied in Greek and not in Arabic; the Dutch Pieter van Foreest cracked the Arabian urine-bottle by his judgment of uroscopy (*De incerto et fallaci urinarum judicio*); the French Pierre Brissot struck the strongest blow by condemning the Arabic method of bloodletting which was then the basis of therapeutics—in the furious disputes that followed, he was denounced by the faculty of Paris, but upheld by the university of Salamanca; Jean Fernel, so often a pioneer, poured scorn on "Arab excrements sweetened with Latin honey" (*faeces Arabum melle latinitatis conditae*).

Ultimately the Arabs were defeated, but the victory was neither easy nor complete. In the latter part of the fifteenth century, the students who gathered amid the wooded hills of the Neckar to attend Duke Eberhard's new university of Tübingen, took it as a matter of course that the curriculum was largely Arabic:

FIRST YEAR

Morning—Galen: *Art of Medicine.*
Afternoon—Avicenna: *Canon,* chapters on fevers.

SECOND YEAR

Morning—Avicenna: *Canon,* chapters on anatomy and physiology.
Afternoon—Rhazes: *Book to Mansur.*

THIRD YEAR

Morning—Hippocrates: *Aphorisms.*
Afternoon—Galen: *Internal Diseases.*

Additional Lectures

Avicenna: *Canon,* surgical part.
Mesuë: *Simple Medicines.*
Constantine: *Viaticum.*
Translation: from the Arabic.

Incunabula or cradle-books—that is, books printed not later than the year MD—have become a special branch of study. In round numbers, about forty thousand separate incunabula were issued, in editions averaging about five hundred copies, which means that in the fifteenth century, the printing-presses of Europe turned out about twenty million books. Aside from the Gutenberg purgation-calender (*Laxierkalender*) of 1457, which is "only a sheet of paper," the date 1467 may be regarded as the birth-year of the earliest printed medical books: there is some question concerning Johann Gerson's tracts on masturbation, printed by Ulrich Zell at Cologne, but on July 20, 1467, Rabanus Maurus' folio of 169 leaves was printed by the R-printer (Adolf Rusch) at Strassburg. The Arabians were well represented in the earliest incunabula. In the single decade, 1470-1480, there appeared various editions of Albucasis, Mesuë the Younger, Avicenna, Rhazes, Serapion and Maimonides.

In the sixteenth century, the Arabians did not lack defenders—as witness, Lorenz Fries' *Defensio Avicennae* (1530) —but this was a Grecian century. Greece lived again in a more spacious realm than she had ever known. Fabius Calvus was the first to translate Hippocrates into Latin, published under papal auspices (Rome, 1525); Franciscus Asulanus prepared the first Greek text, which was printed from the manuscript without eliminating the transcriber's errors (Venice, 1526); the second Greek text, edited by Janus Cornarius, was published by the famous press at Basel (1538), though Frobenius himself was no longer in his shop; the Hippocratic folio of Hieronymus Mercurialis, *Graece et Latine* (Venice, 1588), was more critical than its predecessors; the Metz physician, Anutius Foesius, gave forty years of his life to Hippocrates, his first edition (Frankfort, 1595), in Greek and Latin parallel columns, surpassing all others. Aside from the *Opera Omnia,* there were innumerable editions of one or more of the Hippocratic books. The Father of Medicine was first translated into English by the Scotch army surgeon, Peter Lowe, who chose the work on prognosis (*The Booke of the Presages of the Divine Hippocrates,* London, 1597).

No figure of the Renaissance is more striking or colorful than Aldus Manutius. This printer settled in Venice, where he produced the *editio princeps* of Aristotle (1495-8), and then Dioscorides (1499). He wrote to the Prince of Carpi of his plan, "never to allow scholars to want for good books of literature and science." Through poverty and misunderstanding, hampered by political factors and wars, he carried on his enterprise. Earnest and generous, he issued a pocket series at a cost of only fifty cents a volume. To print these small classics, he devised *italics*—it is believed in imitation of Petrarch's handwriting—and first employed it in Virgil (1500). His life was consecrated to his one great ideal. He married the daughter of Andreas Asulanus, thus amalgamating the publishing dynasties of Venice. He founded an Academy of Hellenists, which numbered a Linacre and an Erasmus among its membership. Savants crowded around Aldus; craftsmen who loved the best in typography, enrolled under him. Aldus spoke Greek in his home and shop, and was answered in Greek. Hellas was resurrected by the Aldine Press. The founder died poor, but with the knowledge that he had rescued the priceless arts and sciences of ancient Greece, and forever placed them within the reach of scholars.

After his death, his work went on. His press published the principal edition of Galen in five folio volumes (1525), edited by Andreas Asulanus and J. Baptista Opizo. On the title-page we see the familiar pressmark of Aldus Manutius—a dolphin entwining an anchor, symbolical of swiftness and stability. The number of editions of Galen in the sixteenth century is bewildering. The Basel edition (1538), edited by Fuchsius, is memorable for the initial letters by Hans Holbein. Galen was indexed by Antonius Musa Brasavolus, and Latinized by such diverse scholars, among many others, as Conrad Gesner, Jacobus Sylvius, Guintherius, Thomas Linacre and John Caius. Galen in Latin was published at Venice in the great Junta editions, Basel, Paris, Lyons, then called by its old Gallic name of *Lugdunum* —how often we meet *Lugduni* in the bibliography of the Renaissance—and London and Cambridge. The original editions were frequently reprinted.

Before the sixteenth century was over, the medical classics were salvaged in beautiful books. There is something about a sixteenth century book, whether bound in genuine dark morocco, in calf with metal clasps, or in embossed hogskin, which is infinitely pleasing. These books, in excellent preservation, are still offered in the catalogues of all important antiquarian booksellers. The men who printed and bound these books need no other testimonial than that their work is a lasting reproach to unworthy successors.

During the sixteenth century it was sacrilege to dispute a verdict that had come out of Greece or Rome. So worshipful of antiquity was the Renaissance that when Rondelet and Pellicier, wandering through the marshes of the Camargue, came across the pink flowers of the water-germander which corresponded to the Scordium of the ancients, all Europe applauded the botanists who found a plant that Dioscorides and Pliny had known. And when the Garum was rediscovered—that classic sauce whose virtues Horace had sung from his Sabine farm—a flood of praiseful poetry followed.

The passion of the Renaissance for the classics was fruitful in results—but evil was mixed with the good. There arose Greekophiles who uttered the commandment, "Beyond Galen thou shalt not go"—then came the harm. The humanists who had overthrown the Arabians in the name of Aristotle and Galen, felt further progress was impossible. Was there any Italian or swaggering Switzer presumptuous enough to think he could know more than the immortal Greeks? Moreover, several of the most distinguished physicians still offered allegiance to the Arabians as well as the Greeks. Michael Angelus Blondus, although an innovator in surgery, declared: "It is more honorable to err with Galen and Avicenna than to be right with others"; his conservatism is also apparent in his other aphorism: "It is better to die at the hands of a regular physician than to be saved by a quack." Galen, who had given wings to the vanguard, now became the rock on which medical orthodoxy stood immovable.

The Renaissance was destined to go beyond the Greeks. Physicians began to make bedside observations, and to use their hands for other purposes than turning the pages of ancient folios. With the new knowledge came heresy—with new knowledge always comes heresy. Leoniceno's veneration for Hippocrates and Galen did not prevent him from wondering: "Why has Nature given us our eyes and other senses, unless that we might rely upon ourselves in the search for what is true?" The Swiss surgeon, Felix Würtz, who railed against the clouts and rags and balsams which were stuffed between the sutures of wounds, jauntily asked: "How much do you suppose I care whether Galen's or Avicenna's or Guy de Chauliac's opinion does or does not agree with mine?" Hieronymus Mercurialis, after quoting Pliny's statement that men have more teeth than women, which he copied from Aristotle, is actually amused at the father of biology: "Truly, how the divine philosopher could have fallen into this childish error, I cannot understand." In his revolt against orthodoxy, Petrus Ramus—he whose life-blood was to swell the crimson flood on the Night of Saint Bartholomew—wrote as his graduating thesis: "All that Aristotle taught is false." The Greeks fell in the Renaissance, but it was with weapons forged in their own fire.

The earliest botanist of the Renaissance was Niccolo Leoniceno, who, against a phalanx of opposition, had the hardihood to call attention to the botanical errors in the *Natural History* of Pliny. Several traveling botanists increased Europe's knowledge of medicinal plants: Pierre Belon and Rauwolf investigated the Orient for ancient and modern materia medica; Prosper Alpino described the plants he found in Egypt; Oviedo y Valdes, who was the Spanish "superintendent of the foundaries of gold in the American continent," had an eye for luxury, for he wrote the best description of the tobacco-plant that had yet appeared, and seems to have been the first to mention peanuts; while his countryman Monardes published the first accounts of jalap, sassafras, cebadilla, sarsaparilla, balsam of Tolu and balsam of Peru.

Notable work was accomplished by the German Fathers of Botany—Otho Brunfels, Leonhard Fuchs, Hieronymus Tragus, Euricius Cordus and his son Valerius. Brunfels, who graduated in medicine at the age of sixty-five, is memorable for the illustrations of plants which accompanied his *Herbarum vivae icones;* this work inspired the *De historia stirpium* of his pupil Fuchs, which contained more and better illustrations; Brunfels published, as an appendix to the second volume of his *Icones*, Fuchs' *Notes on Certain Herbs and Simples not yet rightly understood by the Physician*, a composition which dealt with the right application of ancient names in order to eliminate errors from the materia medica. Fuchs gave digitalis its name. After a lapse of almost two thousand years, Tragus picked up the broken thread of Theophrastus' work—phytography—and carried it forward. Euricius Cordus in his *Botanologogican* showed that through "sheer ignorance a considerable portion of the jars and drawers and packets in the drug shops are falsely labeled." Euricius Cordus was also a poet, and at least one of his quatrains has survived among the medical fraternity:

> God and the doctor we alike adore
> When on the brink of danger, not before;
> The danger past, both are alike requited,
> God is forgotten and the doctor slighted.

In his early days, Euricius had dreamed of being a great scholar, but he fell in love and married a girl without a dowry, so instead of musing over manuscripts he was forced to become a practical man and hustle for a living. But when he found himself a father, his dream was born again, and he determined that his child Valerius should be learned in the sciences. The cradle of Valerius Cordus must have been converted into an herbarium, for while still a boy he became the most gifted botanist of his day; the dream of Euricius was realized in his son Valerius. Brunfels and Fuchs certainly studied plants assiduously—but from the pages of Theophrastus and Dioscorides. Valerius Cordus likewise studied the ancients, and wrote a commentary on Dioscorides, but he described 500 species of plants which were unknown to the father of materia medica. In his search for new plants, he roamed through the forests of Germany; one nation was not enough for him, and among the mountains of Italy he continued his work, and with the ardor of the true botanist he went down into the marshes for his beloved plants. Malaria attacked him, and before he attained his thirtieth year the life of Valerius Cordus was snuffed out. His works were edited and published by the illustrious Conrad Gesner. Valerius Cordus is of further interest to us from his connection with the discovery of ether, as the author of the first accurate description of nux vomica, and as the compiler of the Nuremberg Dispensatorium, which is regarded as the first official pharmacopoeia.

In the battle between the old and the new, one man stood apart. Leonardo da Vinci, of unfathomable genius, "awoke too early in the darkness, while all the others were still asleep." He was the illegitimate son, not only of his parents, but of his age. He was neither Hellene nor Arabic, neither Latinist nor a typical Italian of the Renaissance. Of unknown antecedents, left-handed, unsexed, he surpassed all men in body and mind. In Leonardo's youth, his physical strength and beauty, his charm of manner, his joyous curiosity in life, his unapproachable skill in music and horsemanship, amazed his contemporaries. Leonardo going to the market to buy imprisoned birds, opening the doors of the cages and laughingly watching the birds soar skyward, his dazzling golden hair falling over his roseate cloak, was the pride of Florence under Lorenzo the Magnificent.

Leonardo is remembered by the great public because of the smile he painted on the lips of Monna Lisa del Gioconda, which remains the most provokingly enigmatic smile in the world—but the brush was only one of the many tools he mastered. Isabella Gonzaga, duchess of Mantua, importuning him for a picture, received the information that he was "working much at geometry and was very impatient with the brush." His knowledge of mathematics and physics enabled him, after watching the movements of the birds, to construct the first flying machine; his work on hydraulics and canalization was as original as his observations on the origin of fossils; the hand that painted the Last Supper likewise made the first experiments on capillary phenomena; it is almost incredible that the same man should have been the greatest artist, the chief engineer and the foremost biologist of his time. These superlatives undoubtedly sound uncritical to a modern ear, but how else can we describe Leonardo da Vinci? We know no other individual who was both a creative artist and experimental scientist of the first rank. We must pronounce him the most versatile and intellectually fertile of all the sons of men.

Leonardo was the first of the modern dissectors—that is, he was the first who dissected many bodies for the acquisition of anatomical knowledge, and the first who drew accurate pictures of these dissections. At the beginning, he was influenced by the current views: in his notebook (*Quaderni* I, folio 3) he draws the structure of the heart, intersecting the partition with passageways which Galen and not Nature had placed there. Had Leonardo not believed with Galen that the blood oozes through this permeable septum, he would have paid more attention to his own brilliant conception of "the continuous course of the blood racing through its veins." But his notebooks show us how he advanced in anatomical and physiological understanding. Moreover, his notes—written in reverse so that they could be read only with a mirror—are as wonderful as the drawings. "I do not understand," he writes, "how to quote from learned authorities, but it is a much greater and more estimable matter to rely on experience. They scorn me who am a discoverer; yet how much more do they deserve censure who have never found out anything, but only recite and blazon forth other people's works. Those who study only old authors and not the works of nature are stepsons, not sons of Nature, who is mother of all good authors." With these words, Leonardo steps out of medievalism into the new day.

Leonardo warns prospective dissectors of the qualifications they must bring to their work:

O searcher of this our machine, you must not regret that you impart knowledge through the death of a fellow creature; but rejoice that our Creator has bound the understanding to so perfect an instrument. . . .

And if you have love for such things you may be prevented by nausea; and if this does not hinder you, you may be prevented by fear of living during the night hours in the company of these quartered and flayed corpses, hideous to look at; and if this does not deter you, perhaps you lack the good art of draughtsmanship, which is essential for such demonstrations, and if you have the art of drawing, it may not be accompanied by the sense of perspective, and even if it is, you may lack the order of geometrical demonstrations, and the method for calculating the force and strength of the muscles; or perhaps you lack patience, so that you will not be painstaking. . . .

As to whether all these things have been in me or no, the hundred and twenty books written by me will furnish sentence, yes or no, for in these I have not been hampered by avarice, or by negligence, but only by time. Vale.

Leonardo is the first who drew the human skeleton—the drawings of his predecessors are too contemptible to be considered—and his portrayal of the curvature of the spinal column is as much a masterpiece as the Leonardesque smile. His figures of the muscles, supplemented with philosophical studies of muscular movement, cannot be surpassed. His dissections and delineations of the heart and the cardiac vessels resulted in many discoveries, including the little bundle known as the intraventricular moderator band. The fetal opening between the heart's auricles usually closes, and Leonardo was probably the first investigator to note a persistent foramen ovale. He devised casts with valves, made of glass, to illustrate the action of semilunar valves; by injecting melted wax into the brain which he removed from the cranium, he was the first to obtain impressions of the cerebral ventricles; and he was the first to employ cross-sections, now so indispensable in anatomy. Only Leonardo could have given us such masterly drawings of the generative organs and their blood supply, of the position of these organs during coitus, and of the child in the womb. His work on the mechanism and dynamics of the body, on surface anatomy and morphological relationship was without parallel.

Leonardo followed criminals to execution to observe their fear-distorted features, and likewise in the interests of his Art he studied corpses—until the Pope excluded him from the Roman hospital as "a heretic and cynical dissector of cadavers."

In the interval Leonardo had acquired more anatomical information than all the physicians of his time possessed. He is the real Father of Modern Anatomy, though for centuries he has gone unacknowledged of his children. His wonderful drawings in red chalk, unpublished and unknown to most of his contemporaries, were later scattered and forgotten, and many have disappeared; from the surviving notebooks over a thousand drawings have been recovered and within recent years have been reproduced in exact facsimile showing the various pigments and even the different qualities of the paper. Leonardo da Vinci, disinherited by his father, his country and his time, bequeathed to mankind in his *Fogli* and *Quaderni* the most precious legacy since the Greeks.

In the Renaissance a humanist wore the tiara, for the second son of Lorenzo the Magnificent became Leo X. This Pope was deeply interested in literature and art, and the easiest method of attaining a bishopric in his reign was to be one of the literati. He employed Jewish physicians and artists, and borrowed much money from Jewish bankers. His freedom from religious prejudice was such that he pawned the statues of the apostles. He raised the salaries of professors, and appointed young Raphael custodian of classical antiquities. Under his pontificate, Greek and Hebrew printing-presses were established at Rome. Yet there is an indelible stain upon his reputation; most inconsistently, in 1515, this learned protector of artists, commanded Leonardo da Vinci to discontinue his anatomical studies.

In that very year, Giambattista Canano was born at Ferrara. The child of a distinguished medical family, Giambattista was practically brought up with a book in one hand and a scalpel in the other—his own home contained a library and a dissecting-room. In this room the Canani emancipated themselves from Galen. Canano developed into *anatomicus*, and discovered the muscle known as palmaris brevis, and the valves of the veins. The Canani were as amiable as they were erudite; Antonio Maria Canano—trained at Padua by Leonardo da Vinci's associate, the brilliant and short-lived physician Marcantonio delle Torre—

seems to have stepped down from his chair of anatomy at Ferrara for the pleasure of seeing his young relative Giambattista succeed him.

The new professor was full of ardor. He published a *Dissectio* of the muscles and bones of the arm and forearm, with twenty-seven drawings by Girolamo da Carpi; these oblong copper-plates appeared on the left half of the page, and on the right was Giambattista Canano's descriptive material—brief, clear, authoritative. It was the first printed book in which each muscle was figured separately; the relationship of the muscles to the bones was indicated. Never had twenty leaves carried so much information as Canano's *Musculorum humani corporis picturata dissectio*. In the preface he states that the remaining books of the series are actually in press, but a thick catalogue could be compiled of books that went to press and never were born. Canano, most silent of Italians, never told the story of his literary tragedy. We know, however, that his *liber primus* was also his last, and that he suppressed even this first installment—only eleven copies, upon which the author probably could not lay his hands, are now extant.

Canano was too well-poised to destroy his excellent *fasciculus* without reason. A Flemish anatomist, passing through Ferrara, anxious to see his brother Franciscus who was studying under Canano—and perhaps equally anxious to show the Ferrarese what he himself had accomplished—furnished adequate cause. As Canano looked at the text and illustrations which his visitor placed upon his table, he realized he could not compete with this man. He knew then, what others were to know later, that here was the new master. Despite the praise of Amatus Lusitanus and Fallopius, he disappears from the anatomical arena. We bid Giambattista Canano farewell, and follow Andreas Vesalius.

Vesalius looms so large on the horizon of the Renaissance as the anatomist who dethroned Galen, that we must remember he was not a conscious antagonist of Galen. After studying at Louvain, he came to Paris, most orthodox of universities, and the stronghold of Galenism. Vesalius himself edited portions of Galen and Rhazes, published anatomical plates which were Galenic in conception, and introduced Arabic and Hebrew words into his works, although he did not know these languages. Vesalius had studied Galen too deeply ever to forget his obligations, and he was too much of a humanistic scholar not to realize the greatness of the Pergamene.

What annoyed Vesalius in his student days was the method. Human cadavera were still so scarce that Vesalius found it necessary to climb gallows or rob graveyards for material. So difficult was it to obtain a human corpse during the Renaissance that when the learned Rondolet, noted for his gentleness and piety, opened his anatomical course at Montpellier, he was forced to dissect the body of one of his own children. Even on the rare occasions when a human cadaver was exhibited instead of the usual dog or pig, Vesalius was dissatisfied with the procedure. He had dissected since his boyhood days, but now he saw Sylvius and Guinterius sitting in beautiful chairs, reading the texts of Galen; as the professor expounded a passage, his ostensor pointed to the part with a wand, careful not to touch it with his hand; his barber demonstrator performed the dissection; students in their robes stood around and looked on, or did not look on; only the corpse and the menial demonstrator did not wear robes; the whole scene was academic and medieval. The advantage of this method is that it saved the student's fingers from contact with cadaveric material, and the disadvantage is that the student did not learn any anatomy.

No wonder Vesalius complained that the student acquired less information in the anatomical theater than a butcher might learn in his shop. He said his teacher never used his knife for any other purpose than to cut his steak. Warm blood coursed through the veins of Vesalius; during a demonstration, irritated at the awkwardness of the barber, he thrust him aside and performed the dissection himself. "By Hercules!" exclaimed Guinterius, and looked with admiration at his gifted and impetuous pupil.

All this was in Paris, and Vesalius longed to be in the land where anatomy was cultivated with more zeal than elsewhere—Italy, that interesting country so often destroyed by the rapacity of ecclesiastics and diplomatists, but ever reviving afresh with new beauty. In 1537 Vesalius saluted the Queen of the Adriatic. Between Venice and the Vatican there existed an antagonism of long standing. When the Pope said Yes, the Venetian senators said No. In the Republic of Venice no churchman was permitted to hold a civil post, and throughout the hall of the great council often rang the sentry's warning-cry, *Fuori i Papalisti*. Vesalius never bothered his head about such matters; osteology and myology left him little time for theology. The Paduans, who were then Venetians, soon found room for Vesalius. They created a chair for him, and thus at the age of twenty-three Andreas Vesalius of Brussels established at the university of Padua what was to become the most important of all anatomical traditions.

His enthusiasm in anatomy was infectious. When Vesalius lectured no one thought anatomy was as dry as dust. When the young professor dissected, which he did personally, five hundred auditors—students and teachers, officials and clerics—leaned forward with attention. The fame of Vesalius spread; other cities asked him to come and reveal to them the wonders of the human body. Those who attended these demonstrations began to marvel at the audacity of Vesalius; it was noticed that at times he did not teach according to Galen.

Vesalius decided to write a book on anatomy. Of course every word of the text would be his own, but an artist was needed to make the finest figures that ever adorned a medical work. Vesalius had his troubles, and he often complained that the artists were much more interested in painting Venus than in drawing his dissected carcasses. When we remember that preservative fluids were not used in those days it is not astonishing that the Titians and van Calcars and Coriolanos found less pleasure in decaying viscera than in the lively limbs of a living signorina. Vesalius was certainly exacting; at times the artist grew tired—and then curses were bandied back and forth. More than once the distracted Vesalius envied the peaceful corpse that was safe from the antics of the artistic temperament. But Vesalius generously scattered money—a mystic commodity which inspires even such impractical men as artists—and the work advanced.

During the summer of 1542 a merchant on his way to Basel carried in his train bulky blocks of wood. On these blocks was built the science of modern anatomy—they were the blocks of Vesalius' book. Vesalius had uneasy nights; he had a presentiment that the trader Danoni would not go straight to the printer Oporinus, but would get drunk on the way and lose his precious blocks; or he would be attacked by rival anatomists and the blocks would be stolen. But Danoni attended to his business and brought the blocks into the shop of Joannes Oporinus, the scholarly printer of Basel. Printing was still a new art, and a printer was a man of mark. Vesalius wrote to Oporinus begging him to take extreme care with his work; as Oporinus, professor of Greek literature, already possessed a European reputation for fidelity, he must have considered Vesalius' precaution unnecessary, but probably excused it on the ground of vanity of an author. Vesalius was nervous—he was sure that the shop of Oporinus would burn down—and he came to Basel himself to see that everything was all right.

Vesalius' folio, magnificent in appearance and monumental in contents, came from the press in 1543; it is in seven books entitled *De humani corporis fabrica libri septum* (Fabric of the Human Body). As we look upon the title-page, in the center of which stands Vesalius dissecting a female subject, surrounded on all sides by youths and greybeards, we enter the new world of anatomy. The large historiated initials are evidence of Vesalius' excess of vitality: for example, the first page of the text opens with an O, within which we find cupids engaged in the forbidden practice of boiling a skull; behind an I the cupids, with the aid of a lighted torch, are disinterring a dead body—that is, they are acting as resurrection-men; and squatting over the lower part of an L, we see these mischievous children defecating. The initial letters alone are sufficient for a monograph on medical satire. The vigorous personality of the author is impressed on every one of his 700 folio pages. Vesalius was twenty-eight when his *Fabrica* reconstructed our knowledge of man; in that same year, the Polish physician-astronomer, Copernicus, received on his death-bed a copy of his *De Revolutionibus*, which reconstructed our knowledge of the universe. The year 1543 is therefore doubly epochal in the history of culture.

Galenism was constantly challenged by the *Fabrica*. Galen believed there was no marrow in the bones of the hand; he believed that during parturition there is a separation of the bones of the symphysis; he believed that the inferior maxilla consists of two pieces; he believed that the ascending vena cava arose from the liver; Vesalius proved that in each instance Galen was incorrect. Vesalius showed that Galen was wrong when he assumed the existence of a general muscle of the skin, an imputrescible bone of the heart, the os intermaxillare in adults, a decided curvature to the bones of the thigh and the upper arm. Before Vesalius finished with the Prince of Physicians, he demonstrated and corrected over two hundred Galenian errors. He disposed also of the resurrection-bone supposed to be lodged in the right great toe, and he approached the fagots of the Inquisition when he pointed out that Adam's missing rib was not missing. Pre-Vesalian anatomy is antiquated anatomy; Vesalian anatomy is modern anatomy.

The hypnotic effects of Galenism are apparent in the reaction of Sylvius, a highly trained and competent anatomist of the old school. It is hardly an exaggeration to say that if Galen had claimed the kidney is larger than the liver, Sylvius would have believed it. For instance, Galen had written that our thigh-bones are curved. Now, when even a cursory examination revealed the fact that our thigh-bones are straight, Sylvius still asserted that they were curved in a state of nature, and that their straightness was due to the narrow trousers which men wore. Galen had declared that man, irrespective of age, possessed an intermaxillary bone. Vesalius could not find it, and he said so—he who could tell every bone in the human body blindfolded. But the Galenists refused to be convinced. A human skeleton was brought to Sylvius. "Where is this intermaxillary bone?" he was asked. The faithful Galenist answered angrily, "Man had this bone when Galen lived. If he has it no longer, it is because sensuality and luxury have deprived him of it." Galen confused cardiac anatomy for centuries by his assertion of the opening between the two ventricles, for thereafter every anatomist saw a hole that did not exist. Only Vesalius was courageous enough to admit he could not see it. Back at Paris, old Jacobus Sylvius, untouched by the Italian Renaissance in Art and Anatomy, was shocked by his former pupil. He called Vesalius *Vesanus* (madman), which even at that time was regarded as a very bad pun.

By one stupendous effort, this youth showed us man as nature formed him; after 1543, wherever our bodily framework was studied, the Vesalian spirit was present, but Vesalius in publicly giving birth to modern anatomy, had exhausted himself. In the twenty years that followed, he did nothing. He became court-physician of Spain, and instead of brushing aside harmful legends and opening up scientific vistas, he labored faithfully on the gouty toe of Charles V. He attended pompous dinners, and grew polite in manners and learned in etiquette. He was taught how low to bow to a pilfering bishop, and how far to bend his knees to a luetic marquis. He found his place among the king's dwarfs and his jesters. He took unto himself a wife, made money, and exchanged the intellectual life for the easeful one. There was no dissection in Spain—he could not place his hands even on a dried skull. So the years passed.

Spain was in consternation; dismay was written on the impassive Hapsburg face; alarm hung over the peninsula—as if the commons of Castile were rising again in insurrection under the leadership of young Juan de Padilla and his gallant wife. But it was no second *guerra de las communidades* that now frightened Toledo and spread confusion throughout Tordesillas; it was a calamity of a different sort that threatened the stability of Hispania. The licentious Don Carlos had been chasing a girl, the girl ran away, Don Carlos followed, Don Carlos tripped, Don Carlos tumbled down the steps, Don Carlos broke his head. Don Carlos was not fair to look upon: he was a little fellow, with a lame leg, a crooked shoulder and a twisted brain, but he was the son of King Philip, and heir-apparent to the largest empire on the globe. If he should die, who would rule mankind? Ten days went by and Don Carlos was not yet out of danger; he breathed heavily, and developed high fever and erysipelas. The situation was critical; something extraordinary had to be done; at least that's what the Spanish physicians and prelates whispered together. From the churches of Seville and Alcala and Madrid arose prayers for the recovery of the prince. The miraculous image of the virgin of Atocha, and the bones of St. Justus and St. Pastor were placed upon his pillow. Philip knelt within the Jeronymite monastery, and promised God that if Don Carlos survived, he would heap gold upon every shrine in Spain. The Duke of Alva, that terrible and merciless man who crushed out the liberties of the Netherlands, remained all night at the foot of his bed. But a Netherlander also was in the room —Andreas Vesalius bent over the nasty abortion to see what science could accomplish. Even Miguel de Cervantes, in his most mocking moment, never imagined so preposterous a scene.

Vesalius received a book. It was written by his own pupil Fallopius, a lovable man who never ceased to praise Canano and Vesalius. To Fallopius we owe the terms hard palate and soft palate, vagina and placenta; the discovery of the chorda tympani, semicircular canals and sphenoidal sinuses; the best descriptions of the trigeminal, auditory and glossopharyngeal nerves; and the original accounts of the facial canal (*Fallopian aqueduct*) and oviducts (*Fallopian tubes*). In a leisure moment Vesalius commenced to glance through the volume. A tinge of jealousy crept through his veins. The Father of Anatomy read of anatomical discoveries of which he knew nothing. While he had been dawdling away his days in the performance of petty functions, science had been advancing. Vesalius grew sad. He felt himself a Lost Leader. Old memories awoke. He remembered how, long ago, he had taught anatomy to eager students. He recalled his own enthusiasm, his disputes, his demonstrations, his discoveries. . . . Fallopius even went so far as to point out some errors that Vesalius had made; Vesalius was enraged, but the effect was wholesome. While preparing an answer to Fallopius, his better nature reasserted itself. He determined to quit the pathologic court of Spain, and once again devote himself to the pursuit of knowledge.

About this time, after an obscure illness, a nobleman died, whereupon Vesalius decided to perform an autopsy, to determine, if possible, the disease which carried off this grandee. With his skilled hand he opened the chest . . . but then Vesalius saw, and all present saw, what they had not thought to see—a beating heart. The breezes carried the unpleasant news, the enemies of Vesalius accused him of impiety and murder, and the Inquisition sentenced the great anatomist to death. According to a less-known story, Vesalius was thus condemned because while dissecting the mistress of a priest he discovered unmistakable evidence that Christ's bachelor had not kept his vows as to chastity. But Philip II interceded for his Archiatrus, and the punishment of Vesalius was commuted to a pilgrimage to the Holy Land. There is a story that Vesalius undertook this journey voluntarily, to get rid of the vigorous tongue of his wife. In this multiplicity of versions it is difficult to reach the truth, but it is generally believed—and there is contemporary testimony to support it—that it was to escape the fires of the Inquisition that Vesalius sailed over the waters to Palestine.

Not Jerusalem is the Holy Land, not Sinai's top, nor the Mount of Olives; not the Sea of the Plain, or the Pool of Siloam, and neither the waters of Merom nor the wilderness of Judea can claim the sacred name; neither the valley of Achor nor the fountain near Jericho, not Jacob's well nor where the river of Jordan rolls, but the land where man works for the welfare of man—this is Holy Land.

Fallopius died young, and the Venetian senate invited Vesalius to again fill the Paduan professorship thus made vacant.

So Vesalius left the palm-trees of Cyprus and sailed to the Ionian Sea. A storm arose, and under the Italian sky on the Isle of Zante whose laurels and myrtles were sung by Homer and Virgil, the anatomist was wrecked. A wandering goldsmith entered a wretched hut and was startled to see a corpse on the floor—a corpse that Andreas Vesalius would never dissect. It is believed he succumbed to typhus. Was the central figure of the Renaissance, the most imposing physician since Galen, killed by a louse?

An equally unpleasant fate had befallen Vesalius' classmate, the Spanish Michael Servetus. Whatever subject he touched, he illumined. When he edited the geographical work of Ptolemy, his notes showed that he did not consider geography merely a matter of maps. His intellect was broad enough to grasp the connection of geography with botany, zoölogy and astronomy. In the preface, Servetus, writing as a geographer and not as a panegyrist, said: "Judea has been falsely cried up for beauty, richness, and fertility, since those who have traveled in it have found it poor, barren and utterly devoid of pleasantness." Because of this statement he was accused of attacking the authority of Moses, who had described Judea as a land overflowing with milk and honey!

His theological views, of a unitarian-pantheistic nature, caused him to be equally abhorred by all sects. Michael Servetus did not believe in the Trinity, was tolerant to Moors, and bothered little with Original Sin and Baptism of Infants. Therefore Martin Bucer, who is described as a very moderate man, used very moderate language and said that Servetus should only be torn to pieces and disemboweled. And Philip Melanchthon, whom every one called mild, wished in a mild sort of way that the heretical Spaniard should merely be done to death by sword or fire.

The book in which Servetus first set forth his heterodox opinions was published at Hagenau in 1531 and entitled *De trinitatis erroribus*. It brought him into collision with a theologian who believed strongly in the Trinity. He was an uncanny individual—everything that was human was alien to him. He was a cold soul, and could warm himself only at the flames of hell. His only joy consisted in contemplating the fact that at least nine-tenths of mankind was predestined to eternal damnation. He was not ashamed to declare that the infant, while yet in the mother's womb, was already an abomination to God. He broke away from the tyranny of the Popes, but established a theocracy of his own—including a Protestant Inquisition. Spies eavesdropped among the people; for any nonconformity, howsoever slight or unintentional, the harshest punishments were administered; physical measures were employed, and often the cries of tortured prisoners made Switzerland resemble Spain. He might even be willing to burn a heretic. No doubt this man was sincere, but he was also conceited: he thought an insult to John Calvin was blasphemy against God. Calvin engaged in polemics with Servetus. Servetus defeated him. At least that was the general opinion at the time, and when Calvin heard a laugh at his expense, wounded pride rankled in his unforgiving bosom; furious and malevolent, he waited for revenge.

At Lyons, while engaged in editing scientific works for the firm of Trechsel, Servetus became friendly with the physician Symphorien Champier. Like the other scholars of the period of the Revival of Learning, Champier clamored to see Hippocrates and Galen in their own dress, and not in Arabic trimmings. In those days Lyons was one of the intellectual centers where Athens was born again. Besides Champier and Servetus, Rabelais was there, fresh from his lectures on Hippocrates and Galen at Montpellier, now editing the *Aphorisms* of the former and the *Ars parva* of the latter. But it was not as a physician that the world's greatest humorist was to earn his laurels. At Lyons was also Rabelais' friend, the talented Etienne Dolet, loud in his praises of Cicero, and printing everything interesting that came into his hands—but not for long, for the theological faculty of the Sorbonne accused the young man of atheism, and he was strangled and burnt.

Servetus decided to follow the profession of Champier, and

accordingly registered at the renowned university of Paris. Jacobus Sylvius was the shining light of the faculty—but the light too often sputtered because the teacher blocked the path of his advancing pupils with the folios of Galen, crying: "At this sign, stop; all medical wisdom ends here!" A more tolerant teacher was Guinterius of Andernach whose acquaintance we made through Vesalius. Guinterius was a man who had risen from the depths; he had stood in the streets of Deventer, imploring the passersby for bread. But hunger never prevented Guinterius from studying Greek, and the learned beggar became a professor in the university of Louvain. But even success did not chill his passion for knowledge, and at the age of forty he began to study medicine. After graduation, he remained in Paris, practising and teaching, and translating the Greek physicians into Latin. Other events crowded into his career; when the Reformation came, Guinterius sided with Luther, and his life was endangered; he wandered from place to place, but romance dogged his footsteps, and Guinterius eventually became a nobleman of Strassburg.

Guinterius was delighted with the vivacious Servetus, and linked his name with his other pupil whose scalpel opened up the era of modern medicine: "Andreas Vesalius, a young man, by Hercules! of singular zeal in the study of anatomy; and Michael Servetus, deeply imbued with learning of every kind, and behind none in his knowledge of the Galenic doctrine. With the aid of these two, I have examined the muscles, veins, arteries and nerves of the whole body, and demonstrated them to all the students."

Servetus graduated with the highest honors. He became a lecturer at the university on the medical sciences and mathematics, and his wide and varied culture attracted distinguished visitors, including the Archbishop of Vienne, whose confidential physician Servetus became. A life of peace and much glory and money would have been his, had he been able to keep his critical faculty in abeyance. But this was the one thing Michael Servetus could not do—his propensity for getting into trouble was unsurpassed. He published a learned medical work, *Syruporum universa ratio,* in which from a therapeutic and physiological standpoint he criticized Galenism and Arabism—for Servetus was an all-around rebel.

His book was a distinct advance in the art of prescribing. For the nauseous mixtures—the mere names of which now act as emetics—he introduced more palatable drugs; in these pages we see the first rational attempt to avoid incompatibilities, and we find also the first suggestion of what the pharmacist calls vehicles, that is, pleasant-smelling and sweet-tasting ingredients of no use in themselves, but valuable as carrying other drugs of therapeutic action. In those days people took books seriously, and *Syruporum universa ratio* aroused intense antagonism. The Faculty of Paris attempted to impeach Servetus. Dissensions divided the university, riots occurred in the streets, and some of the students were severely injured. Who today would get excited over a treatise on syrups? It must be admitted that Servetus was not averse to argumentation. He had a ready tongue and a facile pen—and he liked to use both. There must have been a sort of child-like vanity about him, for he sent Calvin one of his manuscripts and asked him what he thought of it.

A stranger rode into Louyset, and the next day wandered into Geneva, where he earnestly asked for a boat to take him toward Zürich on his way to Naples. It was Servetus who had escaped from prison; Calvin heard of it, and demanded his immediate arrest, and the Christian Hercules (as Beza called Calvin) labored for a death-sentence. The trial lasted from August till October, and several passages deemed heretical were read from Servetus' latest book, which had recently been published —*Christianismi Restitutio*. Calvin, tirelessly malignant, was the chief prosecutor. There was no escape from the implacable Genevan. Servetus had defeated him once—it was now Calvin's turn. Yet even without Calvin, Servetus' life was in danger, for during the month of June he had been burnt in effigy at Vienne, and in July the Roman Catholic Inquisition condemned him to death. But as Calvin himself was anxious for the honor of burning a heretic, he would not relinquish Michael Servetus, and on October 26, 1553, his tribunal read the following judgment:

Against Michael Servetus of Villeneuve, in the kingdom of Arragon, in Spain: Because in his book he calls the Trinity a devil, and a monster with three heads; because contrary to what Scripture says, he calls Jesus Christ a Son of David; and says that the baptism of little infants is only an invention of witchcraft; and because of many other points and articles and execrable blasphemies with which the said book is all stuffed, hugely scandalous and against the honor and majesty of God, of the Son of God, and of the Holy Spirit; and because Servetus, full of malice, has entitled his book thus directed against God and the holy evangelical doctrine, *Restoration of Christianity*, and that for the better seducing and deceiving the poor ignorants, and for more easily infecting with this unhappy and wretched poison the readers of his said book, under the shade of sound doctrine: therefore—

For these and other just reasons us hereto moving, desiring to purge the Church of God of such infection, and to cut off from it a corrupt member—having well consulted with our fellow-citizens, and having invoked the name of God to guide us to right judgment, sitting on the tribunal in the place of our ancestors—having God, and his Holy Scriptures before our eyes, saying in the name of the Father, of the Son and of the Holy Ghost, by this our definite sentence which we give here in writing, we condemn thee, M. Servetus, to be bound, and led to the place of Champel, there to be fastened to a stake, and burned alive, with thy book, as well written by thy hand as printed, even till thy body be reduced to ashes, and thus wilt thou finish thy days, to furnish an example to others who might wish to commit the like.

As previously stated, parts of his latest book were read as evidence against him, but there was a certain passage which the prosecution overlooked, so we will quote it here: "The vital spirit," wrote Servetus, "is generated by the mixture in the lungs of the inspired air with the subtly elaborated blood, which the right ventricle sends to the left. The communication between the ventricles, however, is not made through the midwall of the heart, but in a wonderful way the fluid blood is conducted by a long detour from the right ventricle through the lungs, where it is acted on by the lungs and becomes red in color, passes from the arteria venosa into the vena arteriosa, whence, it is finally drawn by the diastole into the left ventricle."

This remarkable passage, which contradicted Galen, was the first account of the lesser circulation There stood Michael Servetus, the discoverer of the pulmonic circulation of the blood, condemned to death for writing the book that contained the most momentous physiological discovery of the time. Not one voice was raised in his behalf. As the fatal day approached, a visitor entered Servetus' cell. It was John Calvin. The prisoner looked at the pale face and burning eyes of the bigot, but remained silent. His passion for discussion had deserted him. The opponents parted forever.

The Lord-Lieutenant rode his horse, and by his side galloped a herald. Behind them came the archers, and in the midst of all walked a proud and taciturn physician whose prescriptions had failed to purge the age of fanaticism. A crowd swelled the rear —poor and unlearned—but not one in all that throng envied him who walked in silence. On a hill—overlooking the graceful half-moon of the Lake of Geneva—was set a stake around which were piled the fagots of green wood so they would burn slowly. Michael Servetus was a devoted believer in God and the Bible, and even warmly attached to the person of Christ, but he spoke of the "Son of the Eternal God," and would not say "Eternal Son of God." His obstinacy cost him his life.

By several twists of an iron chain, Servetus was bound to the stake. To mock him, a crown of straw dipped in sulphur was put upon his head. By his side they tied the child of his brain—the book that should have made an epoch. The torch blazed, and a hot sheet of flame, as if it were the spirit of Calvin, leapt high in air and pounced upon his body. . . . Through the escaping smoke Michael Servetus lifted his unseeing eyes to heaven, and cried in agony. The Renaissance, for all its glory, was a dangerous age for a thinker.

Not only in anatomy and physiology, but in pathology, the

Renaissance is the ante-chamber to modernism. Antonio Benivieni performed post-mortems to learn the hidden causes of disease; Jean Fernel was the first to write a treatise entitled *Pathologia;* and Marcello Donato voiced the thoughts of all pathologists in these indignant words: "Let those who interdict the opening of bodies well understand their errors. When the cause of a disease is obscure, in opposing the dissection of a corpse which must soon become the food of worms, they do no good to the inanimate mass, and they cause a grave damage to the rest of mankind; for they prevent the physicians from acquiring a knowledge which may afford the means of great relief, eventually, to individuals attacked by a similar disease. No less blame is applicable to those delicate physicians, who, from laziness or repugnance, love better to remain in the darkness of ignorance, than to scrutinize, laboriously, the truth; not reflecting that by such conduct they render themselves culpable toward God, toward themselves, and toward society at large."

The earliest and most popular surgical textbook of the Renaissance was John of Vigo's *Practica copiosa,* which reached an unprecedented number of editions and translations. The author was compelled to cover new ground because of the recent discovery of firearms, and the appearance of the first epidemic of syphilis, but he was essentially a medievalist, leaning heavily on Avicenna, and saying more favorable things about ointments and oil of elder boiling hot, than about the knife. History has taken him at his word, and the name of this surgeon survives, not in connection with any operation, but in a diachylon plaster and an orange-red powder.

Among the surgical thinkers of the Renaissance, first place belongs to the abused and abusive Paracelsus, who refused to recognize the cleft between medicine and surgery. Erratic and unbalanced, and often lost in incomprehensible mysticism, he nevertheless enunciated principles—in most vehement vernacular—which furnished an impetus to all the rebellious spirits of the time, and have since been incorporated into modern surgery.

Paracelsus tells us why he became a reformer: "Since I

saw that the doctrine accomplished nothing but the making of corpses, deaths, murder, deformity, cripples, and decay, and had no foundation, I was compelled to pursue the truth in another way, to seek another basis, which I have attained after hard labor." He had a noble conception of the duty of a physician, and was so anxious to cure that he exclaimed, "If God will not help me, so help me the Devil!" In the presence of the sick, Paracelsus was a changed man: his arrogance and bombast turned to humanity and charity. The maimed, the diseased, the suffering, came to him:

A man named Bartholomew who had for two years a pain in his side, a woman who had a great swelling on her thigh, a soldier who was shot in the breast with a forked arrow, a young man who had a crusty ulcer on his chin, one whose stomach was swollen and standing out, a lad whose finger was eaten to the bone with disease, a goldsmith whose skull had been injured, one Jonas who fell in love with one Sabina and then fell beside himself, the daughter of one Oliver who was pale and ate small stones and chalk, a boy of eighteen who had a black bladder appear where a tooth was drawn, a young gentlewoman named Ascania who had pain all over her body, one who had a flux of blood from a severed artery, a knight who suffered a stroke of apoplexy, a man of the country who was stung by an adder, one who was wounded in the tunicle of the heart, a young man who was vexed with a continual and violent cough, a certain woman who was troubled with a disease in her secret parts, one named Vermundus who was so weak in his head that he staggered as if drunk, a fair young man who was infected with the pox through the act of the Sodomites, one named Gallenus who had lost his speech, one who was troubled with a great burning of the urine, one who had a cataract of the eyes, a woman whose courses were so long that she was ready to give up the ghost, a sucking child whose palate was full of pustules, one Gotius who had a bone out of joint for several days, a lawyer who was long sick of the colic, a man of threescore years who was full of melancholy humors, a woman who three months after conception feared abortion, a certain man who had carnal company with his wife but could void no sperm, a certain Queen who through the retention of her menses had her tongue inflamed, a German prince who was sick with the frenzy, a gentlewoman of name who was troubled with a suffocation of the matrix, a certain baron who was sorely afflicted with syphilis.

Because of his famous cures, Paracelsus was made professor at Basel. In this pretty town, near a chestnut-covered terrace that overlooks the hills of the Black Forest, still stands the house where lived two illustrious friends and patients who sought health at the hands of Paracelsus—Frobenius the printer and Erasmus the philosopher. "I cannot," wrote Erasmus, "offer thee a reward equal to thy art and knowledge, but I surely offer thee a grateful soul. Thou hast called from the shades Frobenius who is my other half: if thou restorest me also thou restorest each through the other. May fortune favor that thou remain in Basel."

So Paracelsus came to the University, looking as natural as the portrait of himself, wrongly ascribed to the great Tintoretto. He regarded the students with those strange eyes which have been described as "wild, intense, hungry, homeless, defiant and yet complaining eyes; the eyes of a man who struggles to tell a great secret, and cannot find words for it, and yet wonders why men cannot understand, and will not believe what seems to him as clear as day." The new professor did many astonishing things that day. Instead of using monkish Latin, he lectured in native German, which then seemed "even to the German emperor, suitable only to address horses." Paracelsus had with him a pile of books—the works of Galen, Avicenna, Averroes and other medical masters. It was surprising to see the iconoclast in company with the authorities. But Paracelsus did not quote from them. He placed some sulphur in a brazier, set fire to it, cast in the sacred volumes, and burnt up the idols:

"Follow me," he cried, "not I you, follow me Avicenna, Galen, Rhazes, Montagnana, Mesuë, and ye others! Follow me, not I you! ye of Paris, Montpellier, ye of Suabia, ye of Meissen, ye of Cologne, ye of Vienna and the banks of the Danube and the Rhine, ye islands of the sea, Italy, Dalmatia, Sarmatia, Athens, ye Greeks, ye Arabs, ye Israelites, not one of you shall remain in the remotest corner upon whom the dogs shall not void their urine! How does this please you, Cacophrastus? This dung must ye eat! And ye Calefactores, ye shall become chimney-sweeps! What will you think when I triumph? I am to be the monarch, and the monarchy will belong to me. For I tell you boldly that the hair from the back of my head knows more than all your writers put together; my shoe-buckles have more wisdom in them than either Galen or Avicenna; and my beard more experience than your whole Academy."

The academic career of Paracelsus was brief and stormy; his life was a constant battle, and he would have aroused even greater turmoil if he had published his theological writings, since they contained these sentiments: "Those who stand with the Pope consider him a living saint, those who stand with the Arian also hold him a righteous man, those who hold with Zwingli likewise consider him a righteous man, those who stand with Luther hold him a true prophet. Thus are the people deceived. Every fool praises his own motley. He who depends on the Pope rests on the sand, he who depends on Zwingli depends on hollow ground, he who depends upon Luther depends on a reed. They all deem themselves each above the other, and denounce one another as Antichrists, heathens and heretics, and are but four pairs of breeches from one cloth. It is with them as with a tree that has been twice grafted and bears white and yellow pears. Whoever opposes them and speaks the truth, he must die. How many thousands have they strangled and caused to be strangled in recent years." Had Frobenius put this manuscript into print for its author, the fate of Paracelsus would have been that of Charles Estienne—classicist and scientist, first to demonstrate the spinal canal, whose reward was to perish in the dungeons of religious intolerance. The only man of that age who remained immune while he thrust his pen at fanaticism was Erasmus—the unique monk who scorned a cardinal's hat in his lifetime, and refused a priest's attendance at his death-bed; the unapproachable Erasmus whose wit mocked the wickedness of kings and the corruption of prelates.

The complacent cocksureness of Paracelsus was enough to stir the ire of a turtledove. "Tell me, Galenic doctor," he jauntily asks, "on what foundation you stand? Have you ever cured podagra, have you ever dared to attack leprosy, or healed dropsy? Truly I think you will be silent and allow that I am your master. If you really wish to learn, listen to what I say, attend to what I write." Such vanity overtops the loftiest peaks of his native Alps, but much can be forgiven the man who in the age of polypharmacy was able to say: "Bah! this miserable compounding business! Yet the woman requires only one man to father her child; many seeds only corrupt it. Mix many kinds of seeds and bray them like an apothecary and bury them in the earth; no fruit will come from them. . . . My accusers complain that I have not entered the temple of knowledge through the legitimate door. But which one is the truly legitimate door? Galenus and Avicenna or Nature? I have entered through the door of Nature: her light, and not the lamp of an apothecary's shop has illuminated my way."

He advanced our understanding of syphilis, was the first to point out the connection between goiter of the parent and cretinism of the offspring, wrote an admirable description of hospital gangrene, and truly roared against what he termed "the damnable precept which teaches that it is necessary to make wounds suppurate." His insistence on the cleanliness of wounds is found in various declarations which at that time were revolutionary: "In wounds nature is the real physician. All that is necessary is to prevent infection in wound diseases. The humors and complexions, diet and weather, and the stars have no influence. Only the proper treatment, that which lets nature act in peace, determines the result."

When Paracelsus is in a strange mood, and begins with his aniadum, aquastor, evestrum, erodinium, his hidden iliasters, ultimate essences, astral corpses, haunted houses and poisoned moons, we feel all the superstitions of the age creeping over us. Not only did he accept the occultism of the sixteenth century, with its witchcraft and magic, but he was the father of the *homunculus*—a motherless miniature man produced in a glass bottle by mixing horse-dung with human semen and adding the appropriate chemicals. In spite of his adherence to mysticism, Paracelsus had the luminous intelligence to inform his time: "In Nature's battle against disease the physician is but the helper, who furnishes Nature with weapons, the apothecary is but the smith who forges them. The business of the physician is therefore to give to Nature what she needs for her battle. Nature is the physician. . . . Ere the world perishes, many arts now ascribed to the work of the devil will become public, and we shall then see that the most of these effects depend upon natural forces."

Less regarded at the time than John of Vigo, but held in more honor by modern surgeons, are: Pierre Franco, the first to perform suprapubic cystotomy; Francisco Diaz, author of the earliest treatise on urology; Fabricius Hildanus, who in addition to enriching surgery with an astonishing number of new instruments, was the first to amputate the thigh; and Tagliacozzi, who after restoring noses mutilated by "syphilis and a nose-destroying pope," wrote the first monograph on plastic surgery. Gasparo Tagliacozzi's fate—the fervor with which this Bolognese was hailed by those who required his services, the ecclesiastical opposition he encountered on the ground that he was interfering with the Deity, the insinuation that his success was due to the aid of the Devil, the exhumation of his remains from consecrated ground, because the nuns at night heard a voice declare that Tagliacozzi was damned, and the expiatory statue erected at the anatomical school showing him holding a nose in his hand—makes him the avatar of the restorative surgery of the Renaissance.

The provincial barber's apprentice who developed into the surgical Hercules of the century was Ambroise Paré. He was not born a gentleman, and could not read Hippocrates in the original, nor Galen in a Latin translation, but on many bloody battlefields he learned the language of wounds. During his first campaign he followed the usual method of treatment—he poured scalding oil into the wounds. He had read carefully John of Vigo's chapter on oil of elders mixed with a little treacle. But either he was too enthusiastic in its application, or there was an unexpectedly large number of wounded, for the boiling oil gave out. The inexperienced frightened surgeon could do nothing better than apply a simple dressing. He passed a most uneasy night, fully expecting that when he looked at his non-cauterized patients the next morning, they would be dead. He arose earlier than usual, and vast was his astonishment on finding that those whom he had treated according to authority with the scorching oil were in great agony, suffering with severe inflammation at the edges of the wounds, while the others were quite comfortable, and had neither pain nor swelling. "See," says he, "how I learned to treat gunshot wounds; not by books."

Aside from proving that gunshot wounds are not "poisonous," and popularizing the ligature instead of the red-hot cautery to control hemorrhage after amputations—although the ligature was so well known in antiquity that Galen actually mentioned the location of the shop in which those of best quality could be bought—Paré was famous for the artificial limbs he devised for the victims of the wars. Paré's surgical work was rendered possible by the new anatomical knowledge of the times, due chiefly to Vesalius' *Fabrica*. His quaintness, frankness and naïveté, the racy vernacular of his style, his characteristic maxim, "I dressed him and God healed him," his picturesque battles with the reactionary Paris Faculty, combined with the essential goodness of his character, have contributed to the enduring popularity of Ambroise Paré.

The surgical works of Hippocrates laid the scientific foundation of the art—marred by one baneful rule. The Hippocratic aphorism, "Diseases which are not cured by medicines are cured by iron; those which are not cured by iron are cured by fire; those not cured by fire are incurable," was a surgical calamity.

Subsequent centuries, whose mental equipment was much below that of the Periclean age, were better able to extract the worst features of Hippocratism than understand his teachings of the healing power of nature. To say that the Greek aphorism was derived from the older Hindu dogma, "The fire cures diseases which cannot be cured by the knife and drugs," is rather an explanation than a justification. Hippocrates rationalized medicine by stepping over the hurtful traditions of former ages, but he fell with the cautery in his hand. When we consider that, in the name of Hippocrates, the actual cautery was employed until the advent of Ambroise Paré—and conservatives clung to it long after his time—we realize that in surgery there must be no Holy Writ.

No survey of the Renaissance is complete without reference to the disease which from that time on has cast its sinister shadow over the earth. In the closing years of the fifteenth century, gonorrhea acquired a gruesome companion—syphilis. In the middle of December 1494, when the vain youngster, Charles VIII, was invading Naples, syphilis broke out in the French army. Must we agree with Diaz de la Isla, Oviedo, Fallopius and Montanus, that syphilis was imported by the Spaniards from America? Was it possible for the returned crew of Columbus, even if all its members were immoral, to cause an epidemic of such proportions? Or shall we rather agree with Leoniceno that syphilis is of ancient lineage, and was referred to by Hippocrates himself in the aphorism, "ulcerations of the mouth and mortification of the privy members"?

Syphilis, under the name of evil pocks (*pösen plattern*), was first mentioned in print, on August 7, 1495, in the Edict of the Emperor Maximilian, who believed syphilis was sent by God in punishment for blasphemy. "Formerly," ran the Edict, "as the result of famine and earthquakes, pestilence and other plagues fell upon the earth. But in these days of ours, as is evident, grievous and sundry sicknesses and scourges have ensued. Notably in our time there have been severe diseases and plagues of the people, to wit the *pösen plattern*, (bösen Blattern) which have never occurred before nor been heard of within the memory of man."

Between 1495 and 1498, tracts on the subject were published by Konrad Schellig of Heidelberg, Joseph Grünpeck of Burckhausen, Niccolo Leoniceno of Vincenza, Caspare Torrella of Valencia, Joannes Widmann of Tübingen, Corradino Gilino of Ferrara, Bartholomäus Steber of Vienna, Natale Montesauro of Verona, and Antonio Scanaroli of Modena. The best of this earliest printed literature on syphilis is the treatise by the Spanish Torrella; his practical experience was extensive, for within two months (September and October 1497) he treated seventeen cases of syphilis in the papal court.

If syphilis in Europe existed before Columbus, why are we unable to find a single syphilitic bone of pre-Columbian origin? We may never know the date of the disease which has corrupted the blood of the human race—we know only that at the threshold of the Renaissance a new and terrible malady doomed all Europe, impartially attacking cardinals, kings and peasants. Those writers who were contemporaneous with the first outbreak of the new plague, clearly differentiated between syphilis and its elder sister, gonorrhea. For example, John of Vigo mentions the exact date of the first appearance of the French evil, and does not confuse it with gonorrhea. John of Vigo was among the first to recommend mercury for the treatment of syphilis.

Thirteen years after the publication of John of Vigo's book, mercury was evidently established as the treatment for syphilis, for Jacques de Bethencourt wrote: "The treatment of this disease consists of a rigorous and Lent-like regimen and medicines, chiefly mercury, which by its effects, constitutes a sort of purgatory and chastisement for the patient." He goes on to say: "It was observed for the first time in the French army when King Charles VIII invaded the kingdom of Naples; the Italians called it the French evil, while we French call it the Neapolitan evil. Besides it is known by the name of the great pox, elephantiasis, and more generally under the name of the great disease. It is my idea a disease should be named according to its cause:

consequently the disease which we are discussing should be called venereal disease (*morbus venereus*)." Thus Jacques de Bethencourt seems to have baptised venereal disease.

Then came trouble. In the mid-sixteenth century Brasavolus wrote a book, which was one of those books which should have been left unwritten. For Brasavolus dealt with gonorrhea, not as a distinct disease, but as a complication of syphilis. Other writers, like Thierry de Hery, took up the error; Bernard Tomitan affirmed gonorrhea was the sign preceding syphilis, and the misconception spread everywhere, and not until modern times was it uprooted. To some extent we can conceive of the misfortune: since gonorrhea was now regarded as an initial symptom of syphilis, and since the treatment for syphilis was mercury, it followed that all who had gonorrhea were treated with mercury. Even today there are few things in medicine worse than mercurial gingivitis and salivation, but in those days, their production, like laudable pus, was desired by the physician. In addition, the patient was violently purged and bled. The chief danger of contracting venereal disease at that period was the medical attention that resulted.

The new disease was called by many names, until Girolamo Fracastoro published, August 1530, at Verona, "Syphilis or on the Gallic Disease" (*Syphilis sive Morbus Gallicus*)—the most successful medical poem since the *Regimen Sanitatis Salernitanum*. In Fracastoro's poem, Syphilus, the shepherd of King Alcithous of Hayti, enraged at a prolonged drought which causes his flocks to perish, denounces the sun-god and worships his master Alcithous instead, claiming, "At least he will guard our flocks, will lead them to cool shelter and green shades." It was natural enough for an honest herdsman to speak in this fashion, but Apollo never overlooked an insult to his godhead: "At once upon this criminal earth there arises an unknown plague. Syphilus is the first attacked by it, for he was the first to profane the sacred altars." The disease spreads, and mortals are informed: "This disease shall be eternal, and whoever shall be born on this earth will suffer from its attacks." Finally a compromise is effected, and a sacred tree is born, whose branches bear healing for mankind—"the divine guaiac, the savior tree with luxuriant trunk and generous sap, the pride of the New World."

Fracastoro undoubtedly derived the name Syphilus from Ovid's Sipylus (*Metamorphoses,* vi, 145-312)—Sipylus being one of Niobe's children destroyed by the angry Apollo; in some Ovid manuscripts, he is called Syphilus, precisely the spelling that Fracastoro chose. Fracastoro's poem gave syphilis the name by which it has since been known. Sixteen years later, in his prose treatise on "Contagion" (*De contagione et contagiosis morbis et curatione,* 1546), he devotes considerable space to syphilis. He says his former work was written as a poet, but this one as a physician.

This versatile Veronese was not only poet and physician, but astronomer, physicist, geologist and geographer. He perceived that the fossil mussels found in the rocks of Verona were the remains of animals, anticipated the telescope, and was the first to mention the magnetic poles of the earth. His most important concept and one which places him among the makers of modern medicine, is his contribution to the germ theory of disease. Amplifying the conception of Lucretius (*De rerum natura,* vi, line 1093), "I have shown before that there are many seeds helpful to our life, but also many seeds that fly about bringing disease and death," Fracastoro was the first who scientifically developed the doctrine of infection—and he distinguished between infection by contact, through fomites and at a distance. We may repeat the words of Hieronymus Mercurialis, who was born in the year that Fracastoro published *Syphilis:* "It was Hieronymus Fracastorius who first opened men's eyes to the nature of contagion."

In those pre-microscopic days, Fracastoro could not speak of living bacteria, but his invisible seeds of contagion (*seminaria contagionum*) are capable of multiplication, penetration and infection, and hence correspond to our microörganisms. His analogy between infection and the fermentation of wine was a stroke of genius. His recognition of the contagiousness of tuberculosis, of the clinical entity of typhus, and the specific characters of fevers, make *De Contagione* a clinical classic. Fracastorius, once for all, displaced the ancient humoral theory of disease by the present doctrine of the specificity of disease. Thus the Renaissance, which revealed to man the fabric of his body, also showed him how that fabric is overthrown.

In the early Greek days, we saw Thales rubbing amber, and thus learning the alphabet of electricity. That was about 600 B.C., and for the next two thousand and two hundred years, there was slight advance in our knowledge of that imponderable invisible agent of nature whose conquest is one of the romances of science. By that time, Greece had perished, though its legacy to mankind is imperishable. A woman sat on England's throne, and among her subjects was her physician, William Gilbert of Colchester, the first of the English Copernicans. It is often said that Elizabeth took a keen interest in Gilbert's experiments—but according to the banalities of biographers, all monarchs were the patron-saints of science. It is fully attested that an astrologer who claimed to hold converse with spirits was asked to calculate a propitious day for Her Majesty's coronation, and Elizabeth displayed more curiosity in the magic mirror of this John Dee than in Gilbert's comparisons of magnetic force to a living force.

When a waxen image of Elizabeth, with a pin stuck through its breast, was found in Lincoln's Inn Fields, the terror-stricken queen turned for succor, not to her physician, but to her astrologer. Dee had an extensive library, possessed considerable book-learning, and proved himself an able interpreter of Euclid, yet in spite of the constant tricks and impostures he practised upon others, he was himself so credulous that he was completely victimized by the younger but greater scoundrel, Edward Kelly —who never removed his black skull cap because he had lost both his ears in the pillory at Lancaster. Dee loved his second wife, and was overwhelmed when Kelly calmly informed him that the spirits insisted they share their wives. He could not, however, disobey the divine command, and with his own hand wrote . . . "for indissoluble and inviolable unities, charity and friendship keeping between us four, and all things between us to be common. . . ." Their crystal globe must have been awry in its circumference, for soon after these necromancers had signed the oath of eternal amity, they quarreled so violently, abetted by their wives-in-common, that they parted forever.

Old John Dee carried a shew-stone which he asserted was the personal gift of an angel, he dressed in an artist's gown with hanging sleeves, he realized the value of his long beard as white as milk, and he received numerous visits from his sovereign, for his legerdemain was more congenial to her Tudor intellect than the sober investigations of William Gilbert.

In 1600—the year in which the Italian Copernican, Giordano Bruno, was marched to the stake in the Campo dei Fiori—Gilbert published *De magnete, magnetisque corporibus, et de magno magnete tellure,* which contains the first mention of the word electricity. Summing up the current knowledge of his time in regard to electricity and magnetism, in the manner of modern scientific treatises; showing how little was really founded on demonstrated fact, and how much on inherited superstition; discarding a host of other wonder-tales, picturesque but untrue; scorning the men who fill out bulky volumes by copying pages upon pages, yet know nothing of their own experience; putting down in his book only what he had himself many times explored, performed and repeated; inventing instruments, including the electrical needle, yet capable of such poetic phrases as "Amber holds flies, ants, and other small creatures shining in eternal sepulchres"; conceiving the globe of the earth as a vast spherical magnet; illustrating his experiments with diagrams; never deviating from a rigid adherence to the modern scientific methods of investigation and experimentation; applying the principles of electric and magnetic phenomena to navigation and other practical purposes; declaring again and again that not intuition and inner consciousness, but accurate observation and careful experimentation are the only foundations of true science, Gilbert produced the first systematic classic of physics; like all pioneers, he had his Robert Norman, but alone, he virtually brought forth, by the experimental and inductive methods, the sciences of electricity and magnetism.

Before 1600, these mighty twin forces still slumbered in the womb of darkness; they were aroused, stirred to activity, and modernized by the hand of Gilbert. The belief that the lodestone can reconcile quarreling husbands and wives; that there are northern mountains of such magnetic power that they extract nails from the timbers of passing ships; that when a magnet is rubbed with garlic it ceases to attract iron; that if pickled in the salt of a sucking fish it will pull up gold from the deepest wells—are a few of the fables he laid at rest.

The author of *On the Magnet, Magnetic Bodies and the Great Magnet, the Earth,* never married, and left no heir to mankind except an immortal folio of 240 pages; he died three years after its publication, presumably of plague; he bequeathed his library, globes, instruments and minerals to the Royal College of Physicians, where they were destroyed by the Great Fire. But neither plague nor flame nor the forgetful centuries can obliterate the landmarks he erected on the highway of science. "Gilbert shall live till lodestones cease to draw"; Dryden's prophecy is one of the commonplaces of quotation.

His work opened various currents, and after him the story of electricity flows through ever-widening channels. A piece of sulphur, a silk stocking, a kite among the clouds, the twitching legs of a frog—these were sufficient to create epochs. The invention of the simple Leyden jar was as momentous as the discovery of a continent. Electricity has given us a new world, and almost daily enlarges the frontiers of human understanding: the fundamentals of this knowledge date back to William Gilbert, the First Electrician.

IX

MEDICINE IN THE SEVENTEENTH CENTURY

OUTSIDE of Venice, on the river Bacchiglione, lies the town where the exiled Dante lingered—brown-walled Padua. Of Salerno's lineage, daughter direct of Bologna and mother of Leyden, Padua was the *alma mater* of the Renaissance. With its many arcades and little bridges over the lazy river, the old city is a picture: nature has been lavish in Padua, but man has been greater still—for generations Padua was the nursery of learning.

Even in its formative era, we meet famous names—Pietro d'Abano, sometimes called Peter of Padua, the neo-Averroist of Europe; Witelo, a pioneer of optical science; the encyclopedic Albertus Magnus, whose soubriquets range from the Ape of Aristotle to Doctor Universalis; Giacomo della Torre, renowned for his commentaries on Hippocrates and Avicenna; the balneologist de' Dondi, and his son, Giovanni, who gained the esteem of Petrarch, scorner of physicians; Gentile da Foligno of the *Consilia,* who gave a public dissection at Padua as early as 1341; and Niccolo Falcucci, whose *Sermones medicinales* recapitulated medieval medicine. With the Renaissance, these names become antiquated; the builders of the new medicine now emerge at Padua—Fracastorius, Vesalius, Realdus Columbus, Fallopius, Sanctorius and Volcher Coiter; here Galileo devised a machine to raise water, the first thermometer, one of the first microscopes, one of the first telescopes, and here he saw a new sky.

Padua—the university town of the merchant republic of Venice—was unecclesiastical, and men of all nations and opinions crowded those dark semi-circular lecture-rooms. England's foremost scholars studied at Padua: the medical humanist, Thomas Linacre, who returned to become the founder of the College of Physicians of London; Edward Wotton, the first British physician who devoted himself systematically to zoölogy; John Caius, who lived in the home of Vesalius, the first Englishman to describe an unknown disease—sweating sickness—and distinguished as the re-founder of Gonville and Caius College of Cambridge.

In the records of the College there is still extant this entry in Latin: "William Harvey, son of Thomas Harvey, a yeoman of Kent, of the town of Folkestone, educated at the Canterbury Grammar School, aged 16 years, was admitted a lesser pensioner at the table of scholars, on the last day of May 1593." The registrar wrote history that day. In due course, Harvey received his Bachelor of Arts degree, but of his undergraduate days at Cambridge nothing is known. An invisible bridge stretched from Caius College to Padua, whose fame had already crept into Shakespeare's lines:

> Tranio, since—for the great desire I had
> To see fair Padua, nursery of arts—
> I am arrived for fruitful Lombardy,
> The pleasant garden of great Italy;
> ... for I have Pisa left,
> And am to Padua come; as he that leaves
> A shallow plash, to plunge him in the deep,
> And with satiety seeks to quench his thirst.

William Harvey decided to go to Padua chiefly because a certain teacher was there—Hieronymus Fabricius ab Aquapendente. For four years the young Englishman stood amid the perpendicularly-rising balconies; there are no benches in that interesting amphitheatre, and while leaning over the circular railing Harvey listened to Fabricius' lectures by candlelight. The sun never entered that windowless amphitheatre, but Harvey received the inspiration for his lifework from the old teacher's words and demonstrations. Fabricius, of whose early days we are in doubt, was destined to pass his long life in greatness. Pupil of Fallopius who was the pupil of Vesalius, Fabricius carried on the Padua tradition by numbering among his own pupils a Casserio and a Harvey. The researches and publications of Fabricius are landmarks in embryology, anatomy and comparative anatomy; in physiology he halted and stumbled as did all his contemporaries. The dawn of the new physiology was to be revealed only to the watchers of the next generation, but it is here that Fabricius has his greatest glory: it was by following his master Fabricius that Harvey passed immeasurably beyond him.

On April 25, 1602, Harvey obtained from Padua the degree of doctor of physic, and returned to England to receive the doctorate in medicine from Cambridge. Just at that time a new play was being tried out in London, and proved successful; it was called *Hamlet*, but we do not know if Harvey ever heard of it. There may have been more things in heaven and earth than were dreamt of in his philosophy, but Harvey was wholly absorbed in his own problems.

The usual professional honors were awarded him without too much effort on his part: fellow of the College of Physicians in 1607; physician to St. Bartholomew's Hospital in 1609; Lumleian lecturer in 1615; physician extraordinary to James I in 1618; physician to Charles I in 1631. It is now seen that the honors were to the donors, not to the recipient. We know little about Harvey himself, of his father we know less, and of his grandfather nothing at all. Harvey married the daughter of the physician Launcelot Browne, but he mentions her only in connection with her pet parrot which he post-mortemed. He had no children. In other words, William Harvey was without ancestry or posterity.

The personal life of Harvey, as distinguished from his scientific life, is utterly dry. That is why his biographies—aside from Aubrey's gossipy notes—make tedious reading. Harvey lived in stirring and romantic times, but he was anything but a stirring and romantic figure. Fortunately for science, he was able to live

MEDICINE IN THE SEVENTEENTH CENTURY

in his period without seeing it. He appears to us reserved, uncommunicative, prosaic. What he really thought about his times is another matter.

When Harvey was ten years old, all England was in agitation: the Pious Philip of Spain vowed to God he would smite the heretic queen. Perversely enough, the weather fought on her side, and storms and scurvy destroyed the Invincible Armada. . . . Six years afterwards, there was another commotion: the youthful Earl of Essex—old Queen Elizabeth's handsome kept-boy—accused her majesty's physician of conspiracy to murder her; Essex had no proof, and the charge itself was not plausible, since by his sovereign's death Lopez would lose his high position and privileges. Essex in attack was irresistible: the doctor was pronounced guilty, ballads were sung denouncing his infamy, and drawings were published showing him in the act of concocting poisons. Dragged on a hurdle up Holborn Hill, Lopez was hanged, castrated, disemboweled, quartered. (Long afterwards, among the archives of Spain, documents were found which exonerated him) . . .

In his own last days, young Essex may have remembered Roderigo Lopez, for when Elizabeth grew too aged to be eroticised, she permitted her fascinating favorite to be beheaded. Among those present at his execution was his chief rival, Sir Walter Raleigh. . . . Nature took its inevitable toll, and Elizabeth died. England's secretary, Robert Cecil, was a cripple—"wry neck, crooked back, splay foot"—his cousin, Francis Bacon, with characteristic malignity, embalmed him in his famous passage on Deformity. Little Cecil was a master mind, and even before James I crossed the border, that monarch heard *rawly* a few secrets about Sir Walter Raleigh. The new king plucked the proud feathers from his cap, and Raleigh who sought to roam the globe with sword unsheathed, spent twelve years in the Tower with ink and alembics. He wrote the History of the World and prepared the Great Cordial. *Confectio Raleighana* became official in the London Pharmacopoeia, but its forty drugs could not save its inventor. Raleigh died by a keener medicine.

... The buffoon king passed, and Charles I mounted the throne. As obtuse as he was false, he climbed steadily to the scaffold. ... An innocent Jewish physician, a whirlwind of an earl, a gallant and versatile adventurer, a king—Harvey lived through all these executions and said nothing.

Harvey's connection with the Stuarts has been overstressed by patriotic Britishers. He served the royal family and dedicated his book to the king because he could hardly do otherwise. It is highly significant, however, that although the sovereigns conferred knighthood upon even the most insignificant of their followers, Harvey received no such title. Breathing the air of corruption, the Stuarts rewarded charlatans, and not men of genuine nobility. At the battle of Edgehill, while the king's fortunes were at stake, Harvey read a book, believed to be by Fabricius; after the king's defeat at Oxford, Harvey left his service. It is obvious that he cared no more for royal Charles than for protector Cromwell. He simply could not see his contemporaries because his eyes were fixed beyond. The intrigues of Bacon and the crimes of Buckingham did not exist for him. His neighbors were less real to him than Galen.

A few years after his retirement to private life, Harvey, at the august age of seventy-three, met young John Aubrey. It is surprising he had not met him before, because Aubrey was everywhere and knew every one. As a matter of fact, Aubrey in his sixteenth year had seen Harvey at Oxford, but did not dare speak to him. Aubrey was now twenty-five, preparing for an Italian journey, and he asked Harvey how to proceed. Harvey told him what company to keep, what books to read, how to manage his studies, bidding him go the fountain-head and read Aristotle, Cicero and Avicenna. As for contemporary writers—and here Harvey used a word which Aubrey repeats but which must be omitted here because it belongs to the latrine muse. It turned out that Aubrey did not go to Italy after all, because his mother would not permit him, but the interview had the important result that Aubrey became Harvey's first biographer.

Aubrey was a born antiquarian. His discovery of the megalithic remains at Avebury in his youth, his curios, rare books and documents, his history of the county of Surrey in his latter years, reveal his lifelong inclinations. Aubrey inherited considerable property, but by "several love and lawe suits," one after the other, his estates were taken from him until nothing remained to him except his quill. Such matters as being arrested, or hiding from baliffs, were trifles to a man who for years had faced the lawyers. So genial was the bankrupt Aubrey that it required all the resources of his memory to keep track of his invitations to dinner. He met people of quality at many nocturnal orgies, and in the morning hours while his fellow-guests were sleeping off their dissipation, he was busy with their conversation of the night before. He filled folios with conversation that he overheard at such divergent places as the Royal Society, Commonwealth Club, coffee-houses, taverns and drawing-rooms of drunken lords and ladies. He was the most enterprising eavesdropper of his time.

The man's passion for collecting details that others overlooked turned out to be a most useful talent. Aubrey was insolvent, but all posterity is his debtor. Countless personal traits of the most eminent men of the seventeenth century would be lost, had they not been preserved for us by the prying disposition of John Aubrey. He himself knew this and wrote: "How these curiosities would be quite forgott, did not such idle fellowes as I am putt them downe!"

The easy-going Aubrey could keep neither his estates nor his manuscripts. He wrote many books but published nothing except a collection of ghost-stories, since most of his material went into the books of his friends, especially Anthony à Wood's *Athenae Oxonienses*. Wood was Aubrey's antipodes; like a medieval hermit, he imprisoned himself in a chimney, spending his life in exhuming the antiquities of Oxford—a strange, self-imposed labor of hate, for Wood "never spake well of any man." He was under measureless obligations to Aubrey, whom he swallowed page by page, without gratitude or acknowledgment. Aubrey was indispensable, and never would have slaved for himself as he did for his spiteful friend. Wood, after taking from the good-natured fool the results of his unrewarded industry, remarked that some day while running down stairs after some one to get his story, John Aubrey would break his neck. He called his benefactor "a shiftless person, roving and magotie-headed, and sometimes little better than crased. And being exceedingly credulous, would stuff his many letters sent to A. W. with follies and misinformations, which sometimes would guide him into the paths of errour." These words came with the worst possible grace from Wood, but there was some truth in them. Aubrey had sent him notes about the earl of Clarendon which Wood published: Wood was declared guilty of libel, the uncomplimentary pages were publicly burned, and the antiquarian in the chimney was expelled from Oxford until he recanted.

Aubrey has been censured for his frankness. He thinks nothing of recording that Sir Edward Coke was a cuckold. The pen of Ben Jonson and the brush of Van Dyke keep alive the beauty of Venetia Digby, but within three pages Aubrey set down enough scandal about her to make the fame of a thick novel. In connection with the immortal Harvey, he relates without any ado: "I remember he kept a pretty young wench to wayte on him, which I guesse he made use of for warmeth-sake as King David did, and tooke care of her in his will, as also of his man servant." Aubrey was equally outspoken about himself. Under the general heading of "Accidents," he mentions not only ague, violent fever, "measills, but that was nothing," "small-pox at Oxon," but also, "1656: December: *Veneris morbus.*"

Modern Harveians warn us to accept Aubrey's statements with suspicion, but they do not point out any misstatements. The truth is, if Aubrey errs, he errs unwittingly, not because of pompousness or prejudices. He is altogether devoid of pretense, he does not claim to have verified his references. He put down what he was told and what he saw and heard and remembered. He frequently says, "I thinke," "I beleeve," "I have now forgott," "to the best of my remembrance," "what is one to beleeve?" He queries, leaves spaces and makes dashes when he is uncertain, erases, substitutes, adds notes pell-mell mixed up with marginalia and addenda, and in many places promises fuller memoranda which later he forgets to insert. This is not the way to write history; but we think Clio would rather dispense with many of her formal historians than with such a gossip as John Aubrey.

Here, then, is a selection from Aubrey's notes on Harvey, indispensable as being the only contemporary account:

He was wont to say that man was but a great mischievous baboon.

He would say, that we Europaeans knew not how to order or governe our woemen, and that the Turkes were the only people used them wisely.

He was far from bigotry.

He had been physitian to the Lord Chancellor Bacon, whom he esteemed much for his witt and style, but would not allow him to be a great philosopher. "He writes philosophy like a Lord Chancelor," said he to me, speaking in derision; "I have cured him."

About 1649 he travelled again into Italy, Dr. George (now Sir George) Ent, then accompanying him.

At Oxford, he grew acquainted with Dr. Charles Scarborough, then a young physitian (since by King Charles II knighted), in whose conversation he much delighted; and whereas before, he marched up and downe with the army, he tooke him to him and made him ly in his chamber, and said to him, "Prithee leave off thy gunning, and stay here; I will bring thee into practice."

For 20 yeares before he dyed he tooke no manner of care about his worldly concernes, but his brother Eliab, who was a very wise and prudent menager, ordered all not only faithfully, but better then he could have donne himselfe.

He was, as all the rest of the brothers, very cholerique; and in his young days wore a dagger (as the fashion then was, nay I remember my old schoolemaster, old Mr. Latimer, at 70, wore a dudgeon, with a knife, and bodkin, as also my old grandfather Lyte, and alderman Whitson of Bristowe, which I suppose was the common fashion in their young days), but this Dr. would be to apt to draw-out his dagger upon every slight occasion.

He was not tall; but of the lowest stature, round faced, olivaster complexion; little eie, round, very black, full of spirit; his haire was black as a raven, but quite white 20 yeares before he dyed.

I have heard him say, that after his booke of the Circulation of the Blood came-out, that he fell mightily in his practize, and that 'twas beleeved by the vulgar that he was crack-brained; and all the physitians were against his opinion, and envyed him; many wrote against him, as Dr. Primige, Paracisanus, etc. (vide Sir George Ent's booke). With much adoe at last, in about 20 or 30 yeares time, it was received in all the Universities in the world; and, as Mr. Hobbes sayes in his book "De Corpore," he is the only man, perhaps, that ever lived to see his owne doctrine established in his life time.

Harvey's lecture-notes have recently been found. They furnish a good example of what is meant by rough notes, for it is a task to read this medley of bad Latin, crabbed English, and abbreviations, hastily written in a notoriously difficult hand. One partly-filled page reveals that the fellows of the Royal College of Physicians who attended the Lumleian lectures in 1616, heard this small, young, raven-haired, quick-speaking doctor read from these notes: "It is plain from the structure of the heart that the blood is passed continuously through the lungs to the aorta as by the two clacks of a water bellows to raise water. It is shown by the application of a ligature that the passage of the blood is from the arteries into the veins. Whence it follows that the movement of the blood is constantly in a circle, and is brought about by the beat of the heart." Thus William Harvey first announced the most important physiological discovery in the history of medicine.

As we turn from the daily life of Harvey to his mental processes, we feel at once the presence of a master-mind. Harvey has left us no immature compositions, no juvenalia over which we may smile indulgently; his works are few and all of the first rank. He allowed twelve years to elapse before giving to Wilhelm Fitzer of Frankfort-on-Main his manuscript on the circulation of the blood. Printed in a foreign country—did he fear the British censor?—by an undistinguished press on thin paper which readily foxed, this little quarto teeming with typographical errors—did Harvey read proof?—is a wretched-looking production, and except for the title-page and two plates borrowed from Fabricius, it is unillustrated. It is not size that counts, nor appearance; many beautiful books printed on paper as tough as vellum have disappeared from consideration, and Harvey's seventy-two pages ultimately changed the medical world. His "Anatomical Exercise on the Motion of the Heart and Blood in Animals" (*Exercitatio anatomica de motu cordis et sanguinis in animalibus*, 1628), usually referred to by its short title, *De motu cordis*, modernized physiology.

In the first paragraph of the first chapter, Harvey explains some of the riddles which confronted him:

When I first gave my mind to vivisections, as a means of discovering the motions and uses of the heart, and sought to discover these from actual inspection, and not from the writings of others, I found the task so truly arduous, so full of difficulties, that I was almost tempted to think, with Fracastorius, that the motion of the heart was only to be comprehended by God. For I could neither rightly perceive at first when the systole and when the diastole took place, nor when and where dilatation and contraction occurred, by reason of the rapidity of the motion, which in many animals is accomplished in the twinkling of an eye, coming and going like a flash of lightning; so that the systole presented itself to me now from this point, now from that; the diastole the same; and then everything was reversed, the motions occurring, as it seemed, variously and confusedly together. My mind was therefore greatly unsettled, nor did I know what I should myself conclude, nor what believe from others; I was not surprised that Andreas Laurentius should have said that the motion of the heart was as perplexing as the flux and reflux of Euripus had appeared to Aristotle.

Harvey's experiments eventually solved the problem: "I began to think whether there might not be a motion, as it were, in a circle"—this thought, fermenting in his mind, overthrew the old doctrine and established his own which can never be overthrown. Aristotle's comparative method aided him; he quotes Aristotle by name twenty times, and Galen much oftener; in fact, he fathered some of his most significant observations and experiments upon Galen. Evidently, in this respect he was more conservative than his younger contemporary, the Paduan Sanctorius, whose genius for devising instruments of precision made him the pioneer of experimental metabolism; writing to Galileo of his new art of measuring the insensible perspiration, Sanctorius neatly adds, "But even if Galen did not know it, it matters little, since it is true."

That Harvey anticipated opposition is apparent from the remarks in his eighth chapter: "What remains to be said upon the quantity and source of the blood which thus passes, is of so novel and unheard-of character, but I not only fear injury to myself from the envy of a few, but I tremble lest I have mankind at large for my enemies, so much doth wont and custom, that become as another nature, and doctrine once sown and that hath struck deep root, and respect for antiquity influence all men: Still the die is cast, and my trust is in my love of truth, and the candour that inheres in cultivated minds."

For two years nothing happened. Then James Primrose cast the first stone, the same Primrose whose qualifications to practise medicine were less than a year old—and among the examiners who had passed him was William Harvey. Primrose was a pupil of Riolan, who induced the Paris Faculty to prohibit the teaching of Harvey's doctrine. Although the ink on his license was hardly dry, Primrose prepared to demolish Harvey according to the method of the Paris Faculty: he locked himself in his room, and quoted all the ancient authorities. Harvey's book was the result of years of research, but within two weeks Primrose wrote a much bigger book in refutation—and he did it without looking at a heart or taking a scalpel in his hand.

"This is the end of little Dr. Harvey," thought Primrose, as he emerged pale but triumphant from his dialectic labors. Others took up the cry, and Harvey was called Circulator—in the Latin sense of the word which means quack. In the face of widespread detraction and decreasing practice, Harvey preserved a silence which today is almost as much admired as his demonstration of the circulation of the blood. He could afford to wait, for he lived to see himself vindicated. The dramatic feature of his discovery was his concept of a circuit moving uninterruptedly within us; instead of pools of stagnant blood, we now conceive of a continuous life-stream. From this viewpoint began the reading of the cryptograms of function—heart beat, tissue changes, metabolic processes, glandular activity, blood transfusion, mechanism of respiration—and physiology as a working science was born, changing the outlook of Medicine.

Much continues to be written on the question of Harvey's priority and his numerous predecessors. It is obvious that every fighting savage who struck with club or spear, that every butcher who slit an animal's throat, realized that blood spurts or flows from the wounded vessels. The passages on the pulse from the Egyptian papyri; the old Chinese dictum, "The heart has jurisdiction over the blood, and the blood in the vessels never ceases"; the Hindu description, "The disease called panduroga (anemia?) is sometimes caused by swallowing of clay which blocks the lumen of the veins and stops the current of the blood"; Plato's picture of the heart, as "the fountain of the blood, which is rapidly carried around through all the limbs"; and the Salernitan Copho's reference to the blood passing through the capillaries (*pars in sanguinem transit per capillares*), exhibit some knowledge of the circulation and of the invisible anastomosis.

It is not surprising, therefore, that the anatomists of the Cinquecento should have been on the trail. His teacher Fabricius taught him that the venal valves are always directed toward the heart; Colombo, perhaps echoing Servetus, again propounded the lesser circulation; Andrea Cesalpino not only visualized the pulmonary and systemic circulation, but actually used the term "circulation of the blood" (*sanguinis circulationi*); had he stopped in time, Caesalpinus might have been a more serious contender for the Harveian laurels, but his last published book (*Praxis universae,* 1606) declares "the blood goes forth from the heart not only through aorta and pulmonary artery, but also through vena cava and pulmonary vein," which proves how confused was his understanding of the circulation, valves and anastomosis. The claims that have been advanced for the two great laymen—the lawyer Carlo Ruini of Bologna, whose magnificent book on the horse founded the science of veterinary anatomy; and Fra Paolo Sarpi, the "terrible friar" who saved Venice—belong to the same class. Sooner or later, the student of medical history realizes the essential difference between scattered quotations, howsoever brilliant, and a consistent experimental demonstration. The forerunners of Harvey were many and sagacious, and in comparing their work with his, we see that while they groped for the truth stumblingly, he went forward, step by step, and saw what the others had overlooked.

In 1616, the year of Shakespeare's death, many could repeat the poet's lines in Coriolanus:

> I send it through the rivers of your blood,
> Even to the court, the heart,—to the seat o' the brain;
> And, through the cranks and offices of man,
> The strongest nerves and small inferior veins;

or the words that he put in the mouth of Brutus:

> As dear to me as are the ruddy drops
> That visit my sad heart;

but only Harvey could trace the movement of these ruddy drops from the instant they left the heart until they returned from their circular journey.

The curious theory of telegony—the first male who fecundates a female makes such an indelible impress upon her that subsequent offspring by another man bear the characteristics of the first father—was well known in the seventeenth century. Long after Aubrey helped to carry Harvey to the vault at Hempsted, the body "lapt in lead," he deemed it expedient not to let the bailiffs know his address at Broad Chalk; in his enforced leisure, Aubrey amused himself by composing a comedy known as *Countrey Revell*, "written in the blank spaces and between the lines of a long legal document." Harvey is mentioned in the

MEDICINE IN THE SEVENTEENTH CENTURY

scene in which the sowgelder, on scientific grounds, argues with Sir John Fitz-ale never to marry a widow:

Sowgelder. To see, Sir John, how much you are mistaken; he that marries a widdowe makes himself cuckold. Exempli gratia, to speake experimentally and in my trade, if a good bitch is first warded with a curre, let her ever after be warded with a dog of a good straine and yet she will bring curres as at first, her wombe being first infected with a curre. So, the children will be like the first husband (like raysing up children to your brother). So, the adulterer, though a crime in law, the children are like the husband.

Sir John. Thou dost talke, me thinks, more understandingly of these matters then any one I have met with.

Sowgelder. Ah! my old friend Dr. Harvey—I knew him right well—he made me sitt by him 2 or 3 hours together discoursing. Why! had he been stiffe, starcht, and retired, as other formall doctors are, he had known no more then they. From the meanest person, in some way, or other, the learnedst man may learn something. Pride has been one of the greatest stoppers of the advancement of learning.

Reference has already been made to the Paris Faculty, and we shall meet it again, but always as one of the most malign influences that blocked the progress of medical science. Insisting on its infallibility, it is difficult to discover a single instance in which its influence was not deleterious. Congenitally incapable of entertaining a new idea, it issued a decree in the seventeenth century that none may deviate from Hippocrates and Galen upon pain of excommunication. Day-long disputations were propounded to the candidate, and during the weary hours that he was forced to pit his wits against the assembled professors, men trained and exercised in subtle dialectics, he was also required to furnish food and wine for his adversaries—the final result depended upon the faculty's state of digestion. Characteristic disputations were: Is it well to get drunk once a month? Are women imperfect works of nature? Are bastard children brighter than those which are legitimate? Should the phases of the moon be considered when we have our hair cut?

The Paris Faculty excluded surgery from the curriculum,

and pursued with incredible malignity every one who dared suggest that surgery was of equal rank with regular medicine; it expelled, with bitter rancor, any member who prescribed the new drugs, such as antimony, cinchona and ipecac; it railed at Servetus because of his rational treatise on syrups; it announced when the Collected Works of Ambroise Paré were translated into Latin by his able pupil and son-in-law, Jacques Guillemau, that as no one but themselves were capable of writing Latin, it was over-presumptuous for surgeons to attempt such a thing, and it was decreed that this edition be torn up and kept for a vile purpose; not only did it forbid Harvey's demonstration of the circulation of the blood to be taught, but it opposed Pecquet's discovery of the thoracic duct, and denounced Aselli's discovery of the lacteals.

The Paris Faculty was consistent in refusing to recognize any discovery or to permit experimentation. The Paris Faculty believed in interminable discussions and not in demonstrations, and when the candidate—after infinite mental torture—finally received the cap and accolade, he was a full-fledged doctor, but had never seen a patient. Under its auspices, medicine marched backward to the Dark Ages. What would have happened, had it not been for the genius of Molière? More than any other factor, the laughter of Molière was the savior of medicine in the seventeenth century.

It was now many years since Vesalius and Fallopius had exposed the mistakes of Galenism, but a university is sometimes the last refuge of ancient error, and several of the professors in the university of Bologna still clung to the old doctrines. Bartolommeo Massari was the radical of the faculty: not only did he expound the new learning, but like a true Vesalian he dissected human bodies in his own home. Among the favorite pupils who were admitted into this circle was Marcello Malpighi, and the discussions, the dissections, and the experiments stirred his mind mightily. The pursuit of knowledge by the experimental method was still novel, and what its devotees lacked in numbers they made up in fervency. Real enthusiasm is the privilege of the minority.

Malpighi was born in 1628, always remembered as the year in which Harvey's *De motu cordis* appeared; in 1653 he graduated in medicine and philosophy, his thesis being a defence of the Hippocratic method of unprejudiced observation as opposed to the dogmatism of Galen; in 1656 the Bolognese senate nominated him as public lecturer in medicine, and he had no sooner undertaken his duties than Ferdinand, grand duke of Tuscany, created for him the chair of theoretical medicine at the university of Pisa. So the twenty-eight-year-old professor journeyed to Pisa by the sea, its university famous as one of the hobbies of the Medici family. It is said that during one of his first lectures the new doctrines which he expounded so offended the members of his audience, that they gradually withdrew until only one listener remained.

If this story is true, it was no misfortune for Malpighi, for that one man was Giovanni Alfonso Borelli of Naples. Borelli was the medico-mathematician who viewed the human organism as a machine, treating muscular motion, respiration and digestion as mechanical processes, explaining physiological problems by the laws of physics. An irascible man, of a morose and quarrelsome disposition, assertive, aggressive, antagonistic, usually unpleasant and often unbearable, Borelli was nevertheless a profound thinker who not only did important scientific work himself, but inspired others to achieve and accomplish. It was under Borelli's direction that Auber discovered the structure of the testicle, and Bellini, a youth of nineteen, discovered the uriniferous tubules, and it was while working with Borelli that Malpighi made his first discovery—the spiral nature of the fibers of the bullock's heart. Borelli was twenty years older than Malpighi, and the younger man looked upon him as a father, consulting him almost every day. Borelli taught Malpighi the physics of Galileo, and Malpighi instructed Borelli in biology.

The relationship between them indicates how modest and lovable Malpighi must have been, for few could get along with the fierce Neapolitan. Together they performed dissections which were attended by dukes and princes, thus giving rise to the Academy of Experiment, which was soon removed to Florence, the Academicians meeting in the Ducal Palace, where the royal host and his family mingled freely with them. Galileo was a Pisan, but Malpighi was not even Pisa-plated; he claimed the humid climate did not agree with him, for although brought up in the country he was always in delicate health, and after three years he returned home, meeting and studying with Fracassati and Buonfigluoli, lifelong friends.

The riddle of respiration had puzzled philosophers at least since the days of Aristotle, and surely it is interesting to know how we breathe. Many of the acute minds of the mid-seventeenth century—Boyle, Hooke, Lower, Mayow, and Borelli—tackled this problem, and in 1660 it became the object of Malpighi's inquiry. Up to this time the lung had been regarded as a sort of porous parenchyma—Fabricius compared it to tow—and it was believed that somewhere within its substance the smaller divisions of the pulmonary artery lost themselves, pouring out their blood into the open spaces, where it was later gathered up by the pulmonary veins, while the minuter parts of the windpipe were also supposed to terminate in this fleshy tissue. But now, with the lungs of a dog, a tortoise, and a frog, Malpighi began that series of observations which have caused him to be regarded as the greatest of microscopists and the founder of histology.

He showed that instead of a perforated mass in which the blood was poured and then sucked out, the lung was vesicular in nature, the bronchi being continuous with the air vesicles, the air and blood of the lung never actually in contact, but separated by a membrane, and that the blood was constantly within channels, even when crossing from the arteries to the veins—for he observed the capillary circulation. This momentous discovery bridged the one remaining gap in the Harveian hypothesis—for Harvey, unfamiliar with the microscope, could never explain where or how the interchange occurred between arterial and venous blood. Malpighi wrote:

I saw the blood, showered down in tiny streams through the arteries, after the fashion of a flood, and I might have believed that the blood itself escaped into an empty space and was gathered up again by a gaping vessel, but an objection to this view was afforded by the movement of the blood being tortuous and scattered in different directions and by its being united again in a determinate part. My doubt was changed to a certainty by the dried lung of a frog which to a marked extent had preserved the redness of the blood in very minute tracts, which were afterwards found to be vessels, where by the help of a glass I saw not scattered points but vessels joined together in a ring-like fashion. And such is the wandering about of these vessels as they proceed on this side from the vein and on the other from the artery that the vessels no longer maintain a straight direction, but there appears a network made up of the continuations of the two vessels. This network not only occupies the whole area but extends to the walls, and is attached to the outgoing vessel, as I could more abundantly and yet with greater difficulty see in the oblong lung of the tortoise, which is equally membranous and transparent. Hence it was clear to the senses that the blood flowed along sinuous vessels and was not poured into spaces, but was always contained within tubules, and that its dispersion is due to the multiple winding of the vessels. . . . From the simplicity which Nature uses in all her works, it may be concluded from these results that the network which I once thought to be nervous in character is really a vessel attached to the vesicles and sinuses carrying thither the mass of the blood or carrying the same away, and that although in the lungs of the more perfect animals a vessel seems sometimes to leave off and gape in the middle of the network of rings, yet it is probable that, as in the frog and the tortoise, the vessel in question is prolonged further into very small vessels after the form of a network, although these on account of their exquisite fineness escape our senses.

These discoveries were announced in two epistles which Malpighi dedicated and sent to Borelli, who was very much pleased with them, and urged that they be published. Thus his first book, "On the Lungs" (*De pulmonibus*), appeared in 1661 at Bologna, establishing the anatomical foundation for a true conception of the respiratory act. In the following year, scientific circles heard that the chair of medicine at Messina had become vacant through the death of Pietro Castelli; before coming to Pisa, Borelli had taught in the Sicilian university, and he immediately wrote to its senate, recommending the appointment of Malpighi.

In a temperate region, nature is garbed as a respectable matron, but in Messina she is arrayed as a wanton, in many colors and odors—the spectrum suffused in perfume; languorous and passionate, she is warmed by the sun of Sicily and bathed by the waters of the Mediterranean; with her extravagant and uncurbed beauty, in each generation she allures afresh the tribe of Theocritus. But Malpighi did not watch the tints of azure blend with the smell of myrtle; this poet's paradise was to him a workshop; he took out his tools and began his labors. The sea at his feet teemed with life; in the shark he found the spiral intestinal valve, and in the swordfish saw the twisted optic stalk. Of course he wrote about his researches to Borelli, who answered, "I was astounded by the drawings of the optic nerve of the swordfish, of which observations you should make great capital, and should easily find traces of this in other larger animals, such as the ox. If it proves to be so I should advise you to compose a treatise upon the subject and have it published."

The years at Messina were fruitful ones; Malpighi was in his early prime, and activity was a joy and a necessity. He thought of writing a great work on anatomy, reviewing the whole subject, and in accordance with this plan he completed a chapter on the circulation and on the lungs, but when Borelli and Fracassati heard of it, they objected loudly, telling him that such a task was for second-rate men, and that a Malpighi must not become a compiler; Malpighi's Sicilian patron, the enlightened Viscount Ruffi, joined in the protest, and Malpighi agreed to devote himself to original work exclusively.

He studied the brain, discerning the cortical cells and their connection with nerve fibers, and showing that the fibers of the white matter form tracts which connect the surface of the brain with various regions of the spinal cord. The papillae of the tongue were believed to be secretory in nature, but Malpighi merely stuck his tongue out, which soon became dry, and thus again an unpretentious fact overthrew an elaborate theory. Malpighi was able to demonstrate their provision of nerve filaments, and from this he deducted their gustatory function. He studied hair and feathers and skin; he discovered the papillae in the skin, and as they were most abundant where the sense of touch was most developed, he correctly announced that he had discovered the organ of touch. He further discovered the lower layer of the epidermis, the rete mucosum, since known as the Malpighian layer, and he pointed out that here accumulates the pigment that makes the negro black. The pigment in the white man's skin is the same as in the black man's skin, only the latter has more of it, but this simple anatomical fact has made the black man an outcast on the white man's earth.

While investigating fat, he made microscopic examinations of the mesenteric blood-vessels of the hedgehog, and in recording one of his observations, wrote, "And I myself in the omentum of the hedgehog in a blood-vessel which ran from one collection of fat to another opposite to it, saw globules of fat, of a definite outline, reddish in color. They presented a likeness to a chaplet of red coral." But like the Genoese sailor who discovered a new continent and knew it not, it was more than globules of fat that Malpighi saw—it was the red blood corpuscles; and his simple words were the first published record of the minute structures which have since been studied in infinite detail in every physiological laboratory. His discoveries in the liver, spleen and kidneys added greatly to our knowledge of glands; his fundamental work was so accurate that several structures in the body are still named after him.

Later, Malpighi began to cultivate and study the silkworm. He hatched them, watching them day by day, dissecting them at various stages. He described their external form, musculature, tracheae, nerves, heart, intestines, their habits, generative organs, egg-laying and silk-spinning apparatus—and he drew pictures of all that he saw. To prove the respiratory nature of the tracheae, he clogged up these organs with a drop of oil or honey, and the animal died in convulsions—while a monk might say a paternoster. He compared the silkworm with the locust, the pine-caterpillar and the firefly. Concerning his work on the silkworm, Malpighi has an interesting note:

> I tried to show not only the external mutations but the relations and structure of the viscera. This was a most tedious and laborious task, and fatigued by months of toil I was seized with a fever and an inflammation of my eyes in the autumn. Still, notwithstanding these difficulties, there was a mental delight in this work—in finding so many and puzzling miracles of nature that I cannot describe them with my pen. My collected observations, with drawings, I sent in the beginning of the year 1669 to the Royal Society.

Malpighi's next venture was in the vegetable kingdom. He had been interested in plants and trees at least since that day in Messina, when strolling with Giacomo Ruffi in the Visconte's garden, the friends found their path blocked by the overhanging branch of a chestnut tree; Malpighi snapped and broke the bough; the way was cleared, but Malpighi did not walk on: he stood there, looking at the vascular bundles which jutted from the fractured stem. That moment a botanist was born.

After that, Malpighi watched the growth of many plants. He studied the phanerogams and the pteridophyta, the rusts and smuts, the sporangia and the mosses, mucor and other molds. He made drawings and examinations of wood and bark, of medullary rays and tracheid vessels, of sclerenchyma and rings. He was not content to deal only with the architecture of plants: he tried to explain their physiology, and their laws of development. His views on the function of leaves in nutrition were correct. He was among the first to detect sexual differences in plants. He was the first to describe the tubercles that are produced by nitrifying bacteria on the roots of legumes. He worked out the development of ovum into seed, and of ovary into fruit. Malpighi's *Idea anatomes plantarum* was presented to the Royal Society of London in 1671, and the first sketch of it was read just as Nehemiah Grew's work on the same subject came from the press, and thus the names of the Englishman and the Italian are inseparably linked as the founders of plant morphology.

Malpighi next turned his sagacious eye upon the barnyard chick, and made it biologically famous: with it he created the science of embryology. He floated off the embryo in water and spread it on a glass slide, viewing the developing organs under his microscope. He described the changes he observed hour by hour. He saw and drew the formation and closure of the medullary groove, the primitive metameres, the formation of the cerebral vesicles, the appearance of the optic vesicles with their stalk, the development of the heart from a single bent tube to the arrangement of auricles and ventricles and aortic arches—and generation after generation of medical students have followed his eye and drawn as he has drawn. His work "On the Formation of the Chick in the Egg" (*De formatione pulli in ova*, 1672) is its history from the time that "the little opaque spot in the egg becomes a living, breathing, feathered bird."

Malpighi was now forty-four years of age, and was to do no more great work; but he rested on fadeless laurels. Even during his own lifetime, his name was honored wherever science was known. He saw his books published, not only in Bologna, but in London, Venice, Copenhagen, Leyden, Frankfort, Naples, Amsterdam, Paris and Geneva. Among his pupils were Baglivi, whose epigrams deserve to rank with those of Henri de Mondeville; and Lancisi, who demonstrated the syphilitic etiology of aneurysm; and Valsalva, whose name is preserved in Valsalva's sinus, and whose method of inflating the middle ear is still used.

It must not be thought that Malpighi's new ideas went altogether unchallenged. The obscurantist Michele Liparo wrote a violent tirade entitled the Triumph of the Galenists, which brought forth a response from Malpighi—the Apology of the Modernists. One of Malpighi's own pupils, Mini, backslid to Galenism, and lambasted his former master with a reactionary tract. His hereditary enemy, J. Hieronymo Sbaraglia, attacked him with arguments which have been thus summarized:

Of what use is the knowledge of the structure of the lung and the streaming of blood through it? Everyone knows that animals breathe, but no one knows why, and it may be said even that in this modern seventeenth century, with all this new knowledge at our command, we are not even quite as successful in curing pneumonia as were the fathers of old. Everyone thought, until the work of Wirsung, that the pancreas was just a cushion to support the stomach. What better off are we to know that it has a duct? Above all, of what use to cut up plants and study the hatching of eggs? Can we cure the troubles of women, knowing how the hatching of eggs goes on?

In these words we hear the immemorial voice of reaction, familiar in every age. Posterity has answered Sbaraglia's questions by answering: With Vesalius we stand on the threshold of modern biology; the work of Harvey unbolts the door; and with Malpighi we pass within.

One of the most versatile men of the century was the great Dane, Niels Stensen of Copenhagen. At the age of eighteen he became a pupil of Thomas Bartholin, a famous member of a famous family. Two years later the Swedes besieged the Danish capital, and Stensen was one of the students who defended the city. He was faithful in building ramparts and fighting the invaders, and during the intermission, in order not to waste time, he attended lectures at the university. Later we find him at Amsterdam, studying under Blasius. One morning, while dissecting the head of a sheep to examine the parotid gland, the point of his knife slipped down an opening and struck with a sharp click against the teeth, and the fortunate youth knew he had discovered the duct which has since been known as Stensen's duct. This observation was embodied in his *Observationes anatomicae*, published at Leyden, in 1662, in the twenty-fourth year of his age.

It may be mentioned that Blasius attempted to gain credit for this discovery, probably because it had been made under his roof, and he had the effrontery to present his claims to Bartholin, who answered him, "Farewell, and control yourself." To Stensen, Bartholin wrote a letter which was less epigrammatic and more hearty:

Your assiduity in investigating the secrets of the human body, as well as your fortunate discoveries, are highly praised by the learned of our country. The fatherland congratulates itself upon such a citizen, I upon such a pupil, through whose efforts anatomy makes daily progress and our lymphatic vessels are traced out more and more. You divide honors with Wharton, since you have added to his internal duct an external one, and have thereby discovered the sources of saliva concerning which many have hitherto dreamed much, but which no one has (permit the expression) pointed out with the finger. Continue, my Steno, to follow the path to immortal glory which true anatomy holds out to you.

When Stensen read this letter from his teacher, no doubt he vowed to follow the paths of science all his life; alas! it is easier to battle against the Swedes than to fight Fate. It is true that Stensen's first discovery led him to speculate brilliantly on secretory glands, and he added to his renown by his cerebral studies, and by proving that the heart is a muscle; later he wrote a book which won for him equal fame in an entirely different science —statigraphic geology, of which he is considered the founder; he was an accomplished linguist, speaking Hebrew, Greek, Latin, French, German, Dutch, English, Italian—but many languages could not save him.

Destiny waited for that fine brain, and at last beclouded it. Stensen, whose father was court jeweler at Copenhagen, had been brought up as a strict Lutheran, and it is said that at Paris when the distinguished Bossuet tried to make a Catholic of him, Stensen scornfully informed him that he had no time for such things. But Fate has time. In Italy, a chance conversation with an obscure monk—a nun, according to others—achieved what Bossuet had failed to accomplish: Stensen became a zealot. Such a convert was received most willingly by the Church; he was appointed Bishop of Titiopolis in Greece, and as Vicar Apostolic to the northern nations he traveled from place to place on a tour of proselytism. The nerves of the heart had never been satisfactorily delineated; many thought that the coagulation of blood was due to its cooling, but was this really the case? Glisson claimed that irritability was a specific property of all organized tissue, but no one had proved it. Here were problems for the sagacious Stensen, but they no longer tempted him. Clad in bishop's robes, he walked other paths, sorrowing for the souls of heretics. The apostle of physiology became its apostate.

An interesting and important worker, of similar fate, was Stensen's lifelong friend, Jan Swammerdam of Amsterdam. After Jan Swammerdam graduated in medicine, his father insisted that he practise, but the boy was too much of a scientist for that. They quarreled, and it was the father who yielded. Jan Swammerdam never wrote a prescription, but he observed the red blood corpuscles before Malpighi, although his observation was not published until many years later; he discovered the valves of the lymphatics, and was the first to announce that a lung which has once drawn the breath of life will not sink in water; also, he described 3,000 species of insects. When Swammerdam drew the finer anatomy of a mayfly or a bee or a worm, it was a work of art in miniature, and its richness of detail and delicacy of craftsmanship made the drawings of others look like rude sketches—he was able to correct some of the mistakes of Malpighi. His patience had no limit; in summer he began his task at dawn, and worked in the open as long as he could see; in order not to interrupt the light he wore no hat, and paid no attention to the sweat that streamed down his face.

There came an evil day for science and for Swammerdam—he read the books of Antoinette Bourignon. One would suppose that a noble intellect would turn in contempt from their irrational rant—frenzied statements actually raving against reason. But the mind of Swammerdam succumbed to the mystic jargon; the woman convinced him of the sinfulness of science: he joined her fanatical sect, and for the remainder of his life repeated its delirious babble. The hand that had been so cunning, no longer injected wax in the vessels of the queen bee; the works that he had written he did not publish, nor did they see print until he had long been dead; the long brass table, which Samuel Musschenbroek had made especially for him, and which had been

MEDICINE IN THE SEVENTEENTH CENTURY

so crowded with specimens for study and dissection, now stood empty and idle; upon it lay his scalpel unused—growing dull, like the brain of its owner. Jan Swammerdam, like another Stensen, became a lost leader of physiology.

We do not travel far in the latter seventeenth century before meeting, in one direction or another, Henry Oldenburg, the Admirable Crichton of the Royal Society of London. His versatility and urbanity, however, could not overcome his Bremenish name, and when it was discovered that he was corresponding with forty foreigners, Lord Arlington wrote a little note: "Warrant to seize the person of Henry Oldenburg for dangerous designs and practices, and to convey him to the Tower." Within a few months the government seemed convinced that Oldenburg's correspondence with Spinoza, Leeuwenhoek, Stensen, Swammerdam, and Malpighi, contained nothing dangerous, and he was released, whereupon the Royal Society resumed its meetings.

Who shall account for the remarkable growth of science in England at this time? What connection is there between a nation's political position and its scientific achievements? The student of the seventeenth century will be puzzled for an answer. Germany was despoiled by the Thirty Years' War and fell behind in culture, while Holland, which had thrown off the everaccursed yoke of Spain, could point to many glorious discoveries; but on the other hand, Italy was only a "geographical expression"—the property of Bourbon and Hapsburg, two families that have brought much misery to the human race—and yet at this time Italy produced several of her greatest men of science; while France, which was at the height of its commercial and military power, brought forth that barren medicine which deserved and excited the satire of Molière. Learning is believed to flourish best in the gardens of quietude, but the country that decapitated its king and established the Commonwealth, only to be later ravished by the Restoration, to say nothing of the Great Plague and the Great Fire, will not be accused of enjoying calmness. Possibly the reëstablishment of political tyranny by the son of Charles the First, made men seek an outlet in adultery or experimentation, but whatever the explanation may be, the fact remains that science became epidemic in London.

The poet Cowley wrote an Ode to the Royal Society, and Dryden apostrophized it, declaring it would soon enable us to converse with our celestial neighbors:

> Then we upon the globe's last verge shall go,
> And view the ocean leaning on the sky;
> From thence our rolling neighbors we shall know
> And on the lunar world securely pry.

The poetry is terrible, but the sentiment is there. Thomas Hobbes became a court favorite. To show the taste of the times it may be mentioned that John Locke, the philosopher-physician, received for the Conduct Concerning the Human Understanding, which is hardly more than a pamphlet, thrice the amount that Milton received for Paradise Lost, a poem of over 10,000 lines.

The Duke of Buckingham worshiped the trinity of wine, woman, and chemistry. The valiant Prince Rupert dropped molten glass into cold water, thereby inventing the brittle curiosity that has since been known as Prince Rupert's Drops. The Duchess of Newcastle came to one of the Society's meetings, and for her benefit the Fellows weighed a large receiver from which the air had been exhausted, and after placing it on a scale the air was allowed to enter—and the container weighed more; then they took two cool liquids, and mixed them together, and to the delight of Her Grace, the fluid became hot.

Charles II fitted up a laboratory at Whitehall, and performed amateurish experiments with mercury and phosphorus. In Pepys' Diary we find this: "Charles the Second saw Dr. Clarke and Mr. Pierce dissect two bodies, a man and a woman, with which his majesty was highly pleased." But although the Merry Monarch styled himself the Founder and Patron of the Royal Society, he never once visited its meeting-rooms, and at times when its finances were so low that it was about to disband, he offered no pecuniary aid, but spent much money on the caprices of his mistresses. During the last ten or fifteen years of his reign he did not seem to be aware that the Society existed, and held no communication with it whatsoever. That the Society resented this attitude of indifference need occasion no surprise: when the king died, the Royal Society did not adjourn, and no record of his decease is to be found in the minutes.

A more wide-awake group than these Fellows never gathered together. Whenever they heard of a new book, they read it; whenever they heard of a new experiment, they repeated it. They discussed their observations of Saturn and the history of wax-candles; they were interested in a new star and in the development of clothing; they inquired about Africa and about the man who lived without a spleen; they investigated earthquakes and a double goose-egg; they asked about a key to the Chinese language and whether the venereal disease existed in Numidia; they studied magnetism and the heart of an eel; they paid attention to the ebb and flow of the sea and to the corroding effects of cider on a knife; they were attracted by a new classification of birds and by an individual who could remain three hours under water. Although some of their experiments, as reviving drowned animals, and transfusing blood from dog to dog, and from sheep to man, and from a youth to an old man, produced more wonder than results, both by the universality of their sympathies and by the splendor of their discoveries, the Royal Society of London became the foremost of scientific associations.

That genius of architecture, Christopher Wren, early stated, "The Royal Society should plant crabstocks for posterity to graft on." His own experimental contributions were highly original. Toward the end of his career, if Sir Christopher had been asked what he considered his principal achievement, he would probably have pointed to St. Paul's Cathedral—but physicians remember him because in his twenty-fourth year he suggested to Robert Boyle the possibility of intravenous medication. Wren and Boyle then injected opium and crocus metallorum into the veins of dogs, and Samuel Pepys was much excited by the new wonder. Richard Lower's important work in transfusion was published in the first volume of the Royal Society's *Philosophical Transactions* (1666). The time was hardly ripe for such a method, for when Sigmund Elsholz of Berlin heard of it, he "proposed to reconcile all unhappy marriages by the reciprocal transfusion of the blood of incompatible consorts." Today Wren's suggestion has become a recognized therapeutic procedure.

To think of the Royal Society is to think of Robert Hooke, one of the most amazing names in science. As a child he was too frail to study for his father's profession—a parish minister. Later he was employed by the wealthy Robert Boyle, the foremost chemist of the age. After the great fire destroyed London, Hooke submitted a plan for the reconstruction of the city, and although the model of Sir Christopher Wren was finally adopted, Hooke's idea was much admired, and when a new London was rising out of the ashes, Hooke's services were constantly in demand as a surveyor and builder, an occupation which netted him quite a fortune.

Hooke was early appointed curator of the Royal Society, his duty being to perform experiments, and so inexhaustible were his intellectual resources, that for several years he announced new discoveries at almost every meeting. To whatever path of science we turn, in the vanguard we will find the footsteps of Robert Hooke. He was the greatest of the English microscopists, and his *Micrographia,* published in 1665, contained the first description and drawings of the biologic cell. He was the only man of his century who knew the art of auscultation—he listened to the voice of the heart and lungs. He made a crucial experiment in respiration: opening the chest of a dog and puncturing the lungs, he kept the animal alive by blowing a bellows over the opened thorax, thus demonstrating that the essential requirement of respiration is not movement of the lungs, but a supply of fresh air. He was a wizard in mechanics, and his inventions in flying-machines, air-pumps, watches, microscopes, telescopes, and meteorological instruments were almost countless. With equal ease and ingenuity he could speculate on the movements of heavenly bodies, and make experiments with a bubble of soap and water.

Those who came to see Hooke, attracted by his fame, must have been surprised at his appearance: he had a crooked figure with shrunken limbs, and his uncombed hair fell like a shaggy mane over an ashen countenance—and he grew smaller and more deformed with the years. His character was as unprepossessing as his body: he was too miserly to be immoral, but he was crabbed, sour, jealous, vain, and morbid. All this must be admitted, but behind those unfriendly eyes and disheveled locks burnt the fire of genius.

Hooke was not satisfied to make only half the discoveries of his age—he claimed also the other half. That is why his contemporary, Sir Thomas Molyneux, wrote of him, "Hooke, the most ill-natured conceited man in the world, hated and despised by most of the Royal Society, pretending to have all other inventions, when once discovered by their authors to the world." Hooke was indeed the gadfly of the Society, stinging even the lofty Newton into exasperation. When the *Principia* was in process of publication—at the personal expense of the abused Halley, as the Royal Society had not sufficient funds at this time—Hooke so insistently proclaimed that part of the work was stolen from him, that Newton determined to suppress a third of the volume, and would have done so, had it not been for the earnest and indignant remonstrances of Halley. Later, when Newton completed *Optics*, he ascertained that Hooke had claims upon it, and he refused to publish it during the lifetime of the curator: he kept his work in manuscript until the bitter tongue of Robert Hooke was silenced forever. Hooke had existed so sordidly as practically to deny himself the necessities of life, but upon his death several thousand pounds were found in an old iron chest whose rusty key had been unused for thirty years. His precious money he had kept to himself—only his genius he had flung abroad.

The seventeenth century, looking through the microscope, saw an invisible world hitherto hidden from men. The Jesuit of

Fulda, Athanasius Kircher, foremost German scholar of the age, earliest student of Egyptian hieroglyphics, a worker in linguistic, archeological, mathematical, philosophical and biological fields, was a pioneer microscopist. Kircher was the first to cast a suspicious eye upon recently-revealed microörganisms, already regarding them as the cause of infectious diseases. Examining the blood and pus of plague-patients, he described broods of worms; what he really saw with his low-power microscope—it could not have been the *Bacillus pestis*—is not as important as his realization of the connection between disease and germs. In ascribing contagion to living organisms (*contagia animata*), he went beyond Fracastorius. Such Kircherian observations as "Flies feeding on the juices of the diseased and dying, hurry off and deposit their excretions on food, and persons eating it are infected," and "Struggle and counter-struggle maintain life," were compelled to wait until recent times for biologic confirmation.

The family of van Leeuwenhoek acquired wealth and respectability in the brewing business, and for thirty-nine years, undoubtedly through influence, Antony van Leeuwenhoek was officially the janitor of the city hall of Delft. Untaught, knowing no language but Dutch, obstinate and opinionated, he ground hundreds of lenses of short focal length, and what he saw through his home-made microscopes was an epoch in bacteriology. The Royal Society of London got hold of him, just as it had of Malpighi, and Leeuwenhoek drew for their Philosophical Transactions of 1683 the first published pictures of bacteria. He discovered protozoa, infusoria, rotatoria, and the yeast plant—he tried his microscope on everything. One day the student Johann Hamm asked him to observe what he found swimming under the lens—and thus were spermatozoa first seen.

The first man who shed light on the problem of equivocal generation was the seventeenth century physician-poet, Francesco Redi of Arezzo, who came to the conclusion that the maggots found in decaying meat were not produced spontaneously by the meat, but had been deposited there by flies. His proof consisted in covering meat with a fine gauze, through which the putrescent odor escaped: the flies buzzed around it, but as the meshes were too small to permit their eggs to fall through, no maggots were generated in the meat, but were hatched on the gauze.

In practical medicine there was endless activity. At this period we meet Willis, who differentiated between diabetes mellitus and diabetes insipidus; Walter Harris, who adumbrated what we now term acidosis; Glisson, who published a classic account of rickets; Thuillier, who showed that ergot was due to corn smut; Bontius, who described beriberi; Colle and Musitano, who showed that syphilis could be conveyed by kissing and from drinking-vessels; Guarinoni, who described gummata of the brain; Ramazzini, who opened up new medical territory—the immense field of trade-diseases; and John Floyer, the first to count the pulse with a minute watch.

A century may inherit a feud in the same manner that a family does. The sixteenth century handed down to the seventeenth century the quarrel about antimony: Besnier was expelled from the Paris Faculty for daring to prescribe the proscribed stibium. But Besnier was no hero: he recanted, and was received again into the Faculty and into oblivion. He thus took his place beside John Geynes, who had been censured by the Royal College of Physicians of London "for impugning the infallibility of Galen. On his acknowledgment of error, and humble recantation, signed with his own hand, he was received into the College."

Unlike Geynes and Besnier, Theodore Turquet was not afflicted with weak knees; he prescribed mineral remedies, and when the Faculty growled its disapproval, Turquet went on prescribing mineral remedies—including antimony. The enraged Faculty accordingly issued this proclamation: "All physicians who practise medicine anywhere are admonished to banish from themselves and their thresholds the said Turquet, and all similar monsters of mankind and monstrosities of opinion, and to remain true to Galen."

Turquet was also a Huguenot, and as seventeenth-century

France was not big enough to hold a man with two heresies, Turquet came to England. Every nation exiles her best sons, and often they become the glories of other lands. In England, Turquet rose high: he was knighted, took the name of de Mayerne, was appointed chief adviser to the king and queen at a salary four times as large as that of the ordinary royal physician, while a comfortable annuity was settled upon his wife. These things, however, mean nothing, for several notorious charlatans of the period likewise basked in the sun of royal favor. But Sir Theodore incorporated the Society of Apothecaries, which separated the pharmacist from the grocer; he was largely responsible for the publication of the first London Pharmacopoeia, for which he wrote the preface; with Sydenham and Glisson he made a stand for bedside teaching, and he is the man who introduced calomel into practice.

After Adrian Mynsicht's discovery of tartarated antimony, numerous patients were vomited into health, but antimony remained under the ban until tartar emetic cured Louis XIV of a dangerous illness. The Paris Faculty found it expedient not to condemn a remedy which had helped a king.

The three most popular eponymic salts date from this period. Pierre Seignette, apothecary at Rochelle, introduced the combination of sodium and potassium tartrate known as Rochelle salt; in a mineral spring at Vienna, Johann Rudolph Glauber discovered sodium sulphate, or Glauber's salt; while in the waters of Epsom, Nehemiah Grew discovered magnesium sulphate, and since then few have been able to escape Epsom salt.

Similar progress was achieved in the vegetable domain, both by the appraisal of old drugs and by the introduction of new ones. The therapeutic reputation of opium was established by the foremost physicians. Franciscus Sylvius said he would not practise without opium; van Helmont prescribed it so frequently that he was called Doctor Opiatus; and Sydenham said: "Without it the healing art would cease to exist, and by its help a skillful physician is enabled to perform cures that seem almost miraculous."

In the opening years of the seventeenth century the life of Clusius was closing, but he gave us the original accounts of Winter's bark, canella bark, vanilla, pimenta, bearberry leaves, gamboge and star-anise. Travelers in all parts of the world sent native drugs to the European botanists: Colombo root, ipecac, copaiba, catechu, cimicifuga, cowhage, pareira brava, Iceland moss, cascarilla and serpentaria. But of far greater importance than this collection was a bark that had been brought over from Peru.

In 1638, a lady's ague was responsible for a medical revolution. Ana, Countess of Chinchon, living in Peru which her husband ruled as viceroy, lay ill with malaria. Her physician, Juan de Vego, received a package of powdered Peruvian bark, with the assurance that it cured tertian fever. It proved a specific, and upon her recovery, Ana sent large quantities of the bark to her sick friends. It was spoken of as the Countess' Powder, and within a year its virtues were known in Europe. There the Jesuits popularized the febrifuge—hence called the Powder of the Cardinal, or Jesuits' Powder—but the story that they gave it to the poor for nothing, and sold it to the rich for its weight in gold, is an exaggeration in both directions.

The controversies that were fought over Peruvian bark (*Cortex Cinchonae*) were fully as bitter as the drug itself. Valiant Protestants swore they would rather die than be saved by Jesuits' Powder. Orthodox physicians, with the fear of the Paris Faculty in their hearts, refused to prescribe a remedy unknown to Galen. Fever was regarded as due to a decoction of humors, causing effervescence; to expel the peccant humors, the *materies morbi,* was a matter of months; debilitating medicines were required during the fever and restorative medicines afterwards; bloodletting and evacuants weakened the patient, therefore wormwood and valerian were needed to strengthen him—it was all very logical. But this new bark from the Peruvian wilderness, instead of voiding the "corrupted humors," ended intermittent fever before there was time to read a chapter of

Galen. It was certain, therefore, that by "fixing the humors," it established a disease more dangerous than the original one.

The fear or favor of College or Faculty did not weigh upon a certain apothecary, for he possessed no qualifications they could impugn. At various times he called himself Tabor, Talbor and Talbot, but his baptismal name of Robert was permanent. This man, shrewd enough to see the merits of Peruvian bark, advertised he possessed a secret remedy that triumphed over disease and kept death at bay. His successful treatment of Lady Mordaunt's daughter brought him to the chamber of Charles II, and the apothecary looked at a king in chills and fever. Charles could be generous, and Talbor received an annuity under the Privy Seal, and "for good and acceptable services performed" was appointed royal physician, although he was not any sort of physician. Charles warned the College of Physicians not to interfere with Talbor's medical practice, and His Majesty further showed his gratitude by conferring knighthood upon him—it was a case of one quack honoring another quack.

Sir Robert Talbor, under the name of Talbot, next appears in France. The silly but sprightly letters of Mme. de Sévigné keep us informed of his progress: "Nothing is talked of here but the Englishman and his cures . . . when his remedy is published, all physicians will be superfluous. . . . M. de Hautefort is dead, so there is another blue ribbon vacant. He could never be prevailed on to take the English medicine, because it was too expensive. He was told that at most it would not cost more than forty pistoles. It is too much, said he, and then expired." Talbot's great opportunity came when the Dauphin was sick, but we must let Mme. de Sévigné continue the story:

> The English physician has promised the King, at the price of his head, to cure the Dauphin in four days. If he should fail, I really believe they will throw him out of the window, but if he succeeds I say a temple should be erected to him as to a second Aesculapius.
>
> It is a pity Molière is dead; he would make an excellent scene of D'Aquin [Louis XIV's chief physician], who is driven to his wit's end, at not being possessed of this panacea; and the rest of the tribe,

who are overwhelmed with despair at the experience, the success, and the almost divine prognostications of this little foreigner. The King will have him make up his medicines in his presence, and trusts the management of the Prince wholly to him. The Dauphiness is already much better; and yesterday the Count de Grammont saluted D'Aquin with the following:

> D'Aquin can no longer withstand
> Talbot, victorious over death;
> The princess owns his healing hand,
> Let each one sing with joyful breath, etc.

Talbot was again successful, whereupon D'Aquin insisted the Dauphin had been bilious and never in serious danger; his words were drowned in the flood of praise that greeted "the Englishman's cure." Louis XIV deigned to request him to remain on French soil, as an ornament to the nation. As Talbor declined, the king purchased his formula with the understanding that it would not be divulged during the inventor's lifetime. Aside from an annual pension, Talbor received two thousand guineas, and the title of Chevalier. The world had not long to wait for the "Wonderful Secret for Cureing of Agues and Feavers," for upon the heels of his royal triumphs, Talbor died at the age of forty (1681). Louis XIV ordered his surgeon, Nicolas de Blegny, to publish Talbor's method, which was immediately translated into English "for Publick Good." The official formula consisted of rose leaves soaked in water with lemon juice, to which was added a strong dose of Peruvian bark. Such was the seventeenth-century romance of a disguised infusion of cinchona.

The outstanding figure in internal medicine was Thomas Sydenham of Wyndford Eagle in Dorset. His studies were interrupted frequently by the Civil Wars in which he fought as a Puritan captain of horse. The grant he received from Cromwell, for faithfully serving the parliament with the loss of much blood, enabled him to set up in practice and get married. Sydenham was wholly unaware of the anatomical and physiological progress that his contemporaries were making, and he stood apart from the main currents of his age. Except Hippocrates, whom he acknowledged as his model, he avoided reading any medical books. Perhaps his ignorance of the prevailing theories was an asset, for therapeutics in the seventeenth century required heroic patients.

In fact, some of Sydenham's own cases show us how far we have advanced since then. One January (year not given) the medical student, Thomas Dover of Warwickshire, residing in Sydenham's house, had the smallpox—and years afterwards he told us how the master treated him: "First I was bled to the extent of twenty-two ounces; then an emetic. I had no fire allowed in my room, my windows were constantly open, my bed-clothes were ordered to be laid no higher than my waist. He made me take twelve bottles of small beer, acidulated with spirit of vitriol, every twenty-four hours."

It is not surprising that Dover eventually decided pirateering was as safe as physic, and more lucrative: on an adventurous voyage around the world, he anchored at the island of Juan Fernandez, taking on board its solitary human inhabitant—the immortal Robinson Crusoe; plundered the city of Guayaquil in Peru; combated a plague by making his sailors drink dilute sulphuric acid; sailed past the Cape of Good Hope, and reached home, loaded with wealth, in a Spanish prize. When he grew too old for buccaneering he practised medicine and wrote *The Ancient Physician's Legacy to his Country*, which contains his diaphoretic prescription of ipecac and opium, still popular as Dover's powder (*Pulvis ipecacuanhae et opii*).

Sydenham may have remained aloof from his colleagues, but he could not escape the maladies which afflicted so many of them. He too suffered from gout and gravel, and his self-treatment was as follows: "In the morning, when I rise, I drink a dish or two of tea, and then ride in my coach till noon; when I return home, I moderately refresh myself with any sort of meat, of easy digestion, that I like (for moderation is necessary above all things), I drink somewhat more than a quarter of a pint of canary wine, immediately after dinner, every day, to promote digestion of the food in my stomach, and to drive the gout from my bowels. When I have dined, I betake myself to my coach again and when business will permit, I ride into the country two or three miles for good air. A draught of small beer is to me instead of supper, and I take another draught when I am in bed, and about to compose myself to sleep." We have since learned that this is the way not to treat gout.

When Sydenham sat down at the bedside, his observations were Hippocratic in scope and character. We owe to him the first satisfactory description of acute rheumatism which he separated from gout, and of scarlet fever which he differentiated from measles. His clinical pictures of hysteria and chorea are classic. Had he remained with Thomas Wharton in London at the time of the great plague, and had he survived, he would undoubtedly have left a valuable account of the pestilence. Sydenham looked upon disease, not as a malignant demon to be exorcised, but in the Hippocratic spirit of the healing power of nature. The title of "English Hippocrates," now invariably applied to him, was of posthumous origin, for Sydenham never heard that pleasing designation. He was not a fellow of the Royal Society or of the College of Physicians—a little oversight which the College has never ceased to regret—and he was not buried in Westminster Abbey.

The leading English surgeon of the period, Richard Wiseman, summed up his lifework in *Severall Surgicall Treatises* (1676). He devised a method of cutting stricture in gonorrhea, and was the first to describe tuberculosis of joints as white swelling (*tumor albus*). In many respects he was reactionary: he knew of Paré's method of controlling hemorrhage with the ligature, but preferred the actual cautery and the "Royal Styptic." Wiseman was an ardent believer in the miracles wrought by the blood of Charles I, yet was inconsistent enough to marry a regicide's granddaughter. He was the staunchest advocate of the Royal Touch for the King's Evil—the once universal belief that diseases such as scrofula could be cured if the king touched them. It is not the air, nor the journey, nor the imagination, nor the token hung around the neck that affects the cure, said Wiseman, but the divine power of healing inherent in the sovereign. Wiseman claimed he saw Charles II effect cures, times without number, and it has been estimated that 90,798 invalids sought healing at the degenerate hand of this Stuart.

To question the efficacy of the Royal Touch was infidelity, for the gift had been transmitted to the kings of England from the Great Physician: "Lord, if thou wilt, thou canst make me clean. And he put forth his hand, and touched him, saying, I will: be thou clean. And immediately the leprosy departed from him." The foremost intellectuals of the age, including Sir Thomas Browne, believed in it, and the famous diarists allude to the practice. Pepys wrote: "Staid to see the King touch people for the King's evil. But he did not come at all, it rayned so; and the poor people were forced to stand all the morning in the rain in the garden. Afterward he touched them in the Banquetting House." Later John Evelyn recorded: "There was so great a concourse of people with their children to be touched for the Evil, that 6 or 7 were crushed to death by pressing at the chirurgeon's doore for tickets."

The seventeenth century was notable for improved instruments, yet the surgical achievements are indeed disappointing. The gulf between physician and surgeon was not yet bridged: the physician scorned to think surgically, and the surgeon feared to trespass on medicine. The sterilization of surgery at this time lies squarely at the door of the Paris Faculty. Its dean, that interesting bigot, Guy Patin, proclaimed the surgeons "a race of evil, extravagant coxcombs who wear mustaches and flourish razors."

Toward the end of the century, however, an accident changed the status of surgery. The all-powerful Louis XIV awoke one morning and found himself afflicted with the condition which John of Arderne had described in so masterly a manner. It was a delicate situation, but the truth had to be told: Louis was suffering from fistula-in-ano. Surgical intervention was imperative, and since common hands could not touch the sun-god, policy required that the king's surgeon, Charles-François Felix, be en-

MEDICINE IN THE SEVENTEENTH CENTURY

nobled. Courtiers, healthy enough but eager to prove their loyalty, demanded similar operations upon themselves. Fistula-in-ano became fashionable, and the French surgeon was a social success. In consequence, later on, several chairs of surgery were established, and withstood the assaults of pedantry. The story of the Paris Faculty, arrayed in wrath and their red robes, brandishing a skeleton and parading the streets in protest, defied by the surgeons and teased by a mob that had long cringed at sight of their gowns, the dignity of the doctors finally disappearing in a snow-storm which seemed made to order, constitutes a surgical melodrama.

But if seventeenth century surgery did not advance further than Paré, workers in anatomy and physiology poured far beyond the broad gate that the scalpel of Vesalius had opened: half the structures in the human body are named after seventeenth century men—Graafian follicles, Haversian canals, Glaserian fissure, Pacchionian bodies, Bellini's tubes, antrum of Highmore, Malpighian layer, circle of Willis, valves of Kerkring, Schneiderian membrane, Glisson's capsule, Casserio's artery, Peyer's patches, Lower's tubercle, Pecquet's cistern, Poupart's ligament, Wormian bones, Ruysch's tunica, Spigelian lobe, Ridley's sinus, Riolan's muscle, Tulpius' valve, Vieussens' ganglion, Nuck's canal, Wirsung's duct, Wharton's duct, Stensen's duct, Rivini's duct, Bartholin's glands, Brunner's glands, Cowper's glands, Meibomian glands.

The cultural contributions of the seventeenth century are Periclean. We need only name Shakespeare, Cervantes, Molière, Milton, in literature; the second Bacon, Descartes, Spinoza, Locke, in philosophy; Rubens, Van Dyck, Velasquez, Rembrandt, in art. This is the century of Galileo and Newton, of Kepler and Wallis, of Halley and Flamsteed, of Wren and Petty, of Huyghens and von Guericke, of Napier and Briggs, of Torricelli and Sanctorius—the golden age of mathematicians, astronomers and physicists, when for the first time the heavens really spoke to the earth. "In consequence of the innumerable new books," complained the industrious Leibnitz, "even the greatest literati cannot survey the whole field. Our scientific life has become a mere slop-shop."

The increase in positive knowledge was unprecedented, yet there is no period in history which more truly deserves the designation of Age of Intolerance. Every one was convinced his sect alone was acceptable to God, and equally convinced of the damnation of all other sects. Science was not yet able to battle with this dogma of "Exclusive Salvation." Moreover, the farther science deviated from the cosmography of Moses, the more virulent grew the persecution, and the more conspicuous the religious funerals. The seventeenth century was blood-drenched over myths. Medicine is a child of the times, and is never in advance of its environment. Official medicine subscribed to all current superstitions, and aided in their dissemination. In spite of the profession's reputation for skepticism, enlightened spirits among the physcians were not more numerous than among other classes. Technical knowledge is not the antidote of credulity.

We now approach the ghastliest page in the melancholy annals of the human race—it is headed Witchcraft, and is dated the Seventeenth Century. There were witches in the primitive world, and in the first civilizations; a Jew wrote "Thou shalt not suffer a witch to live," and Christendom obeyed the injunction; in the early middle ages, Augustine declared that witches indulge in sexual intercourse with the devil, and it is impudence to deny it; the two greatest theologians of the latter middle ages, Albertus Magnus and Thomas Aquinas, were firm believers in witchcraft; the Bull of Pope Innocent VIII (*Summis desiderantes,* 1484), followed by the Handbook of the Witches' Hammer (*Malleus Maleficarum,* or *Hexenhammer,* 1486), were powerful weapons in the eager hands of the witch hunters.

Men began to appear in court, charged with kissing Satan under the tail, and in giving him four of their hairs in exchange for diabolical knowledge; women were accused of making men impotent with an ointment, and of riding through the air on a broomstick to attend the Witches' Sabbat; children were compelled to confess they had intercourse with incubi and succubi;

documents signed in blood were exhibited, and witnesses swore they saw the prisoners dancing with demons on barren moors. Torture, death and confiscation of property were the penalties, yet the persecutions were unorganized and spasmodic, and some of the accused were allowed to go home. The mania grew worse in the Renaissance, and in the seventeenth century became furiously pandemic.

Such was the frenzy at Niesse, and so numerous the victims, that the stake was found too costly, and they were roasted in a huge oven. Not the dark ages, not medieval times, but the enlightened seventeenth century was the Era of the Witch Hunt. Then sons went to the authorities and accused their mothers of being witches, and children denounced themselves for their sexual practices with Satan; women were stripped naked by jailers who thrust with needles for anesthetic areas known as devil's marks—an infallible sign of witchcraft—and many women who withstood the torture, begged for a cloth to cover their nakedness. There were villages in which every old woman had been burnt, but the young were not immune. The prince-bishop of Würzburg, who counted that day lost in which he did not kill a witch, has left us this record of one of his holocausts:

> In the twentieth burning, six persons: Babelin Goebel, the prettiest girl in Würzburg; a student in the fifth form who knew many languages and was an excellent musician, instrumental and vocal; two boys from the new minster, twelve years old; Babel Stepper's daughter; the caretaker on the bridge.

The spread of sorcery, fostered by persecution, gave the Inquisition new power, for witchcraft was considered equivalent to heresy, always punishable with death; and more wealth, for the Inquisition never regarded the property of heretics as undesirable. In the seventeenth century, when a pair of inquisitors walked through a town looking for witches, armed with the *Malleus Maleficarum*, there was no possibility of escape; all the accused, man and woman, child and infant, were tortured, driven insane and executed; before death, to escape further torture, they named all acquaintances as accomplices, who in turn were made to name all theirs, for witch hunting was a ceaseless occupation. The Protestants were equally diligent. The jurist Carpzov found leisure, between fifty-three readings of the Bible, to condemn 20,000 witches; among them was the Saxon physician, Viet Pratzel, whom Carpzov tortured and burnt, at the same time bleeding his children to death, since offspring of a witch could not help belonging to the devil.

Victims who died under torture were sometimes declared innocent, but the most stubborn resistance was only additional evidence that the devil was hardening them. "Do you believe in witches?" was the inquisitor's first question. To answer Yes meant forbidden knowledge, to answer No meant heresy, and both answers meant death. Women were thrown into the water, with thumbs and toes tied crosswise—if they floated they were guilty, since the water repudiated their baptism. "God reveals the truth through the thumb-screw," was a favorite expression of the witch hunters. The accused were compelled to kneel on spike-covered prayer-stools, and enter cages so constructed as to render existence unbearable; they were chased up and down their cells until exhausted, or whirled around until reason left them; they were fed on salt fish without water, and bathed in quicklime; the jailers flayed the skin and broke body and spirit; every limb was stretched on the rack and every joint dislocated; no sensitive spot escaped a candle-flame or the red-hot iron; pliers extracted the finger-nails with the roots, and bones were crushed until the marrow spurted out. The written records of inquisitors and judges reveal how thoroughly they relished their work in the name of God—the witch hunt enables us to see human nature unmasked.

In England the witch panic began under Elizabeth, and was continued by her successor who was a witch-killer "with great delight"; in his *Daemonologia,* he condemns the skeptical attitude of the German physician John Weyer, and the British hop-grower Reginald Scot; upon mounting the throne, James I burned Scot's *Discouerie of Witchcraft,* and would have put the author in the same flame if he had been alive. It is difficult, however, to blame a demented monarch for harboring a delusion which was accepted by such a man as Sir Thomas Browne, who wrote in his Religion of a Physician (*Religio Medici,* 1643): "For my part, I have ever believed and do now know, that there are Witches: they that doubt of these, do not onely deny them, but Spirits; and are obliquely and upon consequence a sort not of Infidels, but Atheists. Those that to confute their incredulity desire to see apparitions, shall questionless never behold any, nor have the power to be so much as Witches; the Devil hath them already in a heresie as capital as Witchcraft; and to appear to them, were but to convert them." Years later, "that famous scholar and physitian" expressed his opinion in court that Amy Duny and Rose Cullender were witches, and his testimony helped to convict them. Thus, Sir Thomas Browne, one of the most tolerant and cultivated men of his time, and much admired at the present day, takes his place with Matthew Hopkins among the British witch-finders.

In the English colonies, Cotton Mather reasoned as follows: Satan had been in undisturbed possession of America until the Puritan invasion of Massachusetts, hence Satan is seeking his revenge in this vicinity. Cotton Mather, spiritual guide of New England, abetted by his father, Increase Mather, stampeded the courts and was mainly responsible for the witch craze of Salem and the judicial murders. John Evelyn noted in his diary: "Unheard-of stories of the universal increase of witches in New England; men, women, and children devoting themselves to the devil, so as to threaten the subversion of the government." Satan was now an international figure, his power and sovereignty acknowledged on both sides of the Atlantic. In America the witch disease was sharp but brief, and the Mathers lived to see Samuel Sewall—the judge who had condemned the witches at their bidding—stand in meeting, accepting "the blame and shame" of the Salem delusion and craving pardon.

Germany, in the throes of the Thirty Years' War, suffered beyond any other country from the witch-plague. At Bamberg, for several years, the prince-bishop John George, with his assistant Förner and the lawyers Braun and Kötzendörffer, kept up a witches' revel, the gold increasing with the blood they spilled: these four men indulged in a soul-satisfying orgy of sadism that has never been surpassed. They aimed high, their victims including John Junius, five times Burgomaster of Bamberg. His blameless reputation, the resolution with which he withstood the thumb-screws and Spanish boots, availed nothing, for upon sticking him with pins they discovered a devil's mark. Junius was doomed, and knew that his goods and chattels, coveted by bishop and inquisitors, contributed to his ruin. The torture was terrible, and unable to endure it the next day, he confessed whatever was desired.

Did he have intercourse with a female demon? Yes. Did she turn into a he-goat? Yes. Had he been at the witch-dances? Yes? Where? He did not know what to say, but remembered that Elsa Hopffen swore she saw him dancing on Haupt's moor, so he answered Haupt's moor. Who else was there? They gave him no peace until he named twenty-seven persons they wanted. What did the devil make him do? So he swore the devil told him to kill his children. Did he not take a sacramental wafer and bury it? Yes. He was sentenced to be beheaded and burnt, and as he waited in prison for the inevitable end, he managed to send out a letter, to his daughter, which reads in part:

Many hundred thousand good-nights, my dearest daughter Veronica! Guiltless was I taken to prison, guiltless have I been tortured, guiltless I must die. For whoever comes to the witch prison must either be a sorcerer, or is tortured until (God pity him) he makes up a confession of sorcery out of his head. I'll tell you how I fared. . . .

Then came the executioner and put on the thumb-screws, my hands being tied together, so that the blood spurted from under the nails, and I cannot use my hands these four weeks, as you may see by this writing. Then they tied my hands behind and drew me up. I thought heaven and earth were disappearing. Eight times they drew me up and let me fall so that I suffered horrible agony. All which time I was stark naked, for they had me stripped. . . .

When the executioner took me back to prison, he said to me, "Sir, for God's sake confess something, whether true or not. Think a little. You can't stand the tortures they'll inflict on you, and even if you could you wouldn't escape, though you were a count, but they'll go through them again and again and never leave you till you say you are a sorcerer, as may be seen by all their judgments, for all end alike." Another came and said the bishop had determined to make an example of me which would astonish people, and begged me for God's sake to make up something, for I should not escape even though I were innocent, and so said Neudecker and others. . . .

There, dearest child, you have all my confession, for which I must die, and it is nothing but lies and made-up things, so God help me. For I had to say all this for fear of the tortures threatened me, besides all those I had gone through. For they go on torturing till one confesses something; be he as pious as he will, he must be a sorcerer. No one escapes, though he were a count. And if God does not interfere, all our friends and relations will be burnt, for each has to confess as I had. . . .

Dear child, keep this letter secret so that nobody sees it, or I shall be horribly tortured and the gaoler will lose his head, so strict is the rule against it. You may let Cousin Stamer read it quickly in private. He will keep it secret. Dear child, give this man a thaler.

I have taken some days to write this. Both my hands are lamed. I am in a sad state altogether. I entreat you by the last judgment, keep this letter secret, and pray for me after my death as for your martyred father . . . but take care no one hears of this letter. . . .

Dear child, six denounced me: the chancellor, his son, Neudecker, Zaner, Ursula Hoffmaister, and Elsa Hopffen, all falsely and on compulsion as they all confessed. They begged my pardon for God's sake before they were executed. They said they knew nothing of me but what was good and loving. They were obliged to name me, as I should find out myself. I cannot have a priest, so take heed of what I have written, and keep this letter secret.

Good-night, for your father, John Junius, will see you never more.
24th July, 1628.

Paper outlasts flesh and blood; the bishops and inquisitors, the lawyers and witnesses are dust with their victims. In the library at Bamberg, in broken handwriting, the letter of John

Junius may still be read. The date at the bottom arrests our attention: it is 1628, the year that *De motu cordis* was printed at Frankfort. The medical historian, focusing on William Harvey's book, calls the seventeenth century the Age of Science.

X

MEDICINE IN THE EIGHTEENTH CENTURY

THE story of medicine in the eighteenth century opens with the name of Hermannus Boerhaave, who occupied most of the chairs in the university of Leyden. In 1701, he delivered his inaugural address on the Father of Medicine, urging all his sons to follow in his footsteps. His *Institutiones medicae* (1708), in its various editions, was acknowledged as the medical textbook of a continent; his *Aphorismi* (1709) recalled his Hellenic master, and Boerhaave was indeed known as the Batavian Hippocrates: his pupils, Gerard van Swieten and Anton de Haen wrote volumes of commentaries on these aphorisms, thus becoming his Galens. Thirty years after his first oration, when he signed his name to his last book (*Elementa chemiae,* 1731), he was the world's most famous physician, and Holland was the schoolmaster of Europe. An extraordinary number of professors had either studied under Boerhaave, or were the pupils of his pupils.

His influence was salutary, and we may be grateful for the accident which turned him to science. Boerhaave was the son of a clergyman, and intending to follow the same calling, his first studies were in theology. One day he was sitting in a public boat with a group of passengers who were also students of divinity: at least, they were good and pious men, spending the voyage in denouncing one of their countrymen, a certain Dutch Jew. This Jew had been cursed by his own people for heresy, had died young and was buried like a dog. They predicted his name would soon be forgotten. His name was Spinoza. One of the speakers was unusually abusive, and Boerhaave turned to him with the inquiry, "Have you ever read Spinoza?" The passenger stopped short in his invective, but within a few days there was talking enough. It was said all over Leyden that Boerhaave believed in Spinoza, and the doors of his church were closed. Thus we have the answer to the question which is sometimes asked: "In what roundabout way did Spinoza give Boerhaave to medicine?"

No anecdotes in medical history are better known than those relating to Boerhaave: Leyden found it necessary to pull down its walls to accommodate his army of pupils; returning to the university after an attack of gout, he saw the streets illuminated and heard the town-bells ringing in honor of his recovery; an Englishman gave him a country house because he advised him how to row a boat hygienically; one night he kept Peter the Great waiting because he recognized no distinctions among patients; his practice was so extensive that he left millions of guilders to his daughter; his works were so popular that they were translated into Arabic; a letter mailed in China by a mandarin addressed "Boerhaave in Europe," was placed on his desk.

Boerhaave was generous and devoid of professional envy. He spoke of "the immortal Harvey" and of "the immortal Sydenham"; he installed Albinus in Leyden; he helped Linnaeus in his troubled days in Holland; he published magnificent editions of Aretaeus, Vesalius, Prospero Alpino, Lorenzo Bellini; he purchased Swammerdam's manuscripts which the author himself had rejected, and published them under the title Bible of Nature (*Biblia Naturae*, 1737), thus rescuing from oblivion the remarkable worker whose miniature scalpels had to be ground under a magnifying lens, whose glass tubes were drawn out to hair-like fineness, and whose "nerve-muscle preparations" laid at rest the legend of nervous fluid.

In spite of his mildness and kindness, Boerhaave could assert himself, and not all his axioms were therapeutic. Knowing the

MEDICINE IN THE EIGHTEENTH CENTURY

history of medicine, he felt impelled to say, "Galen has done more harm than good." This of course was the fault, not of Galen, but of those who endowed him with infallibility. In a similar strain, Boerhaave declared: "If we compare the good which a half dozen true sons of Aesculapius have accomplished since the origin of medical art upon the earth, with the evil which the immense mass of doctors of this profession among the human race have done, there can be no doubt that it would have been far better if there had never been any physicians in the world." This reflection did not cost Boerhaave his general popularity, since all physicians believed they were among the six exempted Asclepiads.

Boerhaave was a savant, familiar with classic, oriental and modern tongues, music, poetry, philosophy, history, literature, botany, and the bibliography of the sciences. He developed the chemistry of the carbon compounds, and gave to chemistry the doctrine of affinity. He was not fertile in discovery, nor great in original investigations; his rôle was rather to sum up and interpret the accumulated knowledge of the centuries. Of unblemished character and a great personality, warm-hearted and clear-thinking, he was the medical arbiter of his age. Sanctorius, able to devise a thermometer, was the first to measure the body temperature; it was reserved for Boerhaave to expound to the medical world the principles of medical thermometry. With a few hospital beds available, Boerhaave proved to be the most effective popularizer ever known of clinical teaching. He realized the need of anatomy, physiology, pathology and chemistry; he insisted on post-mortems, and his reputation enabled him to perform autopsies on noblemen.

Hints and suggestions first dropped in faultless extempore Latin from the lips of Boerhaave, were repeated years afterward in lecture-rooms from Edinburgh to Vienna. As a clinician, much of Boerhaave's work was in therapeutics, and therapeutics has been, and of course will remain, the least scientific and satisfactory branch of medicine. Boerhaave's fame has paid the penalty of that condition. Without doubt, his *Institutes* and *Aphorisms* were the most influential texts of the eighteenth century, and now they do not have a single reader. "I have carefully considered the case," wrote Boerhaave to a fellow-practitioner who consulted him by mail; "let her take three pills of prescription A, followed by a dose of prescription B, to be continued for two months." These prescriptions have long been antiquated, and the great Boerhaave is only a name.

The Old Vienna School, growing up under Gerard van Swieten with a thermometer in its mouth, was modeled upon the clinical beds of Leyden. Van Swieten certainly had merits as a medical man: when he was called over from Holland, the Austrian throne had no heir; van Swieten drew the husband aside, and gave him some private instruction, with the result that Maria Theresa became pregnant sixteen times. Van Swieten's successor, the unpleasant Anton de Haen, was a clinician of ability who left eighteen volumes behind him—if we dig amid these paper ruins, we will find de Haen's treatise in defense of witchcraft. This incongruity later struck Virchow, who in his survey of a century of pathology, exclaimed: "With the fanaticism of a monk, de Haen defends magic and miracles, and attacks the philosophers as atheists. He prepared the soil in which soon were to sprout animal magnetism and somnambulism. What contrasts in one man! The same physician who introduced the thermometer into the observation of the sick, and dissection into clinical investigation, believes in witchcraft and persecutes witches."

A modest admirer of "the most illustrious Baron van Swieten," was Leopold Auenbrugger, himself a nobleman of Auenbrugg. Leopold Auenbrugger was no fool; he had read history, and he knew the usual fate of the innovator: the contumelious stone during life, and a monument after death. Therefore, when sending his *Inventum novum* (1761) out into the world, he wrote an explanatory preface:

> I present to the reader a new sign for the detection of diseases of the chest, which I have discovered. It consists in the percussion of the human thorax and the determination of the internal condition of this cavity by the varying resonance of the sounds thus produced.

My discoveries in this subject are not committed to paper because of an itch for writing, nor an inordinate desire for theorizing. Seven years of observation have put the subject in order and have clarified it for myself and now I feel that it should be published.

I foresee very well that I shall encounter no little opposition to my views and I put my invention before the public with that anticipation. I realize, however, that envy and blame, and even hatred and calumny have never failed to come to men who have illuminated art or science by discoveries or have added to their perfection. I expect to have to submit to this danger myself, but I think that no one will be able to call any of my observations to account. I have written only what I have myself learned by personal observation over and over again, and what my senses have taught me during long hours of toil. I have never permitted myself to add or subtract anything from my observations because of the seductions of preconceived theory.

Van Swieten wrote much on the diseases of the chest, but he did not mention Auenbrugger's percussion. The chief of the Old Vienna School saw no use in tapping the thorax. He did not know that his pupil's finger had ushered in the era of physical diagnosis. Anton de Haen complains that it is almost impossible to recognize thoracic diseases until it is too late to help the patient. The obstinate man did not see that in response to the physician's rapping, the door of thoracic knowledge opened. Auenbrugger had anticipated neglect, and was too well poised to permit himself to be embittered or become exasperated. He devoted himself to practice, made money, went to the opera in winter, cultivated a garden in summer, wrote a libretto for the amusement of the empress, appreciated the beautiful Marianne von Priestersberg, and lived to celebrate his golden wedding. Not until he was senile did his work become fruitful, and that was in another age and another land.

Boerhaave's greatest pupil was Albrecht von Haller, scion of an old Swiss family at Berne. He was an infant prodigy, explaining the Bible at four, outlining a Chaldee grammar, compiling two thousand biographical sketches, preparing a Greek and Hebrew vocabulary, and writing a Latin satire on his tutor, before his tenth birthday. George Daniel Coschwitz, the famous professor of anatomy at Halle, was excited over his discovery of a new salivary duct, until Haller in his teens, showed him it was only a lingual vein. In maturity, Haller's activity was prodigious; systematizing medicine and creating physiology as an independent science did not prevent him from attempting to dispute botanical supremacy with Linnaeus; he wrote novels which were read in their time; his long poems on the origin of evil and on the beauty of his native Alps, which thrilled eighteenth century readers, have gone the way of most didactic verse.

Haller's versatile genius revealed itself best in physiology: grappling with Glisson's conception of irritability—the quality by which living matter responds to stimulus—Haller engaged in many vivisections, "undertaken with great reluctance in the hope of benefiting the human race"; cutting the nerve connecting the spinal cord with a muscle, he demonstrated the muscle's capability of contracting without receiving the hypothetical animal spirits from the brain. These experiments proved: irritability is not dependent upon sensibility; irritability is the specific property of muscular tissue and sensibility is the specific property of nervous tissue; muscle exhibits irritability when excised and separated from its nerve supply, hence inherent muscular force is differentiated from inherent nervous force. The animists and vitalists were alarmed, and the new doctrine seemed irreligious in spite of Haller's known piety; after the discussions were over, the old views passed away, and Haller's classification entered physiology.

Facts discovered in the seventeenth century frequently produced theories in the eighteenth. The microscopic spermatozoan divided embryologists into spermatists and ovists, but both groups united in believing a fully-formed miniature embryo existed in the germ-cell, as the flower exists in the bud. They assumed development was an unfolding of these invisible pre-existing parts, and not a growth of new parts. The logical conclusion of this preformation theory meant that each embryo included all succeeding embryos encased within each other, and this process had gone on from the days of Adam, whose generative organs contained the embryos of all future mankind. Leibnitz, gifted, but usually mistaken, thus explained it: "I mean that these souls, which one day are to be the souls of men, are present in the seed, like those of other species; in such wise that they existed in our ancestors as far back as Adam, or from the beginning of the world, in the forms of organized bodies."

Haller brought his mathematical knowledge to bear on the subject. He calculated that on the last day of God's labor He created two hundred thousand millions of human beings in embryo and neatly packed them into the ovaries of Eve, from which they were unfolded generation after generation. He arrived at these figures by multiplying the age of the earth, which was 6,000 years, by the average age of man, which was 30, by the population of the world, which was 1,000 millions. Bonnet's discovery of virgin-birth (*parthenogenesis*, 1745) served only to confuse the problem—he saw a female plant-louse reproduce, without male contact, ninety-five living daughters who were likewise unfertilized but reproductive.

In 1759, a student of twenty-six, a Berlin tailor's son working for his doctorate, attacked the preformation doctrine in his thesis, *Theoria generationis*, which he dedicated to Haller, whom he called "glorious man." Haller was polite, but remained convinced of preformationism. The thesis advanced the doctrine of epigenesis, which had been foreshadowed by Aristotle and Harvey—it maintained that the organs of the embryo do not unfold and enlarge from invisibility, but that there is a progressive formation and differentiation of organs. Between Haller, potentate of physiology, and this unknown Caspar Wolff, there could be no argument. Haller simply laughed, and no one read the young doctor's thesis. There was no room in Germany for Wolff, and he accepted an invitation to Russia where he spent the last thirty years of his life. Oddly enough, Caspar Friedrich Wolff found peace under the turbulent Catherine the Great. At St. Petersburg he produced his great memoir on the development of the intestine (1768), which was also neglected; when the younger Meckel finally translated it into German, he had to wipe from its covers the dust of many years. So effectually was the light of Caspar Wolff quenched by the Hallerian snuffers that today not a single portrait of the discoverer of the Wolffian bodies is extant. Caspar Wolff is now "justly reckoned the founder of modern embryology." So the moral of this story is: in science the young son of a tailor may be right, while all his contemporaries, including the most famous physician of the age, are being led astray by preconceived theories.

Medicine needs a supposition at every step, and cannot advance without the support of theory, but when the theory controls medicine it is like a crutch walking alone. The plethora of facts discovered in the seventeenth century, bewildered the profession, and appeased its hunger for research—there is a pause in experimentation as the eighteenth century begins to weave hypotheses with the accumulated material. Medicine becomes largely metaphysical, and we watch the rise and fall of medico-philosophical systems. Ink-wells were very busy, and committed much mischief. Classifiers led the profession, and produced tons of literature which have long been waste-paper. In the eighteenth century, the most casual observation, or no observation at all, was sufficient for the creation of a theory which included the entire medical art. Johann Kämpf of Hesse-Homburg noticed that an impacted intestine causes certain disturbances: thus arose the "doctrine of infarctus," which grew to such proportions that the clyster-syringe was the most conspicuous article in the household, especially among the upper classes. One cartoon of the times depicts Voltaire himself, with a resolute expression, administering an enema to a child who has overeaten.

The sensitive soul of Stahl, the vitalism of Barthez, the phlogistic system of treatment which naturally produced the antiphlogistic, the Brunonianism of John Brown which convulsed medical Europe—a troop of Hanoverian horse had to disperse the battling students—are now found only in textbooks of medical history where they are reluctantly printed in small type and dismissed with impatience. The eighteenth century is still spoken of as the "Period of Theories and Systems"—it witnessed the origin of Gall's phrenology and of Hahnemann's homeopathy—and just as this word-spinning age was about to end, it gave birth to Schelling's *Naturphilosophie,* whose vagaries overwhelmed medicine in the years to come.

There were so many theories, physicians did not know what to do. This confusion is apparent in Melchior Adam Weikard of Fulda, whose *Philosophical Physician* resulted in his ostracism. Weikard later admitted it was not tactful of him to have written that book, and he likened himself to the young girl who said, when she became pregnant, "But what doesn't one do when one is discontented." Weikard also relates that the wife of one of his professional colleagues remarked with much satisfaction, "How grateful I am that my husband cannot write!" Weikard did not achieve freedom and comfort until Catherine of Russia took him under her ample wing. There he wrote his autobiography (1784), containing these puzzled passages:

> There is no codex of medicine, no complete handbook on which one may base all theory or practice. One may read nonsense in the old and the new. And when someone shouts with emphasis—*Read the ancients*—READ THE ANCIENTS, it is usually a novice with downy beard or someone who himself has never read the old authorities or perhaps a man who wishes to impress particularly because of his praise of authority. I say read the good and the bad. Nothing is infallible. What confusion when we regard the therapy of different nations! The French bleed, use enemas, astringents, purges, water, always want to dilute. The English give salts and herbs, minerals, and if you read one author you know all the rest. The Viennese praise their new remedies, the good effects of which the other sons of Aesculapius never can confirm. The other Germans mill about, try first this and that, and in therapy do as they do in other things, imitate and admire the foreigner, collect and compile what has been done here and there the world over. Almost every province, every university has its own routine. Where shall an impartial physician seek his information?
>
> Of course, I do not mean to condemn an entire nation. I talk of the great majority. There are exceptions everywhere. The French

have their great doctors, and who but admires the simple methods of Stoll of Vienna. England and the rest of Germany have their able clinicians, but God knows they are not many. It's a pity that the younger doctors, and those who have the smallest practice, do the most writing. Doctors who have years and much experience rather take in the guineas or ducats than write books. Therefore, even most of the handbooks are written by young doctors or professors of theory who seldom see a patient, and would stand in utter helplessness at their bedside. It is one of the reasons why our profession makes so little progress. Add to that other sins of authorship that impede the development of the art. The theorizing, the brazen faking of case histories or at least their revision until they happen to suit the author, and copying. We kill so much time with such unnecessary literature. And yet I have read much. Often, truly, with great impatience if it was senseless or useless; with great pleasure when I discover clear reasoning and good sense. The simpler and less complicated the remedy suggested, the greater was its appeal to me. As a matter of fact, I have mistrusted much in the deluge of the German periodicals. I did not believe everything in the English, Swedish, or Dutch journals. The Viennese I trusted even less. Of the French, I believed not a word.

In this era, while Boerhaave was transferring medical supremacy from Padua to Leyden, the fertility of Italian genius had not exhausted itself. Morgagni of Forli, professor of anatomy at Padua for over half a century, carried on the Vesalian tradition with undiminished zeal. Vesalius, first of the great Paduans, described the normal body; Morgagni, last of the line, described the diseased body. The suggestion of the Paduan-trained Harvey, that more can be learned from the dissection of one person who has died from a chronic malady such as consumption than from ten healthy malefactors who have been hanged, found its culmination in the labors of Morgagni. The world was a morgue to Morgagni in his working-clothes. Cardinals and carpenters, lawyers and thieves, princes and servants, matrons and virgins, prostitutes and nuns, infancy, youth, middle life, old age—all crowd the fatal canvass of his "remarkable gallery of the dead." It is strange that his daily contact with the end of man did not teach him the folly of human vanity, and this tall, blonde, blue-

MEDICINE IN THE EIGHTEENTH CENTURY

eyed Italian scientist regretted he was not born a nobleman. In extenuation it must be remembered he lived in the eighteenth century which classified everything, and the common people were classified as cattle.

In the summer of 1740, after completing his Valsalva edition, Morgagni was relaxing in the country with a friend who was not a professional, and hence very curious about medical matters. He asked Morgagni many questions and stimulated him to talk about his dissections and studies; Morgagni mentioned that long ago Théophile Bonet of Geneva had written an enormous book on the discoveries made at the autopsy table (*Sepulchretum*, 1679). The intelligent youth was much interested, and urged Morgagni to write out his own observations on the anatomy of diseased organs. "Upon returning to Padua," explains Morgagni, "I began by sending some letters to my friend. And that he was pleased with them appears from two circumstances; the first, that he was continually soliciting me to send him more and more after that, till he drew me on so far as to the seventieth; the second, that when I begged them of him, in order to revise their contents, he did not return them, till he had made me solemnly promise, that I would not abridge any part thereof." The letters were published in five books, "On the Sites and Causes of Disease" (*De sedibus et causis morborum*, 1761). Morgagni was seventy-nine when his masterpiece appeared, and he saw various editions before he passed away in his ninetieth year.

These letters of Morgagni, written to a correspondent who is never named, created the science of pathology. Morgagni described lesions with such accuracy that he turned medical thinking into channels which it has since followed. Unconsciously the physician of today visualizes disease in "terms of lesion"—in other words, Morgagni introduced the "anatomical concept" into medical practice. The modern pathologist who sends in his report of solidification of the lung, heart-block, angina pectoris, disease of the cardiac valves, aortic aneurysm, visceral syphilis, tuberculosis of the kidney, ovarian tumor, or acute yellow atrophy of the liver, is writing an addendum to Morgagni's original description.

Whether Trotula, or any other woman, was professor of gynecology at Salerno is a subject upon which there may never be unanimity, but no doubt attaches to Laura Bassi, professor of experimental physics at the university of Bologna. Among her numerous pupils was her indolent kinsman, Lazzaro Spallanzani of Scandiano, who was fifteen before he finished his grammar school course. His father was a distinguished advocate, and Spallanzani began to study for the same profession. If Laura Bassi did not actually incite him to abandon law for science, she certainly influenced him in that direction. Together they studied natural philosophy and mathematics, and ancient and modern languages, as in all these subjects Laura Bassi had attained extraordinary proficiency. In the meantime he took orders in the Church, and is usually spoken of as the Abbé Spallanzani. He refused so many professorships that it seems every vacant chair in Europe, from Coimbra to St. Petersburg, was offered him; finally Maria Theresa captured the Abbé for the chair of natural history in her reëstablished university of Pavia. Years later, Padua attempted to lure him away, but Spallanzani remained at Pavia because his salary was doubled and he was granted a year's vacation in Turkey. On his return, as he approached the gates of the university, the assembled students greeted him with acclamation.

Spallanzani is one of the great names in physiology. His early idleness was replaced by an incessant and effective activity. In his experiments on digestion, he swallowed linen bags containing food, perforated wooden tubes, and was enough of a scientific martyr to obtain gastric juice by making himself vomit on an empty stomach. He supplemented his self-experimentation by experiments on a surprising variety of animals. Spallanzani confirmed and extended Réaumur's work by pouring gastric juice, drop by drop, on meat and bread, demonstrating it dissolved foods in a test-tube as readily as in the body. Some beautiful theories died when the stomach ceased to be regarded as a churning-mill, mechanically grinding food by muscular force, and digestion was seen to be neither coction, trituration, putrefaction, nor fermentation. The eighteenth century learned, through Réaumur, Spallanzani, and Eduardus Stevens of Edinburgh, that digestion is the result of the solvent power of the juice manufactured by the stomach.

Spallanzani likewise carried forward the work of Réaumur and others on the regeneration of removed parts: cutting hydras into pieces, lopping off the heads of polyps, severing entire limbs of salamanders, amputating the claws of lobsters and crabs, these observers watched nature renewing the lost organs of her primitive creatures. Perhaps no biologist of the time was as familiar with fertilization as the Abbé Spallanzani. He studied the semen of various animals and proved the English priest Needham was mistaken—Needham's usual condition—in believing the spermatozoa are formed after the fluid has been voided. He found the fertilizing power of the spermatic fluid is lost when it is filtered, though he left the correct interpretation for later workers; by putting male frogs into trousers during cohabitation, he noted the ova remained unfertilized: the investigator who helped to dethrone the ancient doctrine of spontaneous generation, also demolished the subtle theory of the *aura seminalis* by showing that fertilization does not occur unless there is contact between sperm and egg. Spallanzani was the first who artificially fecundated the eggs of frog and toad, and the first who impregnated a bitch by injecting warm semen into the vagina.

Most of the French clinicians of the period have been forgotten with their abandoned theories, and Théophile de Bordeu's "Tripod of Life" collapsed beneath subsequent hypotheses; his name, however, survives in honor, for Bordeu must be considered the precursor of the doctrine of the internal secretions. When Bordeu said, "Examine the blood returning from each principal region, for it is evident that each has specific properties which it has acquired in the tissues of the parts from which it returns," he was pressing close upon a modern truth.

Numerous passages, as the following, attest his anticipations of endocrinology:

> The semen imparts, as it is well known, a firm, masculine tone to all parts, as soon as it can be drawn off and sent into the humours and solids by its natural organs. It sets a new seal upon the animalism of the individual, who is in part subject to the action of this creative liquor. . . . Eunuchs, losing the ability to procreate, lose all that special odor peculiar to the male, their strength decreases, their pulse loses its bound, the activity of their mind diminishes: nevertheless they grow like other men, and even relatively more so; they become fatter; their flesh becomes softer; they are less constipated; their eyesight is less keen. What happens to their voice is well known and about the same changes are observed in animals that have been castrated. On the other hand, in men enjoying all their natural rights and who easily secrete their semen, this liquor penetrates the mass of the humours. . . . It has the property of consolidating the parts and of nourishing them. It excites and stimulates all the fibers. It is the cause of that fetid odor exhaled from vigorous males. It produces wonderful effects; in a word, it must be considered as a special stimulus of the machine which physicians have not sufficiently considered.

Bordeu, expelled by the Paris Faculty, remained in Paris and prospered—obviously the old Faculty was losing its teeth. The French surgeons, finally freed from this same blight, made definite progress through Jean-Louis Petit's screw tourniquet, and his pioneer work in mastoiditis; Dominique Anel's treatment of traumatic aneurysm by ligation of the brachial artery, and his operation for lacrimal fistula, with the probe and syringe which carry his name; Hugues Ravaton's double-flap amputation; Pierre-Joseph Desault's teaching of surgical anatomy; François Chopart's mediotarsal amputation; Jacques Daviel's extraction of the lens in cataract, and his spoon; and Jean-Pierre David's dissertation on the effects of movement and repose in surgical diseases.

It is one of the ironies of history that the medieval edict, "The Church abhors blood"—a statement which impeded surgical education for centuries—should have weighed most heavily on Germany, the land of the Reformation. Throughout the eighteenth century, despite the efforts of Lorenz Heister and August Gottlieb Richter, German surgery was a vast sociological crime. A barber's apprentice, who sought to evade the humiliations inflicted upon him, was hunted like an escaped animal; the regimental surgeon was compelled to shave the army officers; the wandering oculist, the traveling bone-setter, the straying stonecutter, the roving rupture-specialist, preyed upon the credulity of the people; the genuine surgeon who refused to utter a magic formula as he unrolled his bandages, found himself replaced by an adaptable charlatan; the Prussian executioner, experienced in the disarticulation of joints and the breaking of bones, was granted permission to treat wounds and ulcers and to set fractures. Frederick the Great's reply to the complaint of the Berlin surgeons is characteristic: "If you are as skillful as you pretend to be, every one will trust themselves to you rather than go to an executioner; but if you are ignoramuses, the public must not suffer, and rather than remain lame and crippled, let them go to the executioner." This strange decree which was issued in 1744, was perhaps not more extraordinary than the circumstance that for seventeen years (1736-53), Albrecht von Haller was professor of surgery at Göttingen. Haller's learning and versatility were phenomenal, and he will always be placed among the greatest of physicians, but he should never have been professor of surgery for the one simple reason that he never performed a surgical operation.

It is difficult to omit mention of the forgotten Johann Gottlieb Wolstein, a name which does not occur in most textbooks of medical history. Wolstein studied in several European countries, and in London was the pupil of Pott and the brothers Hunter. As the result of his numerous works on veterinary medicine, which were widely translated, and his twenty years of activity as the director of the Vienna Veterinary Institute, Wolstein may be considered the founder of veterinary science in German-speaking countries. After a long career of distinguished service, Wolstein was expelled from Austria—reasons unknown.

No comment is required; we must simply remember that in every age every nation has exiled its best citizens. In his *Treatise on the Internal Diseases of Foals, Army and Civilian Horses* (1787), and especially in *Annotations regarding Venesection of Man and Beast* (1791), Wolstein fought the "bloody Moloch" of medicine. In this era of intensive bloodletting, when physicians shed ceaseless streams of blood in every fever, Wolstein pointed out that fever by itself is not a disease, but nature's best weapon for the combat of disease. "Blood," he said, "is no water—it is the juice of life; a juice which after each venesection nature replaces rapidly, but in a raw, unprepared, watery, spiritless state." Of course the furious bloodletters of the day did not listen to Wolstein, but kept on bleeding their patients white. It was a species of therapeutic vampirism, which sent unnumbered thousands to premature graves. Descartes' cry through the death-room, "Gentlemen, spare the French blood," found many echoes.

Eighteenth-century England is remembered as the Golden Age of Quackery, a situation due largely to the wretched creatures, male and female, who sat on the throne and patronized charlatans. Queen Anne, suffering from weak eyes and a weaker understanding, insulted the medical profession and turned her country into a Paradise of Quacks by transforming a mountebank into Sir William Read, principal oculist to her majesty. As an advertiser, Read was more aggressive than his predecessor John Case, who inscribed under the Sign of the Golden Ball:

> Within this place
> Lives Doctor Case.

The *Tatler* maintained that Case made more money by this couplet than Dryden by all his poetical works put together; Addison wrote also a note about Read: "There was an epigram current, that Sir William could hardly *read*, but he seldom suffered any periodical to make its appearance in public without some testimony under his own hand that he could *hardly write*. It appears he was a very comely person and a man of fashion, rich and ostentatious. . . . He kept an excellent table and was noted for his special brew of punch, which he served out to his guests in golden goblets."

Uroscopy seemed as popular as ever, and love-sickness and female chastity were still diagnosed by a naked-eye examination of a jar of urine held up to the sun. A survey of the medical literature of that time conveys the impression that with the exception of gout, which was as fashionable among gentlemen as the periwig, the most prevalent disorder was stone in the bladder. Alkalis were regarded as the remedies, and the leading scientists concerned themselves with the problem. None was so successful, however, as Joanna Stephens. Dukes and duchesses, mitred bishops and belted earls testified to the virtues of her secret medicine. Joanna had not studied alchemy, and knew little of the transmutation of metals, but she had learned how to change stone to gold. Statesmen who scorned the College of Physicians, took off their hats at mention of her name. She was a celebrity, and an announcement which appeared in the *Gentleman's Magazine* (April 1738), aroused the hope of a suffering people: "Mrs. Stephens has proposed to make her medicine publick on consideration of £5,000 to be raised by contribution." The church and peerage of England responded generously, yet the £5,000 could not be raised.

Joanna Stephens determined to keep her secret, but such was the public clamor that an Act of Parliament appointed a commission of investigation, which included the three leading surgeons of the metropolis: William Cheselden, of Chelsea Hospital, who could incise the bladder and remove the stone in fifty-four seconds; Sir Caesar Hawkins, of St. George's Hospital, inventor of the cutting gorget; and Samuel Sharp, of Guy's Hospital, whose treatise on surgical operations passed through ten editions and a French translation in his own lifetime. Their unanimous decision was as follows: "We have examined the said medicines and her method of preparing the same, and are convinced by experiment, of the utility, efficacy, and dissolving power thereof." Whereupon the British Government gave Mrs. Stephens the

£5,000, and in return—money can buy anything—the benefactress published (June 19, 1739) a "full discovery" in the *London Gazette*. It was thus revealed to a waiting world that her prescriptions were a decoction, containing boiled herbs and soap, with swine's-cresses burnt to blackness, "but this was only with a view to disguise it"; pills, consisting of wild carrot and burdock seeds, hips and hawes, reduced to ashes with alicant soap and honey; powder, composed of roasted egg-shells crushed with garden-snails in the month of May.

For this barnyard rubbish, usually thrown to poultry, England officially paid a fortune, and the "Act for providing a Reward to Joanna Stephens," bore not only the names of the surgeons, but the greater name of Stephen Hales, England's chief physiologist since Harvey. The prime minister, Sir Robert Walpole, outstanding political figure of his time, shrewd enough to extract profit from South Sea Stock, swallowed the saponified snails by the pound. After his death, Sir Caesar Hawkins performed the autopsy, and discovered several stones in his bladder. This then is the story of a widow who fooled a nation.

Medical ethics were less rigid in those days, and every one quacked it a little. Sir Hans Sloane, president of the College of Physicians, and Newton's successor as president of the Royal Society, sold an eye-salve; Richard Mead put down his well-worn copy of Hippocrates in Greek to concoct a secret remedy for the bite of a mad dog. Robert James, whose Medical Dictionary in three folio volumes numbered Johnson himself among the contributors, devoted a lifetime to pushing the sales of his patented James's powder. Goldsmith took a dose of the powder in his last fever, and later it was prescribed for George III. The fame of this proprietary was more than national, and it received a testimonial from George Washington, who called it "one of the most excellent medicines in the world."

Eminent clergymen caught the contagion. Time has hallowed the name of John Wesley, but to his contemporaries he was a disputatious and lascivious bigot, and as a dabbler in medicine and electricity he produced *Primitive Physick* (1747) and *The*

Desideratum (1759). George Berkeley, bishop of Cloyne, did not believe in matter, or in the higher mathematics—"because it led to freethinking"—but he did believe in tar-water. In his *Chain of Philosophical Reflections concerning the Virtues of Tar-Water* (1744), he proclaimed it a panacea, his chain of reasoning being that from the sunlight and air the pine-trees accumulate the vital elements of the universe and concentrate them in the tar which when imbibed by the human system proves capable of curing such diverse maladies as smallpox, consumption, syphilis, complaints of the bowels, ulcers and gravel. The doctors who protested against this universal remedy were suspected of being financially frightened, and their scoffs could not prevent the belief in tar-water from developing into a mania. While Berkeley's treatise was being reprinted and translated into many languages, barrels and barrels of sooty rosin were being consumed all over Europe, and especially in Great Britain, for Berkeley was a prophet in his own country. Testimonials poured in from all sides, and the Reverend Edward Young, the cheerful author of *Night Thoughts*, in alluding to the opponents of tar-water, wrote: "Now give me leave to say that this infidelity may possibly be as fatal to morbid bodies as other infidelity is to morbid souls."

Our own Benjamin Franklin, whose sound sense kept him free from the entangling quackeries of the age, was the unwitting godfather of as picturesque a pretender as ever caused the multitude to gape. James Graham, a saddler's son, born in the Cowgate, Edinburgh, got inside the university, but was so vivacious that even Monro primus, Cullen, Black, and Whytt could not keep him on the benches long enough to graduate. He traveled in America, practising as he went, and in Philadelphia heard of Franklin's discoveries in electricity—later Graham met Franklin in Paris, in much the same way that Casanova visited Haller at Berne, for the eighteenth century was certainly not an era of discrimination. Patronized by the Duchess of Devonshire, and other aristocrats, Graham became the fashion, and established himself on the Royal Terrace, Adelphi, overlooking the

Thames, midway between Blackfriars and Westminster Bridges; his Templum Aesculapio Sacrum was visited by all who could afford the price of admission.

Under the vaulted compartments and by the central arches of the hall were collections of walking-sticks, crutches, eyeglasses and ear-trumpets—Graham explained that these had formerly belonged to his patients, but they no longer required these adventitious aids, and he kept them as trophies of his victories over disease. Marble statues and magnificent paintings, great globes of glass and remarkable plates of burnished steel aroused the wonder of his crowded audience; spectators overwhelmed by the mysterious sphinxes or flame-breathing dragons would insensibly sink into the luxurious couches of the recesses, and recline half hypnotized by the pervading perfumes of the spices burning in the swinging censers.

The adroit Graham informed the town that they had seen nothing unless they entered the shrine of his Great Apollo Apartment. "In this tremendous edifice," he declared, "are combined or singly dispensed the irresistible and salubrious influences of electricity, or the elementary fire, air, and magnetism; three of the greatest of those agents or universal principles, which, pervading all created beings and substances that we are acquainted with, connect, animate, and keep together all nature." His principal apparatus was a Celestial Bed standing on forty pillars of gorgeous glass, embellished with magnets and electric devices: if the young lay in this bed, they would retain their good looks; if the old experienced its effects, they would be rejuvenated; if married couples slept in it, their progeny would be healthy, beautiful, and virtuous. The price for a night in this Medico-Magnetico-Musico-Electrical Bed was £100, and the fee was paid by human beings who were entitled to engrave a crest on their tombstones. The Goddess of Health who officiated at the ceremonies was the bewitching shawl-dancer, later famous as Lady Hamilton and enchantress of Lord Nelson, but even in her early days Emma Lyon was familiar with many beds—all of which proves that Graham was a born showman.

Graham knew how to keep his followers interested, whether lecturing on the "Preservation and Exaltation of Loveliness," or publishing a pamphlet on sex, "as delivered by Hebe Vestina at the Temple of Hymen," or demolishing his accusers with "A Naked exhibition of Asses stripped of their Ermine, namely, of Country Just-Asses, Mares, Alderwomen, and Whippers-in." In only one respect did Graham disappoint those who believed in him. He vended a remedy, so rare and valuable, that he demanded for this Elixir of Life the payment of £1,000 in advance; whoever took it would reach 150 years at the minimum, and in fact would live as long as the medicine was renewed, a process which could go on indefinitely. At this point James Graham showed his lack of mathematical training by dying before his fiftieth birthday.

Franz Anton Mesmer, of Suabia, came to Vienna to study medicine under van Swieten and de Haen. His graduating thesis, "The Influence of the Planets in the Cure of Diseases" (*De planetarum influxu*, 1766), promulgated the theory that the sun and moon act upon living beings by means of the subtle fluid known as animal magnetism, analogous in its effect to the properties of the lodestone. Mesmer thus revealed himself a belated medical astrologer, a congenital mystic. He claimed he could magnetize trees, so every leaf contributed healing to all who approached. Vienna knew him and did not believe him, and Mesmer went to Paris. He erected a temple to the god of health, and here thronged the afflicted. They trod the halls in silence broken only by the sound of an aeolian harp from a distant chamber. The light that shone through the richly-stained windows fell on walls lined with mirrors. From the corridors floated the odor of orange-blossoms, and from antique vases on the chimney-pieces arose the rarest incense.

The patients sat around a magnetic *baquet*, and waited; the majority were women, and for them a special set of handsome young men had been provided. Slowly and solemnly these assistant magnetizers marched forward; each selected a woman and stared her in the eye; no word was spoken, but from somewhere softly sailed the music of an accordion, and the voice of a hidden opera-singer sweetened the incense-laden air. The young Apollos embraced the knees of the women, rubbed various spots, and gently massaged their breasts. The women closed their eyes, and felt the magnetism surge through them. At the critical moment, the master magnetizer, Mesmer himself, appeared on the scene. Clad in a lilac gown, with lofty mien and majestic tread, he advanced among his patients, making "passes" and accomplishing miracles. If a lady had a "crisis," Mesmer lifted her up and carried her to his private crisis-chamber. Nor were male visitors lacking at these seances, though as a rule they came not for Mesmer's medicine, but to observe the fainting girls, who often fell into convulsions. It must have been a pleasant form of hypnosis, for as soon as a patient recovered from one crisis, she begged for another.

Mesmerism became a sensation. Other systems were deserted for Magnetic Medicine, with the flux and reflux of an incomparably subtle, universally diffused fluid, so continuous as not to admit of a vacuum. "This doctrine," declared Mesmer, "enables the physician to decide upon the health of every individual, and of the presence of the diseases to which the patient may be exposed. In this way the art of healing may be brought to absolute perfection." It seemed as if all the world wished to be magnetized. The French government offered Mesmer a pension and the Cross of the Order of St. Michael for his secret; he refused, because he was already making a fortune, and he could not divulge the essence of his secret (women pay well for sexual excitement in disguise). Mesmer's disciple, Charles D'Eslon, a leading member of the Faculty and physician to Comte d'Artois, received a visit from a man in uniform: "In my capacity as lieutenant-general of police, I wish to know whether, when a woman is magnetized and passing through the crisis, it would not be easy to outrage her." D'Eslon answered in the affirmative, but explained that only the colleagues of Mesmer, physicians of probity, were entitled and privileged to produce a crisis.

Finally a commission was appointed to investigate the phenomenon; among the commissioners were some of the most illustrious scientists of the eighteenth century: the first name signed to the report is Franklin, and the last is Lavoisier. They reached the verdict that magnetism is due to the imagination. They prepared also a secret report, "not adapted for general publication," which is more curious than the official version. In the subjoined extracts, perhaps the reader can recognize the hand of Benjamin Franklin:

> It has been observed that women are like musical strings stretched in perfect unison; when one is moved, all the others are instantly affected. Thus the commissioners have repeatedly observed that when the crisis occurs in one woman, it occurs almost at once in others also. . . .
>
> Women are always magnetized by men; the established relations are doubtless those of a patient to the physician, but this physician is a man, and whatever the illness may be, it does not deprive us of our sex, it does not entirely withdraw us from the power of the other sex; illness may weaken impressions without destroying them. Moreover, most of the women who present themselves to be magnetized are not really ill; many come out of idleness, or for amusement; others, if not perfectly well, retain their freshness and their force, their senses are unimpaired and they have all the sensitiveness of youth; their charms are such as to affect the physician, and their health is such as to make them liable to be affected by him, so that the danger is reciprocal. . . .
>
> The magnetizer generally keeps the patient's knees enclosed within his own, and consequently the knees and all the lower parts of the body are in close contact. The hand is applied to the hypochondriac region, and sometimes to that of the ovarium, so that the touch is exerted at once on many parts, and these the most sensitive parts of the body.
>
> The experimenter, after applying his left hand in this manner, passes his right hand behind the woman's body, and they incline towards each other so as to favour this twofold contact. This causes the closest proximity; the two faces almost touch, the breath is intermingled, all physical impressions are felt in common, and the re-

ciprocal attraction of the sexes must consequently be excited in all its force. It is not surprising that the senses are inflamed. The action of the imagination at the same time produces a certain disorder throughout the machine; it obscures the judgment, distracts the attention; the women in question are unable to take account of their sensations, and are not aware of their condition. . . .

The commissioners' experiments, showing that all these results are due to contact, to imagination and imitation, while explaining the effects produced by M. D'Eslon, equally explain those of M. Mesmer. It may, therefore, reasonably be concluded that, whatever be the mystery of M. Mesmer's magnetism, it has no more real existence than that of M. D'Eslon, and that the proceedings of the one are not more useful nor less dangerous than those of the other.

The electrotherapeutic quackeries of the period were of course the result of the numerous discoveries in electricity: charlatans have a flair for exploiting scientific progress. Various physicians, taught by the wife of Fabricius Hildanus, learned to draw iron particles from the eye with a magnet; the elder Francis Hauksbee, replacing Otto von Guericke's mounted sulphur globe, devised the first electric machine, "a pretty large glass cylinder, turned by a winch and rubbed by the hand"; Stephen Gray, eccentric citizen of the Charterhouse, found how to electrify non-electric substances; Priestley wrote the *History of Electricity* and added to our knowledge of conduction; John Hunter experimented with the electric organ of the torpedo; toward the end of the century, Luigi Galvani, while working in his laboratory on frogs, was prepared to stumble on the electric properties of excised tissues; then his countryman, Alessandro Volta, built that enduring monument, the Voltaic Pile. While the conservative members of the profession were ridiculing Galvani as "the frog's dancing-master," quacks made much money by fascinating their patients with electric shocks.

Venereal disease is no respector of persons, and the learned Astruc compiled a long list of kings who wore the familiar scars of Venus. Then as now, venereal disease was a fertile field for exploitation, and the dreadful doses of mercury put patients at the mercy of those who promised speedy relief either from the malady or from the treatment. Among those who lashed the "venereal specialists," none was more vigorous than Joseph-Jacques de Gardane of Provence; for this reason alone, his name should be rescued from the oblivion into which it has fallen. "There is nothing more surprising," he says in one of his prefaces (1774), "than the methods hitherto followed. In all the seasons of the year, all subjects presenting themselves, without regard to their sex or their age, and without any other preparation than that given to everybody, go through the same trials: all are bled, purged, bathed and rubbed. In such a case the application of the grand remedy becomes a business affair, a money matter. He who treats makes a bargain, pledging himself to cure the patient in the space of a short and often limited time, with the result that, when the time of treatment has expired, the patient is pronounced cured. It is in vain that the sequelae of the disease give evidence against the supposed success; one tries to persuade the patient that he is well, and reassuring him with further promises, discharges him: in such a manner the majority of those much vaunted cures are brought about."

The indignant Gardane continues in this strain for several pages: "It is true that such conditions are demanded by the patient himself who negotiates for his health within a fixed time, but they are never fulfilled by those who do not blush to receive his money in advance. Hence arises that quackery so characteristic of those who treat venereal diseases. In the end, one always resorts to trickery, because one has promised more than one can do. But enough of those who in fear of losing their prey, snatch a fee from the hand of a patient in pain. A physician should promise nothing to his patient. . . . But who would believe it! those factors which should aid us in our combat with disease, often make the gate wider for the admittance of charlatanism. Genuine physicians deem it their sacred duty to publish the discoveries which are useful to their fellow-men. They are ever in arms against the Monster of Quackery, but charlatans know how to profit from the progress of therapeutics. As soon as the profession recognized that a radical cure could be effected by the internal administration of remedial agents, the spirit of cupidity aroused certain men to found their fortunes on discoveries not their own. These harpies deceive the populace by means of advertisements, by extorted affidavits, by surprising cures which often are imaginary, and they never fail in catching victims. This epoch, perhaps the most glorious for the medical art, is so pregnant with misery for afflicted humanity."

The irresistible and insatiable Giacomo Casanova, ripest and rottenest fruit of the eighteenth century, denounced for his passions and envied for his seductions, has left us a dialogue which throws light on the spread of venereal disease:

Surgeon: Yes, captain, I have been practising surgery in this place for twenty years, and in a very poor way, for I had nothing to do except a few cases of bleeding, of cupping, and occasionally some slight excoriation to dress, or a sprained ankle to put to rights. I did not earn even the poorest living. But since last year a great change has taken place; I have made a good deal of money, I have laid it out advantageously, and it is to you, captain, to you—may God bless you!—that I am indebted for my present comforts.

Captain: But how so?

Surgeon: In this way, captain. You had a connection with Don Jerome's housekeeper, and you left her, when you went away, a certain souvenir which she communicated to a certain friend of hers, who, in perfect good faith, made a present of it to his wife. This lady did not wish, I suppose, to be selfish, and she gave the souvenir to a libertine, who in his turn was so generous with it that, in less than a month, I had about fifty clients. The following months were not less fruitful, and I gave the benefit of my attendance to everybody, of course, for a consideration. There are a few patients still under my care, but in a short time there will be no more, as the souvenir left by you has now lost all its virtue. You can easily realize the joy I felt when I saw you; you are a bird of good omen. May I hope that your visit will last long enough to enable you to renew the source of my fortune?

Morality in the eighteenth century must have been in a low state, for men did openly what is now done secretly. It was known that Voltaire visited a certain house at Porte du Roule, for the cultivation of pornography was not deemed incompatible with the pursuit of philosophy. A letter from Diderot to his benefactress, Catherine the Great, introduces us to the encyclopedist himself; to Montesquieu, author of "one of the most important books ever written"; to Buffon the naturalist, who first discussed the origin of species by development, and when the shadow of the Bastille fell athwart his teaching, ended his arguments, "No, it is certain from revelation that every species was directly created by a separate fiat"; and Charles de Brosses, the real hero of the letter, the magistrate-savant famous for his translation and restoration of Sallust, and as the author of the first book upon the ruins of Herculaneum. Of course the "Semiramis of the North" roared in reading Diderot's letter:

When we were young we sometimes went to the brothel, Montesquieu, Buffon, de Brosses, and myself. Of all of us, President de Brosses was the one who, when he was well prepared, presented the most imposing figure—and his merit was a strange contradiction to his miniature stature of four and a half feet, thin and delicate; but as every little man is vain, so he boasted before the nymphs of the place of the only means which gave him some superiority over the rest of us. One of them turned him around and said: "That's very fine, but where is the foundation for all this?" Whenever now I see a sketch for a painting, subject for a poem, a plan for a tragedy, or for a political undertaking, I remember this devil of a woman; I look at the man and I say: "That's very fine, but where is the bottom for it all?"

A perverse papal nuncio, who saw no need for concealment, is revealed in the following social portrait:

Mgr. de Branciforte, papal nuncio, made his entry into Paris in the month of June 1753, carrying a blessed swaddling-band to M. le duc de Bourgogne. He actively frequented the worldly ladies, particularly the house of Beaudoin, rue Saint-Thomas-du-Louvre. One day, he repeatedly sent his valet-de-chambre for Demoiselle Duchenois, who did not think it proper to go, because, she said, he had already summoned several women from various districts who did not have the reputation of being healthy, and besides, he had on several occasions tormented her to serve him in a fashion which is not natural according to the custom of her country. . . .

In the eighteenth century, faith in pharmacology was as strong as belief in religion. When a girl was married, she received as portion of her dowry a big medicine-spoon, and it was taken for granted that it would be filled frequently. Fortunately, there were some dissenting voices. William Heberden of London, who first described angina pectoris, and the fingers in arthritis deformans still known as Heberden's nodules, finally succeeded in terminating the ancient reign of Mithridatium and Theriaca. William Cullen of Lanarkshire was among the few who wanted to know what went into the medicine-spoon. Cullen's comments on the uses of drugs are worth reading even today, for the spirit of criticism is modern, and as we turn the writings of this Edinburgh professor we find suggestions that the use of this drug be restricted and the use of that drug be abandoned. Cullen's century witnessed the origin of American medicine, and before this country wrote its own manuals of materia medica, Cullen's works were gospel. Even that terrible southerner, the most peppery of all physicians, Charles Caldwell, edited one of Cullen's books, though it was inevitable that the additions of the loquacious Carolinian should occupy more space than the original text.

An imposing character of the eighteenth century who also served as a link between European and American medicine, was nature's great classifier, the Swedish Linnaeus. For years, eclipsing all contemporaries, Linnaeus loomed across the scientific horizon. There was much chaos in those days, and more honor was given to Nature's cataloguers than to her interpreters. Several of the early American physicians were botanists, and they sent American plants to Linnaeus for description. In return for this compliment, Linnaeus frequently immortalized his correspondents by naming the plants after them: thus the checkerberry, *Mitchella repens,* was named after John Mitchell; the spring beauty, *Claytonia virginica,* commemorates John Clayton; and the name of Adam Kuhn lives in *Kuhnia eupatorioides.* Linnaeus, who completed his medical studies in order to wed the daughter of a practitioner who would accept only a physician as a son-in-law, wrote a work on materia medica, but like Theophrastus, his heart was in the science of botany, and not in its application to disease.

A less fortunate but equally significant investigator was the Swedish apothecary Scheele, the foremost chemist of the North until the coming of Berzelius. Miserably poor in purse and health, working with only such apparatus as he could manufacture with his own hands, forced to earn his livelihood as a druggist in an isolated town, the modest Scheele amazes us by the wealth of his achievements. Independently of Priestley, he discovered oxygen; independently of Rutherford, he discovered nitrogen; and he alone is the discoverer of chlorine and fluorine; besides his investigations of alum, ether and hydrogen sulphide, he devised methods of preparing phosphorus and calomel, discovered glycerin and barium oxide, and such acids as mucic, citric, gallic, mallic, oxalic, tartaric, and the terrible hydrocyanic, known to the public as prussic acid. More money has been expended upon his statue at Stockholm than the living Scheele saw during his brief, pathetic and glorious career.

Castor oil seeds have been found in the tombs of the Egyptians, allusions to their purgative properties occur in the writings of Dioscorides, and Albertus Magnus cultivated the plant, yet for centuries the profession wasted its ingenuity in devising outrageous purgatives while oleum ricini was neglected to such an extent that even after Peter Canvane's eulogistic essay the demand for it was so slight that the entire European trade was supplied from the island of Jamaica, and in 1777 the stock of a well-known wholesale druggist in London was two small bottles. In the eighteenth century some ranked cod-liver oil with cinchona, opium and mercury, but the status of oleum morrhuae is still being discussed. Other substances which were introduced during this period were Fowler's solution, Hoffmann's anodyne, Gregory's powder, Prussian blue, potassium chlorate, phosphoric acid, quassia, oil of cajuput, pareira brava, senega root, rhanaty root, angostura bark, Canada balsam, kino, logwood, and spigelia —note the influence of the American Indians. At the urging of Störck, hemlock, clematis, pulsatilla, stramonium, hyoscyamus and colchicum were recalled from therapeutic exile; Störck had a passion for rehabilitating the reputations of discredited drugs —if he lived today he would be the busiest of men.

The most important addition to the materia medica of the eighteenth century was foxglove—"the opium of the heart." It is one of the curiosities of medical history that the purple foxglove, growing throughout the greater part of Europe, is never mentioned by Dioscorides or any other ancient writer. This common and beautiful plant received its familiar name from the Anglo-Saxon foxes-glew or foxes-music, because of its supposed resemblance to an ancient instrument consisting of bells hanging on an arched support. In the Middle Ages, the Welch Physicians of Myddvai employed foxglove for the preparation of external remedies; in the Renaissance it received its scientific baptism: Leonhard Fuchs, of the university of Tübingen, called the plant digitalis, this being the equivalent of the German popular name of finger hood. In the seventeenth century, the London apothecary, John Parkinson, director of the Royal Gardens at Hampton Court, recommended digitalis in his Theatrum botanicum. Digitalis became popular and was frequently employed without discrimination; admitted into the London Pharmacopoeia, it was later omitted and reinstated.

Accurate knowledge of digitalis begins with the publication at Birmingham of William Withering's *Account of the Fox-glove* (1785). Withering was not a gallant, but women played an important rôle in his scientific career: he began to collect plants for a young woman patient, and by the time he married her, he was a leading botanist; he confesses he received his hint about digitalis from an old woman's recipe, and the result was his pharmacological classic on the most valuable drug since the discovery of Peruvian bark. Withering's international hobbies consisted in furnishing scientific notes for a book of Spanish travels, analyzing Portuguese mineral waters, playing the German flute, raising Newfoundland dogs, and breeding French cattle. Withering was a consumptive who did admirable work in half a dozen branches of science. As this gifted botanist lay on his deathbed, some one uttered the unforgettable phrase: "The flower of physicians is indeed Withering." He lies buried in an old churchyard in the suburbs of Birmingham, with the foxglove fittingly adorning the monument over his grave.

In the eighteenth century, aside from the work of the Hahn family on the use of the cold-pack in exanthematous fevers, the chief hydrotherapeutic landmark was a little book by James Currie. This Scotsman spent several years in America, where he had been informed it was easy to acquire a fortune. Ill-luck in business and the Declaration of Independence drove him home, where he graduated in medicine, studied the Scotch peasantry, edited the official edition of the poems of Robert Burns, and in his spare time introduced cold douche-baths of sea-water in typhoid, including verification and tabulation of results with the clinical thermometer—an innovation then, a routine procedure now. Currie never came across Circe, but he met and survived more accidents than ever befell Odysseus; man and nature seemed to conspire against the benefactor who taught us the Effects of Water. Valvular disease of the heart ended a career of constant misfortune and glory; he sleeps beneath the appropriate epitaph:

> Art taught by thee shall o'er the burning frame
> The healing freshness pour and bless thy name.

It is odd that the English-speaking world has forgotten the country practitioner, Thomas Fuller of Sevenoaks in Kent, for no one in his era had so clear a conception of specificness in infection and immunity. Fuller's *Exanthematologia* (1730), an attempt to give a rational account of eruptive fevers, is remarkable for its anticipations of the modern doctrine: "Many varieties are to be met with in books, of other diseases mixed in with the smallpox, but nobody ever yet saw a miliary fever, or measles, or any of its sub-species beget a true smallpox, or any of its sorts; nor on the contrary; and nobody was ever defended from the infection of any one sort by having had another sort. . . . To every seed its own body; and therefore the pestilence can never breed the smallpox, nor the smallpox the measles, nor they the crystals or chicken pox, any more than a hen can a duck, a wolf a sheep, or a thistle figs; and consequently one sort cannot be a preservative against any other sort." A generation later, that acute thinker, Marcus Antonius Plenciz of Vienna, maintained (1762): all infectious disease is caused by living microorganisms, and a special germ is responsible for each specific disease, hence the period of incubation varies in the different infections. The germ-theory was in travail, and yet another century passed before it was born.

No physiologist of the period exhibited more originality and inventive power than the English clergyman, Stephen Hales, the perpetual curate of Teddington. He was educated at Cambridge, known colloquially as "Newton's town," where he became acquainted with Newton's friend, William Stukeley. To perambulate with young Stukeley, searching for John Ray's plants, was better than a regular course in science. Stukeley was erratic and made mistakes, but his enthusiasm for anatomy, chemistry, medicine and archeology was boundless. Stukeley claimed he cured his gout by long rides in search of antiquities; he followed the entire Roman Wall with an ardor known only to antiquarians; he knew so much about Stonehenge that his contemporaries called him "the arch-druid of this age"; he was both physician and parson, and once postponed the services that his congregation might witness an eclipse of the sun. Stephen Hales was equally diligent as parish-priest, attempting to improve the morals and water-supply of his diocese, and as a fellow of the Royal Society, whose Copley medal he received.

Hales' position in physiology is due to the *Statical Essays*,

MEDICINE IN THE EIGHTEENTH CENTURY 359

devoted to his experiments on the flow of sap in plants (*Vegetable Staticks*, 1727) and on the force of the blood in animals (*Haemastaticks*, 1733). A century after Harvey's demonstration of the circulation, Hales discovered how to investigate its dynamics. When Hales fastened glass-tubes into the arteries and veins of horses, he devised a crude pressure-gauge which in his hands gave remarkable results. He was the first who was able to read the height of a column of blood, to measure its fall, to calculate the velocity of the blood-stream from the volume of the vessels, to ascertain the capacity of the heart and its adjustment to its labors, to understand the resistance of the vessel walls, and to realize the constriction and dilatation of the capillaries. Thus to the old story of the pulse, Stephen Hales added the new chapter of blood pressure. This busy clergyman stands among the pioneers of experimental physiology, and as the Father of Blood Pressure he initiated a method which is now of primary importance in the diagnosis and treatment of disease.

Hales holds also a conspicuous place in sanitary science. In his time a protracted sea voyage meant scurvy, and entailed many other horrors, which Hales sought to alleviate by writing one of the long-titled books of the period, "Philosophical Experiments: containing useful and necessary Instructions for such as undertake long Voyages at Sea; showing how Sea-water may be made fresh and wholesome, and how Fresh Water may be preserved sweet; how Biscuit, Corn, &c., may be secured from the Weevel, Maggots, and other Insects; and Flesh preserved in Hot Climates by salting Animals whole; to which is added an account of several Experiments and Observations on Chalybeate or Steel-waters, with some Attempts to convey them to distant places, preserving their virtue to a greater degree than has hitherto been done; likewise a proposal for Cleansing away Mud, &c., out of Rivers, Harbours, and Reservoirs" (1739). He salted animals whole by passing brine into their blood-vessels.

Perhaps his best-known invention is the artificial ventilator, for conveying fresh air into prisons and hospitals. Eighteenth-century England was cursed by the window-tax. Every window in tenement, poor-house, and prison was taxed, and the burden, as was typical of British statesmanship, fell on those who could afford it least—the tenants; and on those who were wholly indifferent to the fate of prisoners—the jailers. "Blocked up every window to lessen the burden of the window-tax," became a familiar phrase. Light and air were penalized. In order that there might be no loophole, the law, for once, was explicit: "No window or light shall be deemed to be stopped up unless such window or light shall be stopped up effectually with stone or brick or plaister upon laith." Contemporary reports state: "The gaolers have to pay it; this tempts them to stop the windows and stifle their prisoners. . . . This is also the case in many workhouses and farm-houses, where the poor and the labourers are lodged in rooms that have no light nor fresh air; which may be a cause of our peasants not having the healthy ruddy complexions one used to see so common twenty or thirty years ago." The nation which produced Newton, master-worker in light, produced legislators who wrung shillings from the skylights of garrets and from a ray of sunshine stealing into a cellar.

Under these windowless conditions it was difficult to contrive an efficient ventilator for prisons, but the ingenuity of Hales did not falter. In the British Museum is preserved a print of the Windmill Ventilator designed by the Rev. Stephen Hales, and erected by order of the Aldermen of the City of London, on the roof of Dick Whittington's Gate at Newgate Prison. His artificial ventilator was applied also at Savoy prison, and in his efforts to avoid noxious air in French prisons containing English captives, he entered into negotiations with distinguished Frenchmen; it is said "the venerable patriarch of Teddington was heard merrily to say he hoped nobody would inform against him for corresponding with the enemy." It is to the glory of Hales that the installation of his ventilator in any prison was followed by a considerably decreased death-rate.

At that time, to die in a British prison for a trivial offense, or for no offense at all, was a natural method of dying. Oglethorpe had a friend whose poverty led him to Fleet Prison, where he succumbed to disease, a tragedy which caused Oglethorpe to investigate the debtors' prisons; his experience as chairman of the parliamentary committee induced him to establish in America the colony of Georgia as a refuge. The findings of Oglethorpe's committee, revealing the human animal fattening on the misfortunes of his brothers, are thus reported by the historian of epidemiology:

> The committee found a disgraceful state of things:—wardens, tip-staffs and turnkeys making their offices so lucrative by extortion that the reversion of them was worth large sums, prisoners abused or neglected if they could not pay, some prisoners kept for years after their term was expired, the penniless crowded three in a bed, or forty in one small room, while some rooms stood empty to await the arrival of a prisoner with a well-filled purse.
>
> On the common side of the Fleet Prison, ninety-three prisoners were confined in three wards, having to find their own bedding, or pay a shilling a week, or else sleep on the floor. The "Lyons Den" and women's ward, which contained about eighteen, were very noisome and in very ill repair. Those who were well had to lie on the floor beside the sick. A Portuguese debtor had been kept two months in a damp stinking dungeon over the common sewer and adjoining to the sink and dunghill; he was taken elsewhere on payment of five guineas. In the Marshalsea there were 330 prisoners on the common side, crowded in small rooms. George's ward, sixteen feet by fourteen and about eight feet high, had never less than thirty-two in it "all last year," and sometimes forty; there was no room for them all to lie down, about one-half of the number sleeping over the others in hammocks; they were locked in from 9 p.m. to 5 a.m. in summer (longer hours in winter), and as they were forced to ease nature within the room, the stench was noisome beyond expression, and it seemed surprising that it had not caused a contagion; several in the heat of summer perished for want of air.
>
> Meanwhile the room above was let to a tailor to work in, and no one allowed to lie in it. Unless the prisoners were relieved by their friends, they perished by famine. There was an allowance of pease from a casual donor who concealed his name, and 30 lbs. of beef three times a week from another charitable source. The starving per-

son falls into a kind of hectic, lingers for a month or two and then dies, the right of his corpse to a coroner's inquest being often scandalously refused. The prison scenes in Fielding's *Amelia* are obviously faithful and correct.

The eighteenth century is incomplete without the Quaker physician, John Coakley Lettsom, principal founder of the Medical Society of London, and one of the busiest and best of men. It is astonishing to contemplate the correspondence he answered and the literary work he accomplished in his carriage. His practice was so varied that he "habitually knocked up three pairs of horses a day," and yet most of his time was devoted to benevolent enterprises. His *Medical Memoirs of the General Dispensary* contain these case-notes, dated May 1773:

Rowell, an industrious, sober workman, who had supported for many years a wife and three children; some of these having been lately sick, he fell behind with his rent, a little over three guineas; he offered all he had (more than enough) to the landlord, but the latter preferred to throw the man and his family into the Compter, where Rowell died of fever.

Russell, once a reputable tradesman on Ludgate Hill, fell into a debt of under three guineas, sent to the Compter with his wife and five children, took fever and died; attended in his sickness in a bare room by his eldest daughter, elegant and refined, aged seventeen; his son, aged fourteen, took the fever and recovered.

In the year that the philanthropic Lettsom recorded his experiences with jail-fever, a small, sick, thin, sallow-faced, middle-aged man, teetotaler and vegetarian, accepted the position of High Sheriff of Bedfordshire. His name was John Howard, and he took his duties seriously. Howard always did that; in youth he had been nursed through an illness by a sympathetic landlady, and although she was more than a quarter of a century his senior, he felt it his duty to marry her. Former sheriffs had sat at the trials in open court, but had not visited the jail. Howard passed through the prison-gate, and saw what happens to men at the mercy of other men. He learned that persons against whom there

MEDICINE IN THE EIGHTEENTH CENTURY

were no accusations, and those who were declared not guilty, were kept in prison for indefinite periods, until they paid the jailer his fees. The solution seemed easy to this queer matter-of-fact officer, and he asked the justices why the jailer did not receive a fixed sum instead of fees from prisoners. "Precedent! my dear sheriff, where is the precedent to charge the county with the gaoler's salary?" So this English Don Quixote mounted his horse, and went from shire to shire, looking for a precedent. He found no precedent, but everywhere he found indescribable cruelty and typhus.

For the rest of his life, John Howard was the inspector of the prison-world of Europe. Without government aid he traveled fifty thousand miles, and visited more prisons, workhouses, hospitals and lazarettos than all the lawmakers in England. He saw more men, women and children chained in dungeons, dying from foul air and lice on putrid straw, perishing from thirst and starvation on bare floors, than a faculty of physicians. He eluded spies, obtained forbidden information, and subjected himself to quarantine. His itinerary was almost incredible, and everywhere he carried his notebook. It cost him £30,000 to fill up these notebooks which exposed Europe. In Russian Kherson, attending a young woman stricken with camp fever, he was infected. John Howard lies buried in a walled field in Southern Russia, and the memory of this man does much to redeem a brutal age. "He lived an Apostle and died a Martyr."

The biologic Titan of the time was an uncouth and ungrammatical Scotchman. John Hunter labored a lifetime among spiteful and uncomprehending contemporaries who flatly informed him a surgeon had no business to engage in physiological investigation. By collecting his Museum—and it was plastered plentifully with the criticism of eminent colleagues—he saw form and function spread before him, and deduced fundamental principles by which he not only solved many riddles himself, but mapped out problems for the coming generations. This comprehensive Museum has served as the mold from which all subsequent museums of natural history have been patterned;

his collection, illustrating the development of organic life from the most primitive to the highest types, affording an unequaled exhibition of structure in connection with vital phenomena, is a permanent workshop for biologists. We have seen with what avidity the British Government purchased Mrs. Stephens' snail-shells to cure calculus; the time came when the same Government was asked to purchase the Hunterian Museum, and Pitt exclaimed indignantly: "What! Buy specimens! why, I have not money enough to purchase gunpowder." The opinion of his contemporaries, "His museum is as much use as so many pigs' pettitoes," has been replaced by the verdict of posterity: "The road to medical education is through the Hunterian Museum, and not through an apothecary's shop."

In Hunter's time, physicians were still discussing whether syphilis and gonorrhea were two manifestations of the same disease, or different diseases. To settle the problem, John Hunter, on a Friday in May 1767, inoculated himself on the prepuce and glans with gonorrheal pus; unknown to him, the subject from whom he took the poison had also a hidden chancre within his urethra, and Hunter contracted not only gonorrhea but syphilis. He was now convinced that "matter from a gonorrhea will produce chancres," and there is but a single venereal virus. It is one of the tragedies of science—the master of the experimental method being led hopelessly astray by an heroic experiment.

Hunter described the hard chancre so well that it is named the Hunterian chancre, but his venereal mistakes were many. He erred in thinking he had cured his syphilis by rubbing his leg and thigh with mercury. "I knocked the disease down with mercury, and I killed it," is a specimen of Hunterian syntax. Hunter wrote, "I have not seen that the brain, heart, stomach, liver, kidneys, and other viscera have been attacked by syphilis, although such cases have been described by authors." On account of this flippant and careless remark, nothing further was said of visceral syphilis for over half a century. The real pathos of the statement is that he was a victim of the condition which he claimed could not exist. Hunter was thirty-eight when he inoculated himself with syphilis, and though he continued to do a giant's work, his health was never good again.

John Hunter, having the privilege of making experiments on the deer in Richmond Park, caught a buck and tied one of its external carotid arteries; he was not perplexed when the half-grown antler, which had received its blood-supply from the imprisoned vessel, became cold to the touch. But a week or two later, when the wound around the ligated artery healed, Hunter again examined the antler and was surprised to observe that it had regained its warmth and was growing. Thinking that perhaps the artery had not been sufficiently bound, Hunter killed the buck to ascertain if this was really the case, but he had done his work well: he found that the external carotid was tightly secured. But he found also that certain small branches of the artery, both above and below the ligature, had enlarged and by their anastomoses had restored the blood-supply of the developed antler. "Oho," said Hunter, "I see that under the stimulus of necessity the smaller arterial channels quickly increase in size to do the work of the larger. I must remember that."

Not many months later there lay in St. George's Hospital a patient who was looked upon as doomed: either he would succumb to popliteal aneurysm, or he would perish under the surgeon's knife, for few who underwent this operation lived to undergo anything else. So frequently fatal was this operation that the profession began to adopt Percival Pott's method—amputation of the limb above the tumor. But the physician in Hunter revolted against this idea of mutilating a man. He never regarded an operation a success if the patient rose from the operating-table a cripple. Hunter thought of his experiment with the buck—recalled that when the passage through a main trunk is arrested, the collateral vessels are capable of continuing the circulation; if, he wondered, far from the seat of the disease he fettered the artery in the sound parts where it is tied when amputation is performed, would not the absorbents be able to cope with the tumor? So in the lower part of its course in the thigh, in the fibrous sheath since known as Hunter's Canal, he ligated his patient's femoral artery. In six weeks the patient left the hospital, walking on the legs that Nature gave him and that Hunter saved for him. And following in his path, on healthy limbs, have trod thousands of men, rescued from deformity or death by this discovery of John Hunter.

Destiny was in an ironic mood when she fathered the birth-control movement upon Thomas Robert Malthus. This clergyman was a timid bird in the sociological aviary, and turned in despair from the daring eagles he hatched. Malthus was not a Malthusian, but despite his repudiation, the birth-control agitation emanates from him and bears his name. As Malthus was not born in a log-cabin, but in the lap of comfort; as his father was not a hard-headed farmer, but a man of culture who appreciated his son; and as the boy was not sent to a boarding-school where he finally licked the class-bully, but was educated at home by private tutors, it may excite surprise that he achieved eminence: according to the traditions, genius has a different history. Father and son passed many pleasant hours together in friendly debate. The elder Malthus was a correspondent of Rousseau, and a follower of Condorcet and Godwin, echoing their belief in the perfectibility of society, but the son argued that "the realization of a happy society will always be hindered by the miseries consequent on the tendency of population to increase faster than the means of subsistence."

Impressed with these views the father asked the son to write them out, and when he saw the manuscript he urged that it be published. As a result of this encouragement, in 1798 appeared the first edition of an *Essay on the Principles of Population*. A year previous, Malthus had taken charge of a small parish in Surrey, where he expected to lead the undisturbed and uneventful life of an English pastor. But fame came with his book, and he studied deeper to see whether he was right, and traveled abroad, everywhere acquiring information that substantiated his discovery of the law of population. Whether the doctrine of Malthus is mathematically correct, or scientifically tenable from the viewpoint of biology or political economy, matters comparatively little—of real importance is the impetus his Essay gave to the study of many problems.

The ink that lay in Malthus' horn ultimately produced a biologic revolution. Praise and obloquy were showered upon the author in profusion, for supporters and opponents began a controversy which is still mooted. The "much-misrepresented Malthus" possessed a character of unusual nobility. Unswayed by the adulation, and untouched by the abuse, he quietly kept on revising successive editions of his epoch-making book. Malthus was a keen diagnostician; with clarity he saw the evils of an excessive and uncontrolled birth-rate, but as a therapeutist he was a clergyman. For a serious disease he proposed an impossible remedy. In Malthus' day, not so much was known of sexual pathology; perhaps he knew little of the effects of sex repression; perhaps it is a parson's privilege to avoid looking at facts too closely if they conflict with his moral precepts—so he tried to solve the sphinx-riddle of reproduction by advising celibacy and late marriages. There was only one weak link in Malthus' chain of reasoning—he forgot human nature, and placidly urged human beings to abstain from sexual intercouse during the years when the sexual instinct is most imperative.

According to Malthus, only when time had cooled the passions and partial impotence supervened, should man and woman repair to the altar. He looked upon the lusty bridegroom and the blushing young bride as a menace to society—his ideal was the decorous middle-aged couple content with Platonic relations. It is to the eternal merit of Malthus that he opened up a new path and found himself face to face with a great problem—and it is equally to his discredit that he attempted to solve it by robbing life of its ecstasy. Yet Malthus' theory of competition, as exemplified in the phrase which he himself used, "struggle for existence," was the nucleus of the most important biologic concept of the next century which, more than any other one factor, modernized science.

For many centuries the ghost of smallpox terrorized our forefathers. Plagues came and plagues disappeared, but smallpox was never absent. It was the vastest horror that decimated the human race. No mother counted her children until all had passed through smallpox. In those days the young men sighed, "Oh, for a mistress who is not pock-marked." It granted no favor to the old, it smote the middle-aged, it struck down the young, it scarred the babe in the womb. None were so lowly as to be passed by without notice, none so powerful as to enjoy immunity. It lay on the toiler's cot of straw, and parted the purple curtains of the emperor's bedstead. Elfrida, Alfred's daughter, the wife of Baldwin the Bald, was attacked by smallpox, and her grandson succumbed to the malady. It touched the fifteenth Louis of France, and the king rolled from his throne to the grave. It maimed and crippled William the Third of England, and ended the life of his young and beautiful Queen. On the same day it ordered coffins for Mary in the almshouse and Mary in the palace—pauper-woman and royal-lady equally speckled with pock-holes.

After the Spaniards brought the scourge of smallpox to America, the empire of the monarch of diseases was universal. No corner of the earth was now safe from the pock-mark. Everywhere it excited a common fear that made the whole world kin. With swift feet that traveled from household to household, with many-fingered hands that clutched the passer-by, with its impalpable poison carried by the atmosphere, and blown abroad by the winds, smallpox seemed like an eternal biblical curse. When its pimpled visage appeared in the untamed forest an Indian father would call his family together, speak to them of the evil spirit which was torturing the tribes, and pointing to the dehumanized features of those already attacked, would exhort his children to escape a similar fate by falling upon their own daggers, promising them if they lacked the courage, that he himself, as a last proof of his devotion, would do the deed of mercy, and at once follow to the happier land. Falling upon the natives of Mexico, it destroyed six million inhabitants with the same fury that it had decimated China in the pre-Christian era. The naked savage squatting on the equator, and the fur-clad Eskimo of the arctic circle, were equally apprehensive of its approach. It entered the wigwams that dotted our western prairies, and emptied the straw-thatched huts of the African. It thinned the population of Ceylon, and in many districts of Iceland there were not sufficient survivors to bury the dead. In the course of ages the human race accumulated such consternation of this eruptive fever that at times when the cry of smallpox was raised, sick infants cried in vain for mothers who had fled in madness.

A young apprentice at Sodbury overheard a country-girl say, "I cannot take the smallpox, for I have had the cowpox." Edward Jenner pricked up his ears with interest, for he remembered that the farmers and dairy-girls of his native Gloucestershire had the same notion. He never forgot the remark, and later on, mentioned it to his teacher, John Hunter. A country doctor from first to last, Jenner was so lacking in ordinary ambition, that in his youth he refused an offer to accompany Captain Cook around the world as naturalist, but to save the face of mankind from the papule, vesicle, pustule and crust, became the engrossing purpose of his life. After reflection and experimentation extending over a long period, Jenner was ready for the test. A dairy-maid named Sarah Nelmes, who had been pricked by a thorn, and became infected with cowpox while milking her master's kine, was his medium. On the fourteenth of May 1796, Jenner took matter from her hand and inserted it by two superficial incisions into the arm of James Phipps, a healthy boy of eight. This was the first vaccination. On the first of the following July, virulent smallpox matter that would have killed any unprotected lad in the world was introduced into his arm, but without the slightest effect, for Phipps had been vaccinated. This was the crucial experiment. The work of twenty-five years was over, and Jenner knew he had closed a gate of death. That day the gossips of Berkeley who lingered by the village pump greeted Jenner as he passed, but did not know that their fellow-townsman had made the world a safer habitation.

In 1798—the year in which the first edition of Malthus' Essay appeared, and John Haslam in his work on insanity gave the original description of general paralysis—Jenner published his *Inquiry into the Causes and Effects of the Variolae Vaccinae*. It is a small pamphlet, with three engravings of arms, and the picture of the hand of Sarah Nelmes, showing the position and development of the pustules. It is a rather delicate hand, with tapering feminine fingers. Were it not for the pustulous sores on it, a poet might write a sonnet to this hand—the hand that helped to halt the disaster that in the eighteenth century alone wiped out sixty million human beings. Jenner's drop of variolous pus has expanded into the far-reaching science of Immunology. Many triumphs of medicine are written in that word, and it uncloses ever-widening vistas to biology. At the point of Edward Jenner's ivory lancet, the medical dream of a Diseaseless Future moved a step nearer its realization.

XI

MODERNIZATION OF MEDICINE

On January 1, 1801, the birth of the Nineteenth Century was celebrated at the court of Weimar. Across the Ilm came the strains of Haydn's *Creation,* and the ducal actors produced a play written by Goethe for the New Age—Goethe himself being crowned as Olympian Jupiter, as we may still see from Kaulbach's painting. That night there was a masquerade ball, and among the maskers were Schiller, Wieland, Herder, and numerous other poets and philosophers who indeed made little Weimar the German Athens. The festivities were prolonged and gay, but over them hung the lengthened shadow of that phenomenon who emerged from the wreck of the French Revolution. Napoleon Bonaparte everywhere accomplished the impossible, and only his ailments proclaimed him of clay. Napoleon had a cold and coughed like a mortal; he was informed there was a doctor who diagnosed troubles in the chest by examining that part of the body. This directness appealed to Napoleon, and he said, "Send him to me." Corvisart came, and tapped the imperial thorax with his finger-tips.

Corvisart learned about percussion from the forgotten *Inventum novum,* and decided to translate it. "I know very well," wrote the generous Frenchman, "how little reputation is allotted to translators and commentators, and I might easily have elevated myself to the rank of an author, if I had elaborated anew the doctrine of Auenbrugger and published an independent work on percussion. In this way, however, I should have sacrificed the name of Auenbrugger to my own vanity, a thing which I am unwilling to do. It is he, and the beautiful invention which of right belongs to him, that I desire to recall to life." Corvisart, in seeking to rehabilitate the name of Auenbrugger, really established his own: although he was the first to call himself a heart specialist, introduced the term carditis, showed sufficient understanding of the problem to remark, "Upon the muscular efficacy of the heart depends life itself," and wrote an important treatise on the organic lesions of the vascular system (1806), he is cited today chiefly for his revival (1808) of Auenbrugger's discovery. Before Corvisart, percussion was the secret of a few; after Corvisart, percussion became the common property of the profession.

While Auenbrugger was growing old in Vienna, a child was growing up in Brittany. He was sickly-born, the offspring of a frail, probably tuberculous, mother, and he himself was asthmatic, thin-chested, and all his life looked like a consumptive. This was Laennec, who arrived in Paris in his nineteenth year, and was soon a favorite pupil of Corvisart. The young Breton was particularly interested in diseases of the chest, but no one yet knew that Laennec was to be Auenbrugger's spiritual heir.

Besides Corvisart, Laennec's name is associated with that of Broussais, but in a very different manner. With Corvisart he came into loving contact; with Broussais he was in angry conflict. Laennec had no use for Broussais, and Broussais saw no good in Laennec. Broussais was a master of sarcasm, and Laennec was not backward in bandying scorn. No doubt Broussais was more talented in this respect—he handled words as he had handled a cutlass in the republican navy—but then he had numerous and varied hatreds, while Laennec could concentrate. When he spoke of Broussaisism his voice became acid, and his eyes shot sparks of indignation through his tortoise-rimmed spectacles. What must have added special piquancy to the warfare between Broussais and Laennec was the circumstance that both were Bretons, and of all people in the world none are so chauvinistic as the folks that hail from Brittany. Broussais was the medical theorist of the hour, but Corvisart and Laennec accepted only the Hippocratic watchword, Observation. The theories of Broussais are now as obsolete as his hirudinomania, which was carried to such an extent that within a calendar year it became necessary to import forty-two million leeches into France. At one time there was hardly a French belly which had not given nourishment to these blood-suckers.

In 1816, Laennec was transferred to the Necker Hospital. During this year a woman who was suffering from heart trouble consulted him. Laennec questioned her, but was puzzled how to proceed with the examination. There was no use in thumping her thorax, for the patient was too stout; neither could he put his ear directly upon her breast, for she was still young. We may argue that physicians have privileges, but Laennec himself claims that immediate auscultation was inadmissible. In his dilemma he happened to recollect a fact in physics. Acting on the idea, he rolled a quire of paper into a kind of cylinder and applied one end of it to the region of the patient's heart and the other to his own ear. This was the first stethoscope. Then René Laennec heard the language of pathology. A diseased heart appealed to him for aid. Injuries that for centuries had been inaudible, now found a voice. A sick organ murmured its tale of woe into the ear of the listening physician. Mediate auscultation, the crowning glory of physical diagnosis, came into existence.

During his too brief career, the undersized Laennec dissected an army of the dead. Had he never invented the stethoscope, or his method of hearing disease, his dissecting-room discoveries were sufficiently numerous and significant to place him among the foremost pathological anatomists. Laennec's forerunner in this field was Bichat, who demonstrated that "the different organs have membranes and tissues in common, and the seat of disease is in the constituent tissues and not in the individual organs"—a concept which simplified anatomy and physiology, and revolutionized pathological investigation. Bichat, after editing the surgical works of his teacher and foster-father Desault, published in rapid succession a treatise on membranes, physiological researches on life and death, and his masterpiece on general anatomy. In the following summer (1802), Bichat, in his thirty-first year, succumbed to his dissecting-room labors. Corvisart wrote to Napoleon: "Bichat has just fallen on a battlefield which numbers more than one victim. No one has done so much and so well in so short a time." By Napoleon's orders, a bust of Bichat, who has been called the "Napoleon of Medicine," was placed in the Hôtel Dieu.

Across the Channel, men plied the scalpel with equal avidity, but under peculiar conditions. Dissection was not legalized in Great Britain, and the quest of the human cadaver was still unlawful. Yet every anatomical teacher worthy of the name, whether lecturing in a university or in his private school, found it essential to secure cadavers for his students. The greater his anatomical zeal, the more bodies he needed. In the celebrated murder trial at the Warwick assizes, to which John Hunter was called as a witness, he was asked: "You have been long in the habit of dissecting human subjects. I presume you have dissected more than any man in Europe?" Hunter answered, "I have dissected some thousands during these thirty-three years." The court purposely refrained from asking a more searching question: "Where did you obtain these thousands?"

The answer is one of the most gruesome in the history of medicine. Since anatomists required bodies, and since the need was not supplied by the authorities, the anatomists followed the example of Vesalius and stole the bodies. At times a lecturer gathered his strong-armed assistants, and under cover of night rifled the churchyard. These excursions were not without danger, and bullet-marks are still visible on the Kilgobbin tombstones near the Dublin Mountains. The student Robert Liston, later the eminent surgeon, led many such parties because of his immense strength.

Of course an anatomist who dissected every day, or a teacher who demonstrated to hundreds of pupils, could not do all his own stealing: hence arose in London, Edinburgh, Glasgow, Manchester and Dublin, a new professional class known by the various names of fishermen, body-snatchers, sack-'em-up men, and resurrectionists. These resurrection-men became absolutely indispensable to the anatomists, for they were practically the only source from which subjects could be procured. The law made the elegant Sir Astley Cooper and the industrious Joshua Brookes the bed-fellows of such body-snatchers as Crouch and Murphy.

If a resurrectionist was imprisoned, the anatomists helped him and supported his family. If an anatomist refused to traffic with them, or protested at their frequent extortions, not only was he deprived of material, but he was marked for vengeance. The stronger gangs, by intimidation and bribery, by employing sextons, watchmen, grave-diggers and undertakers, monopolized the cemeteries, and dictated terms to the men of science. Corrigan, who described the waterhammer pulse which is still called by his name, thus summed up the situation: "The absurdity still existed that while the law punished any one found procuring a dead body for dissection, the educational laws required that every candidate should possess a practical knowledge of it." In the early nineteenth century, Englishmen could become physicians and surgeons only by violating the law.

Another oddity of this law consisted in the provision that to steal a dead body constituted a misdemeanor, but to steal an inch of the dead body's grave-clothes meant felony: naturally the resurrectionists left the grave-clothes behind in the coffin, though on rare occasions haste made them careless. For example, the well-known body-snatchers, Vaughan and his wife, after attending two funerals in one day at Plymouth, exhumed the bodies at night-fall. Detected, they were sentenced to one month's imprisonment; they were then tried for a stocking which had clung to one of the dead legs, and were transported for seven years. Men who make laws are different.

The resurrection-men boldly entered work-houses and poor hospitals, claiming to be relatives of the recently deceased; usually they secured their prey, for the authorities welcomed the opportunity of saving the expense of a pauper's funeral. At times they sold a body to one anatomist, stole it from him, and resold it to another; at other times they delivered drunkards, instead of subjects, in their sacks, and pocketed their pay before the deception was discovered. A gang would demand a large bonus from a school on the ground that they would not supply material to any other school, and by this device received bonuses from every school. The resurrectionists suffered far more from rival resurrectionists than from the police. They were men of skill and cunning, and as restrictions tightened, the price of the cadaver increased. In the season when there was no dissection in England, they traveled to France or Spain in the wake of the armies; after a battle they extracted the teeth of the fallen soldiers, and realized fortunes from the London dentists. The resurrectionist Butler, upon being asked where he got his teeth, replied, "Oh, Sir, only let there be a battle, and there'll be no want of teeth. I'll draw them as fast as the men are knocked down."

At the university of Edinburgh are still preserved Darwin's cards of admission to the anatomical courses, signed by the third Monro. The Monro dynasty lasted for one hundred and twenty-six years, and Monro primus and Monro secundus were men of originality, but Monro tertius read his grandfather's anatomical lectures in a lifeless voice, without altering a syllable, even repeating, "When I met Boerhaave. . . ." That is why Charles Darwin wrote in his Autobiography: "Dr.—— made his lectures on human anatomy as dull as he was himself, and the subject disgusted me." Had the last of the Monros not dragged Boerhaave into the nineteenth century, Charles Darwin might have completed his medical course. He had not the temperament, however, to follow in the ancestral footsteps, since his Autobiography contains this admission: "I also attended on two occasions the operating theater in the hospital at Edinburgh, and saw two very bad operations, one on a child, but I rushed away before they were completed. Nor did I ever attend again, for hardly any inducement would have been strong enough to make me do so; this being long before the blessed days of chloroform. The two cases fairly haunted me for many a long year."

After Darwin spent two sessions at Edinburgh, his medical father perceived he would never be a physician; the next step was to send him to Cambridge to become a clergyman. At Cambridge, Darwin completely wasted three years—the expression is his own—except that he walked with Henslow the botanist. An incident during one of these historic walks is recorded in the autobiographical reminiscences of Darwin:

> I once saw in his company in the streets of Cambridge almost as horrid a scene as could have been witnessed during the French Revolution. Two body-snatchers had been arrested, and whilst being taken to prison had been torn from the constable by a crowd of the roughest men, who dragged them by their legs along the muddy and stony road. They were covered from head to foot with mud, and their faces were bleeding either from having been kicked or from the stones; they looked like corpses, but the crowd was so dense that I got only a few momentary glimpses of the wretched creatures. Never in my life have I seen such wrath painted on a man's face as was shown by Henslow at this horrid scene. He tried repeatedly to penetrate the mob; but it was simply impossible. He then rushed away to the mayor, telling me not to follow him, but to get more policemen. I forget the issue, except that the two men were got into the prison without being killed.

The dexterity of the resurrection-men with crowbar and chain was nothing short of marvelous. With utmost speed, without a sound they removed a body in the darkness, put back the death-clothes, and restored the grave so skilfully that many flowers were planted and thousands of tears were shed over empty coffins. Mourners watched the burial-ground, spring-guns were set in the church-yards, strong bars known as mortsafes surrounded the tombs, prudent relatives purchased Bridgman's patent wrought-iron coffins, and still the bodies disappeared. As Astley Cooper informed the Committee of the House of Commons: "There is no person, let his situation in life be what it may, whom, if I were disposed to dissect, I could not obtain. The law only enhances the price, and does not prevent the exhumation." Sir Astley also explained that the anatomical teachers of England were entirely "at the feet of the resurrection men." It was not pleasant to be at the feet of such men, because they were not gentlemen: for example, a typical resurrectionist, the tall, pale-faced Merrilees, sold his sister to the surgeons. The legislators, more interested in fox-hunting than in anatomical educators, waited for a national calamity before deciding to act.

In Surgeon's Square, Edinburgh, six rivals lectured on anatomy and bought stolen bodies. In Tanner's Close in the West Port, two Irishmen lived with their women: William Hare and Margaret Laird kept a lodging-house where a bed could be procured for a few pence; William Burke and Helen M'Dougal resided near by; Burke, who pretended to be a cobbler, was the pleasanter of the men, and danced a jig well; Margaret was the more vivacious of the women. All four drank constantly. Among Hare's lodgers, an old army pensioner named Donald, dying before his quarterly pension arrived, owed his landlord £4. The parish officer came and placed Donald in a coffin. Hare wondered how to recover his debt, and talked the matter over with his friend Burke. Neither had ever been a resurrection-man, but they knew that bodies could be sold to the doctors. The parish undertaker returned and took away the coffin, which was now filled with tanner's bark, for the corpse of Donald was lying in Hare's bed. Burke and Hare went to the college quadrangle, and asked a student to show them the rooms of the professor of anatomy. As this student was a pupil of Robert Knox, the most popular of the Edinburgh lecturers, he directed the pair to Number 10, Surgeons' Square. That night Donald's body lay in Knox's dissecting-room. They received for it twice the amount of the debt, no questions were asked, and they were urged to come again as soon as they had another subject. The date on which this occurred—November 29, 1827—is of deep significance in medical annals.

Another of Hare's lodgers, Joseph the miller, lay sick with fever. He was going to die anyway, and his continued illness might be bad for the business of the house, so Burke and Hare smothered him and sold his body to Knox for £10. After that, "Sold to Dr. Knox for £10," became a frequent item in the accounts of the new firm. A nameless Englishman "who used to sell spunks in Edinburgh," suffering from jaundice, was next on the list. The partners now began prowling the streets for subjects, noting the friendless men and women who haunted the neighborhood. Every week, Abigail Simpson, who sold salt and camstone, walked from Gilmerton to Edinburgh to collect eighteen pence and a can of kitchen fee which Sir John Hope allowed her as a pension: Hare and his wife invited her in for a drink, and the next day she was sold in a tea-chest. Knox was pleased at the fresh state of the body, but he asked no questions. Mrs. Hare offered several others the hospitality of her whisky, and they went straight from Tanner's Close to Surgeons' Square. One morning Burke saw two policemen dragging a drunken creature to the watchhouse. "Let her go," he said, "I know where she lives and will take her home." After sunset, Knox owned her. Burke enticed old Effie, the cinder gatherer, to Hare's stable, made her drunk, and smothered her—or as we now say, burked her. Mrs. Hare suggested that Mrs. Burke be turned into merchandise, but Burke was too fond of his Nelly for that.

Ann M'Dougal, a relative of one of Nelly's other husbands, traveled from Falkirk to Edinburgh to visit her kinswoman. She was welcomed with all the whisky she could drink. Burke turned to Hare and explained the situation: "You must have most to do with her, as she being a distant friend I do not like to begin first." Hare commenced the stifling, Burke completed it, and Knox's doorkeeper sent a fine trunk for the country cousin. Mary Haldane, a stout old street-walker, never refused a drink, and the women of the firm gave her plenty. She was escorted to Hare's stable, and falling asleep among the straw, was carried to Knox. Within a day or two, her daughter Peggy called at Hare's house, saying the grocer had seen her mother there. Mrs. Hare damned her impudence, but Hare came out of the "little back room" and said her mother had come and gone. He offered her a drink, Burke joined the party, and the quarrel was forgotten. Peggy got so drunk that Burke placed her face downwards, and pressed her until she stopped breathing. Mother and daughter who in life had walked the same streets, were joined together in death on the same dissecting-slabs.

This catalogue has several other entries, and the procedure was similar: one lay on the victim, and the other placed his hands over the nose and mouth—death came without leaving a mark. At times fortune favored the firm. Burke was about to bring in a forlorn old man, when he was greeted by a hearty Irishwoman, who was holding on to the hand of her grandson, a boy dumb since birth. She knew Burke, and told him she had come in search of some friends, but did not know their address. As two bodies brought more than one, Burke dismissed the old man, and informed his countrywoman he knew the "whereabouts of the folk." She followed him home, and gladly shared the proffered bottle, while the women watched the child. The grandmother drank until she could offer no resistance, and was burked. The next morning the dumb boy showed by his actions that he was alarmed at being left alone; Burke himself said that he looked up at him with frightened imploring eyes, but Burke knew he could not cry out, and taking the dumb thing on his knee he broke his back. The tea-chest, which had sufficed for the remains of Peggy Haldane, proved insufficient for two subjects, and they were stuffed into a herring-barrel. Knox paid £16. Did Knox and his assistants know they were buying murdered bodies? The blundering law made them so eager for bodies they could not afford to ask any questions—otherwise the trade would have been diverted to their rivals.

The thriving firm of Burke and Hare, plus their silent partners who shared the profits, realizing the truth of De Quincey's phrase, "murder being one of the fine arts," naturally grew bold with success and expert with experience. Every one in Edinburgh knew James Wilson, because this lad of eighteen was always on the streets. His one vice was snuff, and a brass snuff-box and copper snuff-spoon were ever in his pockets. He was an "innocent," though not an imbecile; he resented his nickname of Daft Jamie, and his apt replies in his thick Scotch brogue often showed considerable sense. He was strong and agile, but so gentle and timid that when little children mocked and tormented him, he ran away. Adults never molested him, and Daft Jamie trusted all grown-ups.

When Mrs. Hare asked him to come home with her, he meekly followed. As Burke declared, "Mrs. Hare led poor Jamie in as a dumb lamb to the slaughter, and as a sheep to the shearers." The men soon appeared, and insisted that Jamie drink with them. He took one glass, and not all their cajolings could induce him to take another. He was invited to lie down in the bed and rest. Hare stretched out behind him, Burke sat in front, and the unsuspecting Jamie closed his eyes and slept. Suddenly Hare gripped his mouth and nose, whereupon Jamie fought so hard that both fell out of bed. Jamie was getting the better of the fray, but Burke tripped him up from behind, and held his hands and feet until Hare smothered him. They went through his pockets, and Hare kept the brass snuff-box and Burke took the copper snuff-spoon. Knox took the body and the £10 that he paid for Daft Jamie was more than Daft Jamie had ever seen in his life.

When Canongate was the court-end of Edinburgh, the dames were haughty, and their admirers sang:

> The lasses o' the Canongate,
> Oh they are wondrous nice;
> They winna gi'e a single kiss
> But for a double price.

When Canongate became the slums of Edinburgh, the price of kisses dropped, as Mary Paterson well knew. This Venus of the pavement was locked up over night in the Canongate watch-house, and early the next morning refreshed herself at a shop with a gill of whisky. There stood Burke with the publican, drinking rum and bitters. He invited her to his lodgings for breakfast, and Bonny Mary, eighteen, alone and fearless, went with him. Burke's brother, Constantine, a scavenger for the police, lived in the Canongate, and to this room Burke took the girl. As Constantine and his wife were still in bed, Burke drove them out to give Mary a "good Scots breakfast of tea, bread, eggs, and Finnan haddocks." The brother and his wife disappeared, Burke offered Mary a bottle of whisky, and she drank until she lay across the truckle bed, still holding twopence halfpenny fast in her hand. Within a few hours the body of Mary Paterson was at Surgeons' Square.

One of Knox's assistants was sufficiently impressed by her beauty to inquire where they obtained her. This was young Fergusson, later famous as Sir William Fergusson, creator of conservative surgery, professor at King's College of London, and Serjeant-Surgeon to Queen Victoria. Another pupil, Henry Lonsdale, afterwards Knox's biographer and defender, has described the sensation produced by Bonny Mary: "The body of the girl Paterson could not fail to attract attention by its voluptuous form and beauty; students crowded around the table on which she lay, and artists came to study a model worthy of Phidias and the best Greek art. A pupil of Knox's, who had been in her company only a few nights previously, stood aghast on observing the beautiful Lais stretched in death, and ready for the scalpel of the anatomist. . . . Knox, wishing for the best illustration of female form for his lectures, had Paterson's body put in spirit, so that when he came to treat of the myological division of his course, further publicity was given to her remains."

In the first footnote to his *Halloween,* Scotland's poet explains that "Halloween is thought to be a night when witches, devils, and other mischief-making beings are all abroad on their baneful, midnight errands. *R. B.*" The firm of Burke and Hare was ready for business that day. Burke was drinking in Rymer's shop and sizing up prospective "subjects." A little old woman came in, begging for alms; she had come all the way from Ireland in search of her son, and her name was Docherty. Burke approached, and said his mother's name was Docherty, and since they must be related he would help her find her son, and of course she must stay in his house. It happened that Burke's house was full at the time, a laborer named James Gray, his wife Ann, and their child occupying a pallet. Burke told them they must make way for his kinswoman, but Mrs. Hare solved the difficulty by giving them a bed in Tanner's Close. The Grays left Burke's house with the understanding that they would return next morning for breakfast.

With the fall of night, the Halloween was celebrated. Neighbors came in and out, and the merrymaking rose high. The animated old woman drank and sang and danced, but as she was barefoot she "got a scratch on the foot with the nails in Hare's shoes." It grew late, and the other guests departed. The Burkes and Hares remained with the little old woman who thought she would find her son next day. There was a shout, and then all was still. The Grays arrived for breakfast, and inquired about Mrs. Docherty. Mrs. Burke answered she had been too friendly with Burke and was so noisy that she turned her out. "Well," added Burke, "she's quiet enough now." Mrs. Gray had lost her child's stockings, and went to the straw to find them. "Keep out of there!" roared Burke. More than once he kept her away from the bed, and sat there watching it. Mrs. Gray smoked her pipe, and wondered about the forbidden straw. No one moved from the room until "about darkening"; Burke then ordered Mrs. Burke and the lad Broggan not to let any one come near the bed. Burke went out for a drink, and his faithless sentinels deserted their post. Gray and his wife were alone in the room. Without further delay, Mrs. Gray lifted up the straw which covered Mrs. Docherty. They gathered their few belongings and left the house. Mrs. Burke met them in the passage, and offered £10 a week for their silence; the Grays walked to the nearest police station and told their story. At eight o'clock a sergeant entered Burke's house; he lifted up the straw and nothing was there; he saw some blood, and Mrs. Burke said she was menstruating. The sergeant did not believe the Grays and thought they brought the charge because they could not pay the rent and Burke had put them out. Nevertheless, he took the accused to the station-house.

The next morning was Sunday, and Edinburgh rested from her labors. Surgeons' Square was deserted, except for the police who visited Dr. Knox's empty rooms. The porter brought up from the cellar a tea-chest which had been delivered the night before, "in the ordinary course of business." The police opened the tea-chest, and saw the face of a little old woman. James Gray came over, and identified her as Mrs. Docherty. A public subscription was later started for James Gray, and not even £10 was collected—less than Knox would have paid for a single corpse. Gray died within the year, leaving his widow and child destitute. Such was a nation's gratitude to the man whose unshakable honesty broke up the copartnership of Burke and Hare.

The Crown bungled from the beginning. The advocates for the defense were more aggressive than the prosecutors. The excitement throughout Edinburgh was intense, and the lawyers cared more for the correct etiquette of the trial than for the truth. Hundreds of useless questions were asked, and the facts were concealed in too great a punctiliousness for legal ceremonies. Above all, the eminent counsel determined to show the howling mob outside that they were deaf to its cry for vengeance. Finally Hare was promised immunity if he would give king's evidence, and he smilingly admitted sixteen murders. The *Edinburgh Evening Courant,* in the teeth of the law, published a fuller confession from Burke than the Crown, with all its machinery, was able to obtain. The prisoners were tried only for suffocating Mrs. Docherty, and nothing was said of their numerous other victims—there was some technicality about that. Hare, Mrs. Hare and Mrs. Burke went scot-free, and Burke was condemned: "To be hanged by the neck, by the hands of the common executioner, upon a gibbet, until he be dead, and his body thereafter to be delivered to Dr. Alexander Monro, Professor of Anatomy in the University of Edinburgh, to be by him publicly dissected and anatomized. And may Almighty God have mercy on your soul."

The short squat skeleton of William Burke still hangs behind glass in the Anatomical Museum of the University of Edinburgh. Peacefully reposing by his side we see the skeleton of one of his victims, Daft Jamie. Burke is not out of place in this scientific institution, for in nine months of murder he accomplished more for anatomy than all the anatomical teachers in the British Isles. The efforts of anatomists, "to legalize and regulate the supply of subjects for dissection," were balked by the characteristic indifference and stupidity of the politicians. John Hunter's pupil, John Abernethy, exerted himself in vain; the international reputation of Charles Bell meant little to parliament; Benjamin Brodie accomplished nothing; the eloquent testimony of Astley Cooper fell on bored ears; and Henry Cline might just as well have stayed at home.

Nor were the legislators alone to blame. The Royal College of Surgeons of London—grown into the disgraceful and incompetent oligarchy which Thomas Wakley, at the risk of life, exposed in his recently-founded *Lancet*—petitioned against any change in the laws. The House of Lords refused to consider the matter, since the Archbishop of Canterbury was opposed to recognition of anatomical needs. A national calamity was lacking, and parliament would not act. It required Burke and Hare, with their confessed murders of men, women and children, to overrule an archbishop and to move the sluggish representatives of the people. On July 19, 1832, after stubborn debate, the Anatomy Bill, advised by Macartney, introduced by Warburton, supported by Macaulay, finally passed the House of Lords as the Anatomy Act. On that day, anatomy became a legitimate study, and the resurrection-men ceased to exist.

The nineteenth century is known as the Age of Biology, though its earlier years were far from deserving that distinction. In 1823 the Bohemian Jan Purkyně, candidate for a vacant chair of physiology in Germany, was rejected by the professors; they did not reckon, however, with two great European powers who stood behind the Slav, and since the combination of Goethe and Humboldt was irresistible, Purkyně went to Breslau in spite of the faculty. He found himself an unwelcome guest of the university, and his chair was not lined with velvet. Naturally he spoke German with a tinge of Czech accent, and the anatomist Otto sarcastically informed him that if he wished to be understood, he had better lecture in Latin. Purkyně was not eloquent in expounding theories, and when he hinted that up to the present a lecturer in physiology was "merely a mechanism by means of which the theories of the old masters were repeated again and again," his classes dwindled in indignation and the faculty circulated a petition for his removal.

Purkyně stirred up more trouble by asking for a microscope. The authorities could not understand why a physiologist needed a microscope, and they sighed for the good old days of Bartels. There was the famous Bartels, becoming a Geheimrat and climbing to the Berlin chair; writing many books on *naturphilosophie*, medicine and theology; diagnosing all diseases with the most learned phrases and knowing enough to denounce such newfangled notions as Laennec's stethoscope; and yet he never needed a microscope. If this were permitted to go on, the university would be cluttered up with apparatus and specimens, and the students would be occupied in performing experiments instead of reading van Helmont and Haller and Bartels. Evidently the arguments failed to convince Purkyně—he had "a poor ear for German"—and in an unoccupied corner of the college building he began to construct a physiological laboratory. Immediately he aroused the opposition of his colleagues who informed him that such a laboratory was utterly useless in medicine; moreover, Otto, officious and esthetic, strongly objected to the stench.

Purkyně, with his forbidden microscope, found the germinal vesicle in the chick before von Baer saw the mammalian ovum; he discovered the sweat-glands and their ducts; the interlacing fibers in the young heart-muscle; the flask-shaped nerve-cells, with their axones and branching dendrites, which form the characteristic features of the cerebellum. In microscopy he was the first to employ the microtome, microphotography, Drummond lime light, glacial acetic acid, potassium bichromate, and Canada balsam. Considering the prevalence of mental inertia, it is perhaps not surprising that Purkyně—the first to use the term *protoplasm*—was compelled to establish Europe's first physiological laboratory in his own home. Otto won a temporary victory, and Purkyně lived and dined and slept in the midst of biological equipment, including the unavoidable odors. His wife was not supposed to complain, for she was Rudolphi's daughter.

Carl Asmund Rudolphi, physiologist, comparative anatomist, and pioneer of parasitology, increased our knowledge of intestinal worms, though he nullified his achievements by his conviction that the parasites were the result, instead of the cause, of diseased conditions. Rudolphi died suddenly, and Johannes Müller wrote to the authorities, "With the exception of Meckel no one in Germany can fill this post as well as I." Johannes Müller, on his own recommendation, was appointed Rudolphi's successor as professor of anatomy and physiology in the university of Berlin, thus becoming in his early thirties the central figure of German medicine. Müller, physically unable to experiment upon warm-blooded animals, stated in his eulogy of his predecessor: "Rudolphi looked upon physiological experiments as having no relation to anatomical accuracy, and it is no wonder that this admirable man, who had at every opportunity expressed his abhorrence of vivisection, took up a hostile position against all hypotheses and conclusions insufficiently established upon physiological experiments. . . . We could have failed to share his righteous indignation had we not seen how many physiologists were using every effort to reduce physiology to an experimental science by the live dissection and agonies of innumerable animals, undertaken without any definite plan, and yielding often insignificant results." We do not know which is worse—the antivivisectionist who holds all experimenters in abhorrence, or the experimenter who looks with scorn on all who feel compassion for animals. Nature, the blundering giant, has made it impossible for man to secure certain knowledge except by inflicting pain upon the lower creatures.

Johannes Müller and his pupils almost made biology a German province. These pupils include Helmholtz, who climbed from an assistant surgeonship in a regiment of Red Hussars to the heights of mathematical physics, formulating the principles of thermodynamics, and inventing the ophthalmoscope which opened a new world to medicine; Emil du Bois-Reymond, creator of modern electrophysiology; Claperède, the young Swiss naturalist, who lived for biology's sake on a desolate Norwegian reef; Henle, expounder of the epithelial system; Schwann, who struck an effective blow at the mirage of spontaneous generation, and whose theory that all living things arise from a cell and consist of cells, is the starting-point of modern biology; Reichert, whose work on the development of frog's spawn brought the cell-theory into embryology; Virchow, whose *Cellularpathologie*, applying the cell-doctrine to disease, gave to biology its conception of germinal continuity—every cell from a cell—which is the foundation of the study of heredity; Brücke, who suggested the concept of cell-organization; Robert Remak, whose discovery of nerve-cells in the heart of a frog revealed the cause of the heart-beat; Vierordt, who constructed the first instrument (*sphygmograph*) for recording the movements of the pulse; the great Carl Ludwig, who introduced the graphic method into physiology; Kölliker, founder of the new histology.

Friedrich Wöhler erected one of the biologic landmarks of the century. He graduated in medicine at Heidelberg, and intended to prepare himself for practice, but Leopold Gmelin—the most famous of the many Gmelins who cultivated chemistry—persuaded him to see Berzelius, and thereafter Wöhler never touched a lancet. In the annals of chemistry, the name of Wöhler logically follows Gmelin and Berzelius, for in 1817 Gmelin said it was characteristic of organic compounds that they could not be produced from their elements, while Berzelius in 1827 wrote that "the elements present in living bodies obey laws totally different from those which rule inanimate nature."

In the following year, Wöhler, still in his twenties, accomplished what every chemist had deemed impossible: he created an organic substance from its inorganic elements. Wöhler's preparation of urea demolished the barrier between the organic and inorganic world—and built a bridge instead. He cremated the vital force theory, and from its ashes arose a new conception of the unity of matter. He overthrew an ancient dogma, and cleared the way for the laboratory preparation of complex mineral and vegetable products.

Wöhler began with the synthesis of urea, and modern chemists have ended with the synthesis of proteins from their amino-acid constituents: in this field chemists of the future have only one more problem to solve—the synthesis of albumin, which is protoplasm, which is life. If only we could write the chemical formula of a protein! The white of egg consists of carbon, hydrogen, nitrogen, oxygen and sulphur. If only we could take these five elements and mix them in our beakers or heat them in our crucibles or freeze them in our ammonia tanks till they albuminized, man would become the possessor of the secret of secrets. This is the crux of all biologic problems: to create a bit of protoplasm. A chemist can make butter: when the biologist learns to lay an egg he will have solved the problem of life.

Unable to learn at Edinburgh and Cambridge, Darwin was anxious to accompany Captain Fitz-Roy of the *Beagle* around the world as a volunteer naturalist without pay. Robert Fitz-Roy, father of the weather bureau, happened to be a disciple of Lavater, and was on the point of rejecting Darwin because of the shape of his nose. On such an accident hinged the most momentous voyage in the history of biology. The sailor-scientist of the *Beagle* "did not hear the autumn robins singing in the Shrewsbury garden" for five years, but he was able to write, "The sight of a naked savage in his native land is an event which can never be forgotten." Amid South American fossils and the fauna of Galapagos, the naturalist of twenty-eight began to speculate on the Transmutation of Species. In 1838, the reading of Malthus crystallized his ideas, and he was prepared to realize "that under these circumstances favorable variations would tend to be preserved, and unfavorable ones to be destroyed. The result of this would be the formation of new species. Here, then, I had a theory by which to work." For twenty years Charles Darwin worked on this theory.

By a remarkable coincidence, Alfred Russel Wallace, blanketed and shaking with ague beneath the Malayan palm-trees in 1858, recalled the work of Malthus which he had read years before, whereupon "there suddenly flashed upon me the idea of the survival of the fittest." How Wallace thought out the theory during the fit, drafted it that evening and despatched it by the next post to Darwin whom he had met once; how Darwin was amazed at its identity with his own work on natural selection; how he consulted Lyell and Hooker, who presented the joint-essays to the Linnean Society; how Darwin finally composed the *Origin of Species;* how the entire edition of 1250 copies was sold on the first day of publication, November 24, 1859—are familiar incidents in the greatest of cultural revolutions.

The scientific spirit of the nineteenth century closed the Inquisition and took the *strappado* from the hands of ecclesiasticism. In 1835, for the first time, Copernicus, Galileo, and Kepler were liberated from the *Index librorum prohibitorum.* The times had so greatly changed, that theologians who would gladly have led Darwin to the *auto-da-fé,* compromised by calling him a monkey's grandson. In the nineteenth century religious intolerance lost its thumb-screw, and was obliged to substitute abusive epithets. Darwin in one of his characteristic letters to Lyell, added a playful P. S.—*"Our* ancestor was an animal which breathed water, had a swim bladder, a great swimming tail, an imperfect skull, and undoubtedly was an hermaphrodite! Here is a pleasant genealogy for mankind." This was for private consumption, but with the passing of years the ancestral ape grew less alarming; sophisticates even viewed him with satisfaction: "I take a jealous pride in my Simian ancestry. I like to think that I was once a magnificent hairy fellow living in the trees, and that my frame has come down through geological time via sea jelly and worms and Amphioxus, Fish, Dinosaurs, and Apes. Who would exchange these for the pallid couple in the Garden of Eden?"

Without doubt the work of the Evolutionists is the most

important ever accomplished on earth. In comparison with these truth-seekers, the scientific giants of the previous century appear like superstitious children, afraid of the dark. The Darwinists were the first full-grown men who investigated Nature, and reported their findings without reference to gods and devils. They found no moral purpose in Nature, but they found no ghosts either. Lyell's *Antiquity of Man* (1863), Huxley's *Evidences as to Man's Place in Nature* (1863), Haeckel's *General Morphology* (1866) and Darwin's *Descent of Man* (1871) demonstrated that the world was not created for man—a terrible blow to our vanity, but it set us firmly on our feet where we belong. They did not comfort us with the fairy-tales of Haller and Linnaeus, but they emancipated man from the ghastly shadows that hung over him like brooding bats.

The *Athenaeum* charged, "Lyell's object is to make man old, Huxley's to degrade him," and could not see that their object was simply to know the truth. In modifying, correcting and completing the work of the pioneer Evolutionists, we need no better guide than the spirit of Huxley when he said: "Thoughtful men, escaped from the blinding influences of traditional prejudice, will find in the lowly stock whence man has sprung, the best evidence of the splendour of his capacities; and will discern in his long progress through the Past a reasonable ground of faith in his attainment of a nobler Future. . . . There is no alleviation for the sufferings of mankind except veracity of thought and action and the resolute facing of the world as it is, when the garment of make-believe by which pious hands have hidden its uglier features is stripped off."

In the first half of the nineteenth century, English physicians gave their names to various diseased conditions: Joseph Hodgson described dilatation of the aortic arch (Hodgson's disease, 1815); James Parkinson, paralysis agitans or shaking palsy (Parkinson's disease, 1817); Richard Bright, nephritis, or disease of the kidneys usually associated with dropsy and albumin in the urine (Bright's disease, 1827); Charles Bell, peripheral paralysis of the facial nerve (Bell's palsy, 1829); Thomas Hodgkin, malignant lymphoma, or involvement of the lymph nodes with enlargement of the spleen (Hodgkin's disease, 1832); Thomas Addison, pernicious anemia (Addison's anemia, 1849), and disease of suprarenal capsules (Addison's disease, 1849)— an early landmark in the coming science of the ductless glands.

The Irish School of Medicine included such able clinicians as Robert Adams, who advanced our understanding of rheumatic gout; Robert James Graves, who gave us the pinhole pupil, and requested as his epitaph, "He fed fevers"; Sir Dominic John Corrigan, memorable for his description of insufficiency of the aortic valve; William Stokes, who described the type of breathing in which the respirations increase, decrease, cease, and continue the cycle—this is known as the Cheyne-Stokes respiration, a condition first graphically described by Hippocrates in the phrase, "The breathing throughout, as though he were recollecting to do it." The Irish physicians were noted for outspokenness, and certainly Abraham Colles, the surgeon of the School, did not belie that reputation. During the post-mortem of a former patient, he turned to his class and said, "Gentlemen, it is no use mincing the matter; I caused the patient's death." Aside from the fracture of the lower end of the radius known as Colles' fracture, he is remembered for the endless discussion he caused by his statement of Colles' law: "A newborn child affected with congenital syphilis, even although it may have symptoms in the mouth, never causes ulceration of the breast which it sucks, if it be the mother who suckles it, though continuing capable of infecting a strange nurse."

French clinical contributions include Pierre Bretonneau's study of the disease he named diphtheria (1826); Pierre-Charles-Alexandre Louis' researches on "the malady known under the name of gastro-enteritis," which he named typhoid fever (1829), and his statistics which finally stopped the flood of blood-letting; Jean-Antoine Villemin's demonstration that the tubercular virus is specific and inoculable; Armand Trousseau's suggestion of puncture of the chest for removal of fluid (*thoracentesis*); Gabriel Andral's chemical studies of blood diseases;

Pierre-François-Olive-Rayer's memoir on human glanders and farcy; Henri Huchard's elucidation of arteriosclerosis; Charles-Jacques Bouchard's work in autointoxication; Georges Haymen's development of hematology; Alfred Fournier's life-work in one of the saddest of medical fields—congenital syphilis. French neurology reached first rank through the labors of Duchenne and Charcot.

The nineteenth century was the first that saw an alkaloid —the active principle of the plant, found either in the bark, leaves, seeds, or other parts. The secrets of opium were now revealed: Derosne discovered narcotine, Hesse extracted a dozen alkaloids from the poppy plant, T. and H. Smith spent profitable years within the capsule of this wondrous drug, but the chief treasure fell into the hands of the apothecary Sertürner—he found morphine. Nicotine was discovered by Vauquelin, caffeine and codeine by Robiquet, atropine by German chemists, but the most successful of the alkaloidal discoverers was Pelletier— the last of the great pharmacists; working alone, he isolated narceine; with Magendie, he gave emetine to the world; and Pelletier and Caventou discovered brucine and veratrine, extracted life-saving quinine from cinchona, and strychnine from nux vomica.

In electrotherapy, the nineteenth century opened with William Herschel's discovery, by means of the thermometer, of the invisible infra-red zone, and Ritter and Wollaston's ultraviolet band. Berzelius' division of salts by electricity, Humphry Davy's electrolytic preparation of potassium and sodium—which caused him to dance through his laboratory in ecstasy—Faraday's demonstration of electromagnetic induction, Joseph Henry's discovery of the oscillatory nature of the discharges from a Leyden Jar, von Middeldorp's improvements in galvanocauterization, Julius Althaus' work on the therapeutic possibilities of electrolysis, Duchenne's stimulation of individual muscles by moistened electrodes to the overlying skin, and his application of electrotherapy to neurology, Robert Remak's study of the direct current in joint diseases, von Ziemssen's mapping of the motor points of the surfaces of the body, Apostoli's introduction of electricity into gynecology, the Breslau dentist Bruck's idea of electric illumination for medical diagnosis, Clerk Maxwell's electromagnetic theory of light waves, Heinrich Hertz's discovery of electromagnetic action throughout space, Geissler's production of the vacuum tube, Crookes' researches on the radiant or fourth state of matter, d'Arsonval's investigations of high-frequency currents, are among the forces which blazed new paths.

During the nineteenth century, hydrotherapy had a stormier career than its sister science, for its most successful and conspicuous apostle was neither a physician nor an engineer, but a crude and forceful Silesian peasant. In his boyhood, Vincenz Priessnitz sprained his wrist and crushed his thumb, which injuries he healed by pumping cold water over them and applying wet compresses; later, a cart passed over his body, breaking his ribs, and when he overheard gloomy prognostications from his medical attendants, with characteristic energy he tore their bandages from his body, applied wet ones in their place, and pressing his abdomen against the window-sill, he breathed deeply.

Instead of being carried to the fields, he lived to write his name deep in water. Uneducated, not knowing what Hippocrates had written about hydrotherapy in the years B.C., but gifted with natural clinical insight, and a first-class organizing ability, Priessnitz established an hydropathic institute at Graefenberg, which was soon crowded with health-seekers from all parts of the world. After he amassed his first million, the wrath of the academies grew louder, and legal proceedings were started against the irregular healer. The Austrian Government came to the defense of its famous son, powerful personages intervened in his behalf—and in time many well-known physicians of unimpeachable standing sojourned at Graefenberg to learn from the untutored Priessnitz such practical thermotherapeutic procedures as the douche, the plunge, the dripping sheet, the dry blanket pack, the wet sheet pack, the foot bath, the sitz bath, the warm bath, and much else that was not written in books. To call this farmer a quack may give us a certain satisfaction, but it is futile; Vincenz Priessnitz belongs rather to that interesting group of laymen, who, without the sanctity of a diploma, have penetrated the temple of medicine.

In 1832, the year memorable for the passage of the Anatomy Act, a rabbi's grandson who was destined to become the greatest anatomist of the nineteenth century, signed the name of Jacob Henle to his first contribution. In his college days at Bonn, Henle joined the Burschenschaft, as did all the wideawake students, but he soon resigned because the members consumed too much of his tobacco and ham—having been baptized as a matter of expediency he could enjoy a Mainz ham without difficulty. In due course, when Henle applied to the Prussian authorities for formal habilitation as teacher, he expected a routine confirmation. In reply he received the unpleasant reminder he was an ex-Burschenschafter, and was informed his political past was under investigation. This attitude of the State was entirely unexpected, and filled Henle and his parents with consternation. But a calm review of the situation relieved their panic, for they saw no genuine reason for alarm. Of course, the present misunderstanding was disturbing, but after all, Henle's participation in the Bonn Burschenschaft had been so slight, his exit so speedy, his subsequent devotion to science so complete, and his career so promising, that it was unthinkable he should be condemned to any punishment severer than a reprimand.

But society must be saved, and church and state must be protected, and prosecutors must prosecute—and therefore the criminal inquiry proceeded apace. As the evidence was being sifted, exciting rumors leaked through the sieve: one day the academic circles of Berlin heard that both Müller and Henle had been arrested, but those who sought verification of the story, found the professor and his prosector at work in the Anatomical Museum. After a comparative lull, Henle would persuade himself that danger was over—until the sudden imprisonment of one friend after another, no more guilty than himself, stirred new terror in his heart. During this unsettled period, torn between hope and fear, uncertain whether the morrow would find him a state teacher or a state prisoner, Henle's scientific output was naturally diminished, but he produced at least one essay which won the enthusiastic admiration of Alexander von Humboldt.

In the meantime, there came to Henle, a friendly and highly respectful letter, from the Ministry of Dorpat, offering him the professorship of human and comparative anatomy, zoölogy, physiology, general pathology, and pathological anatomy. However, there was compensation for this work, for the letter explained that after twenty-five years of service, the professor is retired with full salary, "which he may spend where he pleases," and after his death, his widow receives a pension.

The latter item held little lure for a bachelor, and Henle's reply was indefinite. Early in the morning of the second of July, 1835, as Henle lay comfortably in bed, dreaming, perhaps of the Dorpat proposition, unexpected visitors entered his room. In that summer dawn, they affixed seals to the door, and took Henle with them. Throughout the day, Müller waited in vain for his prosector, for he had been transferred to the most famous institution in Berlin—the Hausvogtei. His cell swarmed with vermin, there was nothing to read except the Bible, no one came to see him, and he did not have a cigar.

A landlady is usually ubiquitous, but unfortunately, the sympathetic Frau Hegel failed to live up to the tradition; when the police arrested Henle, instead of being present, she was out of town, and the deed was witnessed only by the servant-girl. Now this servant-girl, in spite of her humble position, possessed a mind corresponding with that of certain eminent jurists—she recognized no distinction between a political prisoner and a common prisoner. She knew that no good man is carried off at dawn by the police, and she shuddered when she thought how often she had swept this criminal's room—unaware of any danger. As the day advanced, callers began to inquire for Henle, but ashamed to acknowledge that an inmate of her house was in the hands of the authorities, she covered the official seals on the door-knob with her apron, and persistently announced that the doctor was out. It was due to the intervention of this well-intentioned servant-girl—truly, a pillar of society—that Henle passed many weary hours in the Hausvogtei without seeing a friendly face. As soon as his new residence became known, numerous friends, with attentions and gifts, made his position as bearable as the authorities permitted.

During this episode, the Dorpat officials pressed for an answer, and were startled to learn that their intended professor was a prisoner. Efforts to have Henle released from his lice-laden cell, pending the result of the Burschenschaft investigation, were long unsuccessful. Johannes Müller, impracticably lovable, did not help matters much by his constant reiteration that Henle was indispensable as a prosector; the Gustav Magnus family rendered more effective aid by their pressure upon the proper authorities, but it was probably due to the powerful intercession of Humboldt that Henle was liberated.

After four weeks of prison-life, the genial young man again joined his many friends, and the rejoicing was great. Unnumbered visits were received and returned, congratulations flowed in from all sides, champagne ran like water for him, Berlin pancakes were stacked in hills before him, men embraced him, women wept with emotion, and in the midst of a large assemblage, a pretty woman came forward and kissed him—and with characteristic male exultation Henle notified his parents that for rewards like this, he would gladly spend another month in prison. Müller informed him that his four weeks in the Hausvogtei brought him more popularity than if he had written a thick book. The climax came when a carriage stopped in front of the released prisoner's door, and a gentleman accompanied by a liveried footman mounted the three flights of stairs that led to Henle's apartment. The caller was one of the European powers—Alexander von Humboldt. His wishes altered the decisions of governments, and kings bored him with their society. To have Humboldt climb three flights of stairs to see you, was an epoch in a man's career. But this drama did not end with the climax

—it was followed by a farce. In the liveliest thoroughfare of Berlin, the prosecutor Kamptz greeted Henle affably, and explained for an hour that he personally was convinced of the innocence of the Burschenschafter and how differently all would have been if he had the sole authority—and passers-by could hardly trust their eyes when they saw this peaceful promenade.

Yet the investigation was by no means over, and in the harassing months that followed, Henle's mother went to her grave without knowing what fate was in store for her son. It must have been the extenuating circumstances of the case which kept the judges so long at their task. The problem was indeed a delicate one, for it required due exercise of the judicial mind to determine a fitting penalty for a student who had joined a students' organization, but instead of remaining to plot against the government, had withdrawn when he noticed his fellow-conspirators were too generous with the food he received from home. It was not until the fifth of January, 1837, that this verdict was delivered: deprivation of state office, and six years' incarceration in a fortress. If the sentence seems severe to us, we may console ourselves with the reflection that in every city throughout civilization today, there are judges eager to impose similar sentences upon those whom they deem guilty of intellectual insubordination.

Had Henle been without protection, his career would have been blasted at its outset, but powerful influences, among them being Humboldt, worked for his pardon, and on the second of March, the shadow was lifted. Henle at once wrote to his father: "With my hat still on my head I write in great hurry that I have just received from A. von Humboldt the authentic notification that through the King's clemency I have been freed from all guilt and reinstated in my official position. Personally, I have not yet received a written notification, however, the truth of it is not to be doubted. I have come home in all haste and am hurrying out again to bring the good news to all my intimate friends."

The life of Henle was a drama. None familiar with his career can forget his disastrous love-affair in boyhood, celebrated in a cycle of songs dedicated to the flames, but which nevertheless survived; his duels, in one of which he was successful, only to pierce his foot when he put down his rapier in triumph; his attempt to fling away his bachelorhood in three cities, including a proposal to Felix Mendelssohn's sister, who was already secretly betrothed; his romantic marriage to Elise Egloff, the beautiful nurse-maid, who was really the illegitimate daughter of a well-to-do Swiss; his friendship with his teacher, Johannes Müller; his professional skill in music and relationships with musicians; his increasing fame as Germany's leading anatomist; his refusal to return to Prussia as the professor of anatomy in the university of Berlin; his antagonism to Bismarck; his inimitable letters, which are among the wisest and wittiest in human annals. His career was dramatically complete, for it began with a prison and ended with a Jubilee.

After Humboldt succeeded in persuading Prussia that its institutions were safe with the conspirator out of prison, Henle at twenty-eight produced his habilitation-thesis. With this treatise begins the modern knowledge of the epithelial tissues—that is, the cellular layers covering all mucous membranes. In these researches, although they were conducted with nothing better than a Schieck microscope, the investigator established names which have become permanent parts of histology, such as pavement epithelium and cylinder epithelium, first defined columnar and ciliated epithelium, and first described the stratum mucosum of the epidermis and the intestinal epithelium. His pronouncement in the following year, that "all free surfaces of the body, and all the inner surfaces of its tubes and canals, and all the walls of its cavities, are lined with epithelium," was one of the most momentous generalizations of the century, and it paved the way for the far-reaching cell-theory of Schleiden and Schwann.

Henle's epoch-making *General Anatomy* (1841) was followed by his three-volumed *Handbook of Systematic Anatomy* (1855-71), the most comprehensive survey that had yet appeared. The drawings—of which Darwin said, "the best I believe ever published"—were by Henle himself, for he handled chalk and pen with rare skill. Henle wrote on the disadvantage of eponymic terms in anatomy, but his own name adheres to numerous structures throughout the human body. When he discovered in the kidney the U-shaped turn of the uriniferous tubule which is formed by a descending and an ascending loop-tube, known everywhere as Henle's loop, he wrote one of his characteristic notes to Pfeufer: "It is about time, my dear friend, that I inform you of the good fortune which has befallen me, of making a discovery in my old years, which is far more surprising and remarkable than any heretofore made by me. Apart from the joy of having found something new in an organ a thousand times investigated and settled, I also enjoy the extraordinary satisfaction that my find is based on injection, and that the colleagues who credit me merely with the gift of the tongue, can no longer look down upon me from their injection-syringe."

Henle's chief contribution to pathology was his *Handbook of Rational Pathology* (1846-53). It is the product of an intellectual revolutionist, and not only did it overthrow antiquated systems, but it brought forward certain speculations whose utility had not been fully established. To those who argued that we should cling to the old dead theories until the new ones proved to be of permanent value, Henle proposed the following parable: "A pedant owned a nightingale for a long time, and had great pleasure in its song. Then the bird died. The pedant found the silence unpleasant, and went out to purchase another bird. There were but a few pilfered nests in the market, and the vendors did not know whether the eggs were fertile, or at least would not guarantee that male birds would hatch; then too, the brood would require much attention before they grew up to be singers. The pedant thought this to be too risky, and he went away saying that he would rather keep his dead nightingale. This was conservative, but to what purpose? That the care might be wasted on the young brood was possible, but that the dead nightingale would never sing again was certain."

Written in the graceful and brilliant style of which he was an acknowledged master, opening with the dictum, "The duty of the physician is to prevent and to cure diseases," studded with such epigrams as "The day of the last hypothesis would be also the day of the last observation," and "An hypothesis which becomes dispossessed by new facts, dies an honorable death; and if it has already called up for examination those truths by which it was annihilated, it deserves a monument of gratitude," laughing the medical devil out of existence and establishing rational concepts of disease, the book created a sensation, and what made it of special importance was its cardinal principle: "The physiology of the sick and the healthy are not different, physiology and pathology are one."

Some years previously, Henle had published in *Pathological Researches* (1840), the essay on "Miasma and Contagia," which contains the first clear statement, in modern terms, that infectious diseases are due to specific microörganisms. Henle himself searched for these pathogenic microbes in typhoid cadavers, in smallpox material, and in the scales of scarlatina. He searched with genius, but without technique, and he searched in vain. He relinquished the quest, but never the idea. Henle maintained that if these germs are invisible, it is not because of their extraordinary smallness, but because they differ so little from the tissues in which they are imbedded that they remain unrecognizable.

In the Berlin days, when Henle and Hirschwald met for the last time, the publisher complained that the entire edition of *Pathological Researches* was still in stock. Yet on Henle's dictum, "Before microscopic forms can be regarded as the cause of contagion in man they must be found constantly in the contagious material, they must be isolated from it and their strength tested," we have built the science of bacteriology. A generation later, when Henle's pupil, Robert Koch, introduced the fixing and staining methods by which he demonstrated bacillus after bacillus, the old Henle, in the year of his Jubilee, was hailed as a prophet.

There was so little money in the large Koch family, that Robert took it as a matter of course when it was decided he would learn the shoemaker's trade. Some improvement in the family finances made it possible for him to go to Göttingen, "the great university in the small town," where Henle was jesting and modernizing medicine. After receiving his doctorate, Robert Koch disappeared from academic circles. Money was still the great problem, and he became a general practitioner in the little town of Rachwiz. After serving in the Franco-Prussian war, he resumed practice as district-physician of Wollstein, in the province of Posen, the most benighted region of Germany, more Polish than German. Driving over the roads, day and night, it seemed that Koch's prize-essay at the university would remain his only achievement—Wollstein is far from Göttingen.

Koch, however, had brought his microscope with him, and Koch sitting at his microscope made an unseen institute of research arise in the province of Posen. During his ten years of silence, he was the first to work out the complete life-history and sporulation of a bacterium. At that time, bacteriology was a department of botany, and Ferdinand Cohn, the great botanist of Breslau, was the leading authority on microscopic plants. Whoever wanted information on the parasitism of Algae and Fungi, applied to Ferdinand Cohn. In the spring of 1876, Koch wrote to Cohn: "After many vain attempts, I have finally been successful in discovering the process of development of the anthrax bacillus. After many experiments, I believe to be able to state the results of these researches with sufficient certainty. Before, however, I bring this into the open, I respectfully appeal to you, esteemed Herr Professor, as the foremost authority on bacteria, to give me your judgment regarding this discovery."

It must be admitted that Cohn was not thrilled at the sight of Koch's communication. He had received too many letters whose similar claims were not followed by proof. More than one man had entered Cohn's institute, confidently carrying a beautiful hypothesis with him, only to depart with the theory battered beyond repair. Cohn answered Koch as he had answered the others, and the country doctor journeyed from the wilds of Wollstein to teach the teachers. The rest belongs to history. Cohn, in his generous enthusiasm, asked leading investigators to witness the new methods of the new master. Among them were Carl Weigert, the first to stain bacteria; Moritz Traube, pioneer of osmosis; Leopold Auerbach, who explained how the nucleus vanishes in cell-division, and described the network in the intestines still known as Auerbach's plexus. Ludwig Lichtheim, then a young privat-docent at Breslau, also watched and wondered.

Cohn likewise sent a messenger to Cohnheim's institute, suggesting it would be worth while for one of the pathologists to be present. Perhaps Cohn did not expect the director to come, for at that period Cohnheim, although only a few years older than Koch, was the leading experimental pathologist of Europe. He inaugurated the method of freezing pathological specimens for subsequent examination; described the mosaic-like areas seen in microscopic cross-section of muscle-fibers (Cohnheim's fields); and largely created our knowledge of embolism and infarction. Early in his career, in a microscopic vigil, watching a frog's transparent mesentery which he had purposely irritated with cantharidin, Cohnheim saw the white cells passing through the capillary walls and accumulating at the place of injury—this demonstration, that the migration of the white-cells of the blood is the origin of pus, revolutionized the whole subject of inflammation. The name of Cohnheim is still heard in the physiological laboratory, for a salt-frog—that is, a living frog from whose vascular system the blood has been entirely removed and replaced by physiological salt solution—is everywhere called Cohnheim's frog.

When Cohn's message arrived, Julius Cohnheim came himself, and his excitement was literally boundless. Returning to his institute, he admonished his assistants: "Drop everything and go at once to Koch. This man has made a splendid discovery which is all the more astonishing because Koch has had no scientific connections and has worked entirely on his own initiative and has produced something absolutely complete. There is nothing more to be done. I consider this the greatest discovery in the field of bacteriology and believe Koch will again astonish and shame us with still further discoveries."

Cohnheim was not forced to wait to find himself a prophet, for the next year Koch described his procedures for the examination, preservation and photography of bacteria. One year later, Koch published his investigations into the cause of traumatic infective diseases, demonstrating the various bacteria responsible, breeding them for generations, and reproducing the diseases artificially. Thus Koch, at thirty-five, was a country doctor and an unsurpassed scientific investigator. His friends, especially Cohn and Cohnheim, realizing the incongruity of this combination, managed to have Koch transferred to Breslau as circuit physician. Cohn and Cohnheim, magnificent in science, were weak in political economy, and failed to comprehend that the salary which sufficed for Koch's growing family in the country, was insufficient for their support in the city. Koch soon thought longingly of his old job, and within three months found himself back at Wollstein.

Cohnheim, however, did not intend to allow Koch to be buried among the villagers, and in the summer of 1880, learning that Finkelnburg, a member of the Imperial Sanitary Commission, had resigned to resume his Bonn professorship, Cohnheim's impassioned advocacy caused Koch to be elected to regular membership in the commission. From this time on, Koch never left Berlin. He traveled in Asia and Africa and America, but his home address was always Berlin. Koch's accomplishments wrought a transformation in the health department, to the discomfiture of some of the elder members, and in 1881 he dwarfed all his associates by his scheme of spreading liquid gelatin with meat infusion on glass plates, thus producing transparent solid media for pure cultures. This poured-plate method may be regarded as Koch's greatest single achievement, for there is no other method by which the bacteriologist can grow, isolate and recover pure cultures.

With these enormous gains in technique at his command, supplemented by improved staining methods which he devised,

Koch was prepared to continue the quest of specific organisms, and on the evening of March 24, 1882, he startled the Physiological Society of Berlin by announcing his discovery of the tubercle bacillus. Because of its direct effects in the study of tuberculosis, and as a result of the impetus which this discovery gave to bacteriologic research, it ranks as one of the most important in the history of medicine. In this paper Koch erected the four postulates that stand like the four pillars of bacteriology: one, the microörganism must be present in all cases of the disease; two, it must be cultivated in pure culture; three, its inoculation must produce the disease in susceptible animals; four, it must, when injected into healthy animals, produce the same disease, thus completing the cycle.

In mid-August 1883, Koch departed from Berlin and in May 1884 he returned—between these two dates the average man had attended to his ledgers, but Koch had been in Egypt and in India studying the cholera, and not only discovered the cholera vibrio (comma bacillus), but was able to cultivate it from drinking-water, food and clothing. These investigations opened a new era in public health. From 1885 on, chairs and institutes were created for Koch. From all parts of Germany, and from foreign countries, men came to learn the new science. They returned to spread the gospel of exactitude and experimentation, and grown into teachers in their turn, taught thousands of students the significance of the four postulates, showed them the poured-plate method, and made them stain bacteria in the manner of the master. Perhaps no disciple gave him sincerer gratification than Kitasato, who carried Koch's technique to Japan, and by its application first cultivated the germ of tetanus and discovered the bacillus of bubonic plague.

Koch's announcement (1890), that he had discovered a remedy for tuberculosis, warmed the breast of Mother Earth with a strange hope and everywhere her afflicted children stretched their hands for the health-bringing vial. Alas, there are no Four Postulates in therapeutics, and tuberculin is looked upon as the one folly of a great scientist. As a therapeutic agent, tuberculin certainly has failed to fulfill the expectations which Koch prematurely raised, but as a diagnostic aid it has proved of immense value. Koch established a landmark in epidemiology by pointing out the relationship between epidemics and polluted water, and demonstrating that these water-borne epidemics can be prevented by filtration (1891). Cattle plague is one of man's major catastrophes, and the British government determined to solve the mysteries of the rinderpest which terrorized South Africa and Cape Colony. In this crisis (1896), England turned not to one of her own sons, but to Koch. He accepted the burden imposed upon him, and remained in Africa until he devised a method which is still employed with success. While grappling with the rinderpest, he conducted valuable researches upon Texas fever, tropical malaria, back-water fever, surra, and studied bubonic plague in East India—mere side-excursions for Koch.

At the London Tuberculosis Congress (1901), Koch set in motion unlimited argument by his contention that the human and bovine tubercle bacilli were not identical, thus deducing the fact that we have little to fear from the bovine type. It required courage on Koch's part to utter these views: because they were opposed to the opinions he had formerly published; because they were contrary to the generally accepted belief; and because they exposed him to the charge of being in the service of meat-dealers. The controversy still rages, but year by year the evidence is more in favor of Koch, and this much is certain: in the battle of mankind against tuberculosis, the chief foe of man is not the infected cow, but his infected fellow-man.

His country sent Koch to German East Africa to study Rhodesian red-water fever, and incidentally he made important observations upon horse-sickness, recurrent fever and trypanosomiasis (1902). At about the same time he established principles for the control of typhoid which have since become standard. The Nobel Prize was bestowed upon Koch (1905), and before a single leaf of these laurels had time to fade, he headed the Sleeping Sickness Commission to German East Africa, English Central Africa and the Victoria Nyanza. In this campaign he caught over a thousand Tsetse-flies, and to his astonishment found in their stomachs the blood of crocodiles. He was thus compelled to hatch young crocodiles under the sun, and to find which of the Glossinae are germ-bearing. One result of this expedition, which lasted eighteen months, was Koch's introduction of atoxyl for sleeping sickness. His published observations of the banana-eating natives are most graphic.

That Koch was human enough is clear from the circumstance that in his latter days he put away the wife of his youth for the charming Hedwig Freiberg. Countless poets and artists—and others—have affected similar transfers without commotion, but Koch's action to a considerable extent robbed his old age of the serenity to which Germany's greatest scientist was entitled. The government was displeased, the inhabitants of Klausthal tore down the tablet which they had once proudly placed upon the house where he was born, and some of his closest relatives refused to speak to him.

Koch and his second wife visited Japan (1908), where they met his former pupil, Shibasaburo Kitasato, now known as "the Japanese Koch." The venerable Koch, in Japanese costume, made a pleasing figure. The Japanese published a post-card illustrated with the various organisms discovered by Koch. The Japanese took a few of his hairs and around them built a temple to Robert Koch. Every nation owes an immeasurable debt to the man who gained victories over typhoid and rinderpest and sleeping sickness, uncovered the source of tuberculosis and cholera and Egyptian ophthalmia, and invaded continents, not for the conquest of his fellow-men, but to lead physicians in the warfare against pestilence and plague.

Louis Pasteur was the son of a tanner in the small town of Arbois in the Jura. The pale-faced sensitive boy gave no evidence of unusual gifts, but he was surrounded by family love, and his childhood was happy. No doubt his most terrifying experience occurred in his ninth year: a mad wolf was running through the countryside, biting animals and human beings, several of whom died from suffocation. Near his father's tannery stood the smithy, and here the boy saw one of the bitten Arboisians seared with a red-hot iron—cauterization was advocated by the Roman physicians of the first century, and the passing centuries had added no wisdom in hydrophobia. The foremost physicians of later ages, from Boerhaave to Hunter, and from Magendie to Virchow, had studied this malady in vain. For about two thousand years the doctor turned over his rabic patients to the blacksmith.

Pasteur's attempt at sixteen to study in Paris, resulted in an alarming illness. He presented a picture of adolescent despair, and his father was compelled to take him home, to give him "a whiff of the tannery yard"—in the subsequent crises of his life, Pasteur always sought peace in the garden of this tannery. In his twentieth year, the provincial again attempted Paris. He began his scientific career by solving problems in crystallography which had baffled all previous chemists and physicists. When Pasteur, breaking a tartrate crystal and plunging it back into the mother liquid, saw the crystal completely restored and compared this trauma to a wound which is healed with the aid of new molecules, he demonstrated how his luminous mind passed logically from physics to the threshold of physiology; when Pasteur, noticing a solution of ammonium tartrate grow cloudy, observed that a drop from the infected flask produced putrefaction in a new flask, he naturally moved onward from chemistry to the inner recesses of biology. Pasteur was a scryer whose crystal-gazing showed vaster horizons for humanity.

To realize the darkness that surrounded the entire subject of fermentation, it is only necessary to recall the prevailing views of the period as enunciated by Liebig:

> Those who attempt to explain the putrefaction of animal substances by the presence of animalcules, argue much in the same way as a child who imagines he can explain the rapidity of the Rhine's flow by attributing it to the violent agitation caused by the numerous waterwheels of Mainz, in the neighborhood of Bingen. Can we legitimately regard plants and animals as the means whereby other organisms are destroyed, when their own constituent elements are condemned to un-

dergo the same series of putrefaction phenomena, as the creatures which preceded them? If the fungus is the agent in the oak's destruction, if the microscopic animalcule is the agent in the putrefaction of the elephant's carcass, I ask in my turn, what is the agent which works the putrefaction of the fungus and the microscopic animalcule when life has been removed from these two organized bodies?

With these picturesque and contemptuous words, Justus von Liebig, the dominant chemist of his day, sought to close the door on that invisible world which the microscope of Pasteur opened to science. In the ensuing battles which were waged between the two champions, Liebig, although only nineteen years the senior of Pasteur, was so hopelessly superannuated that he refused to look through a microscope—and yet he was the father of laboratory teaching in chemistry. He belonged to the premicrobic era of science, and thus seems as antiquated as van Helmont. Bacteriology was the bridge that divided the old land from the new, and only those who crossed that bridge found themselves on modern ground.

After incontrovertible experiments that microörganisms cannot arise anew, but only from former microörganisms, Pasteur turned his attention to the maladies of wine; again pursuing the microbe, he saved from threatened ruin one of the most important industries of his country. This was succeeded by an investigation of the diseases of beer, demonstrating both the cause and cure. The famous process of Pasteurization was born in a brewery. While thus pursuing his studies in putrefactive phenomena, Pasteur was unexpectedly deflected from his path by an ailing silkworm. The South of France lives on the silkworm, and its extermination spells absolute destitution for the people. The microparasitic diseases of silkworms imprisoned Pasteur for five years, but in the end he restored the silkworm to France. In the meantime he had been stricken with a hemiplegia of such severity that all who saw him expected a fatal termination. Slowly the paralysis lifted, but never entirely, and in the years to come the savior of sericulture moved through the laboratories with a stiffened hand and limping foot.

Ever since Pasteur had sent his paper on *Lactic Acid Fermentation* (1857) to the Lille Scientific Society, his mind tended to the conviction that in the world of the "infinitely small" lay buried the secret of contagious diseases. For this reason he felt his place was in the Academy of Medicine; after the Franco-Prussian War, when a vacancy occurred, he became a candidate, and was elected by a majority of a single vote. It would have been better for his peace of mind, if he had been overwhelmingly defeated. Since few men have opened so many new paths as Pasteur, few men have endured so much opposition. Even after a subject had undergone the most rigorous proof, being incontestably settled by the experimental method, rhetorical individuals arose in detraction of Pasteur. Usually Pasteur exhibited superhuman patience. For example, in order to clarify the complexities of molecular dissymmetry to certain noisy contenders who should have seen the light long ago, he called for a cabinet-maker and instructed him to fashion a gigantic set of the crystalline varieties of the tartrates—and Emile Duclaux asked him why he did not conclude the session by hurling these wooden crystals at his adversaries' heads! Pouchet and Joly attempted to block the path of Pasteur for years, and men like Colin and Peter will live in scientific history solely because they were vicious enemies of him who walked continually toward truth. At times, however, Pasteur was a terrible opponent, and his exclamation, "What you lack, M. Frémy, is familiarity with a microscope, and you, M. Trécul, are not accustomed to laboratories!"—was an indictment not easily forgotten.

All the truculent argumentation which hitherto interfered with his onward progress, was as nothing compared with the enmity which greeted him when he came among the doctors. To Pasteur, the Academy of Medicine was an armed camp, bristling with prejudice and surrounded by error. Physicians and surgeons who have gone down to nameless dust, resented instruction from a chemist, a non-practitioner, a layman after all. When Pasteur presented facts, their answer was: Monsieur, where is your M.D.? The leading academicians, men who are still remembered by historians, Chassaignac, Piorry, Pidoux, denounced the germ theory of disease in the most scathing and ironical language of which Frenchmen are capable. Today their words read like chapters out of a medieval book. Jules Guérin raved against vaccines, while Pasteur demonstrated their value: in the angry dispute that followed, Jules Guérin, at the age of eighty, became so enraged that he rushed at Pasteur, challenging him to a duel. Louis Pasteur stuck to his seat at the Academy of Medicine: it was his function to force the germ theory down the throat of medical France.

While Pasteur's opponents were denying that germs bore any relationship to infections, the bacillus anthracis which from ancient times had destroyed cattle everywhere, grew especially virulent throughout France. Entire herds staggered and perished miserably within a few hours, their distended carcasses crowding the pastures. A malignant deity seemed at work, for there were times when a shepherd, seeing his flock quietly grazing, would lie dreaming on the hill-slope; when he arose to take the flock home, death was spread all around him. If the shepherd then scratched his hand on one of his stricken sheep, he died among his flock.

So Pasteur, the master-shepherd, came to the sheepfolds of Chartres. Again he faced the unknown, and after years of effort Pasteur held the answer in a little vial. He announced that by an attenuated virus he could prevent anthrax. Half a hundred sheep were inoculated with an extremely virulent anthrax culture, and half of these were vaccinated and half were not. "The twenty-five unvaccinated sheep will all perish," said Pasteur, "the twenty-five vaccinated ones will all survive."

Pasteur's bold prediction was received with general incredulity; there were some Pasteurians whose faith in him was absolute, but many of his friends were uneasy at the sublime audaciousness with which he risked the reputation of a lifetime, while the Colins were certain that at last he would be discredited. The crucial test occurred, and before long the most disquieting symptoms appeared: some of the vaccinated sheep developed fever and edema, and one lamb was lame. Hour by hour the rumors grew worse. At night he received a note which staggered him: one of the vaccinated sheep was reported dying. The destiny of agriculture and the fate of preventive inoculation depended on that sheep. Pasteur's anxiety was pitiful. The disciples around the master for the first time saw the shadows of doubt in those sad, grave eyes. Would the old magician's last trick fail?

Morning came, and the whole excited veterinary world seemed to be at that farmyard, watching the result. Every one likes to be present when history may be made. Never did the Experimental Method gain a more brilliant victory. Not a single sheep went wrong. The twenty-five unvaccinated sheep lay dead from anthrax, the twenty-five vaccinated ones browsed in perfect health. Jennerian vaccination was surpassed. As Pasteur approached that farmyard at Pouilly-le-Fort, a cheer arose, but the Father of Preventive Medicine did not hear. Among the sheepfolds he beheld a vision of Humanity freed from all infectious diseases.

Word was spreading in all directions that another horror might soon be removed from the earth, for Pasteur hoped to vanquish the dreaded hydrophobia. Peasants and emperors now watched Pasteur's laboratory with interest. In answer to an inquiry from the Emperor of Brazil, Pasteur replied: "I already have several examples of dogs made refractory after a rabietic bite. I take two dogs, cause them both to be bitten by a mad dog; I vaccinate the one and leave the other without any treatment: the latter dies and the first remains perfectly well."

Later he wrote to Jules Vercel of Arbois—the same Jules Vercel with whom, almost half a century previous, he had first set out for Paris:

Alas! we shall not be able to go to Arbois for Easter; I shall be busy for some time settling down, or rather settling my dogs down at Villeneuve l'Etang. I have also some new experiments on rabies on hand which will take some months. I am demonstrating this year that dogs can be vaccinated, or made refractory to rabies after they have been bitten by mad dogs.

I have not yet dared to treat human beings after bites from rabid dogs; but the time is not far off, and I am much inclined to begin by myself—inoculating myself with rabies, and then arresting the consequences; for I am beginning to feel very sure of my results.

While the scientist thus wrestled with his doubt, an agonized mother from Alsace entered his laboratory. She brought to Pasteur her little son, Joseph Meister. Walking unguarded to school along a country road, the helpless child had been pounced upon by a mad dog, who bore him to the ground and wounded him fourteen times. He would have been killed on the spot, had not a bricklayer finally succeeded in driving the animal off. That nameless bricklayer deserves a monument: he not only saved a child, but he hastened the proof of the Experimental Method.

Joseph Meister was nine years of age. What memories must have awakened in Pasteur! He too was just nine years of age when, standing by his father's tannery, he had seen a bitten person seared by the blacksmith's iron. For that ancient ordeal, so terrible and so inadequate, Pasteur now substituted a little rabic marrow in a Pravaz syringe.

As the rabic medulla increased in virulence, Pasteur shuddered at the inoculations. When the patient was injected with marrow of such strength that it produced hydrophobia in unprotected animals within a week, Pasteur could no longer sleep. We love this man for his insomnia. Ghosts haunted him throughout an appalling night that would not end: he saw the look of alarm on the child's face, he saw him in vain try to swallow, he heard the paroxysms of choking as the boy perished from the cruelest malady known to medicine. Would dawn never come again? In the morning, Pasteur was a sick man. Taking his daughter with him, he left his laboratory and fled to the country, leaving little Meister in the care of one of his disciples, J. J. Grancher. Pasteur attempted to rest in Burgundy, and then at Arbois, yet was ever tortured by the conviction that a telegram would come from Grancher announcing the death of the first patient treated by inoculation.

But with a pin-prick, the genius of Pasteur had established immunity. Not only did Meister remain in perfect health, but he imagined himself in the best of luck, for he soon made pets of Pasteur's rabbits, chickens, white mice and guinea-pigs. More than one of these animals, predestined for laboratory purposes, was saved by the pleadings of Master Joseph. After Meister's return to his native Alsace, the blue-eyed lad frequently received letters that were postmarked Paris. About a year later, when funds were being raised to establish a hydrophobic service, Pasteur, while looking over the list of subscribers, was happy to find the name of Joseph Meister.

Upon Pasteur's election, a few years before this, as One of the Forty, he had been welcomed in a remarkable address by the author of *Averroes;* not content with enumerating, in bewitching language, Pasteur's actual accomplishments, Renan had played with prophecy: "Humanity will owe to you deliverance from a horrible disease and also from a sad anomaly: I mean the distrust which we cannot help mingling with the caresses of the animal in whom we see most of Nature's smiling benevolence." Ernest Renan lived to see the truth of his augury.

Pasteur's second case of hydrophobia was fully as interesting as the first. Six shepherd boys, from Villers-Farlay in the Jura, were tending their flock, when an enormous dog, lashing his jaws with fury, charged upon them. The children rose in fear, and it was pathetic to watch their attempt to fly with trembling limbs before a swift-moving terror that gained every moment upon them. Only the eldest of the group did not run. Whip in hand, Jean Baptiste Jupille, fourteen years of age, met the mad animal. In the struggle that followed, the whip fell to the ground. With bleeding hands, the shepherd took off one of his wooden shoes and began to beat the animal upon the head. Chance moved back and forth over the meadow that autumn morning. At length death overtook the mad creature, but his mark was likewise on Jupille, covered with rabid blood and saliva. Only from Pasteur could the young hero hope for life.

Meister had been brought to the laboratory in less than three days after his accident, but six full days elapsed before Jupille received his initial injection of the mitigated virus. Pasteur complimented the boy on his courage, and found that Jupille was embarrassed at being praised. At the Academy of Sciences, Pasteur, after explaining the technique of his treatment, could not refrain from extolling Jupille's deed of self-sacrifice. Baron Larrey, usually the most impassive of men, thereupon arose, and proposed that the Académie Française bestow upon Jupille the Montyon Prize. The young shepherd from Villers-Farlay became a French sensation.

Afterwards, Pasteur corresponded with Jupille, and sometimes complained of the hero's orthography. The following extract exhibits Pasteur as a volunteer supervisor of education: "Your writing is already much better than it was, but you should take some pains with your spelling. Where do you go to school? Who teaches you? Do you work at home as much as you might? You know that Joseph Meister, who was first to be vaccinated, often writes to me; well, I think he is improving more quickly than you are, though he is only ten years old. So, mind you take pains, do not waste your time with other boys, and listen to the advice of your teachers, and of your father and mother."

Statistics quickly accumulated in favor of preventive inoculation. Every case that was not already hopeless, found life and health in Pasteur's sterilized flasks. Against his judgment, and knowing it would jeopardize his method, but unable to resist the entreaties of her parents, and overcome with pity for the victim, Pasteur consented to receive for treatment little Louise Pelletier, thirty-seven days after she had been bitten on the head by a mad mountain-dog. Much affection developed between Pasteur and the patient. He gave her a double series of inoculations, and for a brief time a ray of hope warmed his heart, but it was too late to prevent convulsive spasms. The great laboratory was neglected; Pasteur spent an entire day at the child's bedside. Louise Pelletier died holding the hand of Louis Pasteur. He burst into tears, and his opponents, led by Charles-Felix-Michel Peter, burst into triumphant denunciations of all things Pasteurian. A few other failures, inevitable from the outset—and every one of which caused him the deepest suffering—brought upon him an avalanche of anonymous abuse. Pasteur had discovered the method of preventing hydrophobia of the body—he did not possess a vaccine against rabies of the soul.

In spite of the Peters in the Academy of Medicine, in spite of the attacks in the newspapers, all nations made a path to Pasteur's door. Nineteen Russian peasants from the distant province of Smolensk, badly mangled by a raving wolf, some of them torn beyond recognition, began the journey to seek the talisman that hung by a thread in the mysterious flasks. The only word of French they knew was "Pasteur," and the journey was regarded as their last. Yet sixteen of them returned with laughter to Smolensk. Their restoration was looked upon as a resurrection. The Tsar presented Pasteur a decoration of diamonds, and sent a substantial contribution to his institute.

Through the enterprise of the New York Herald, four American children, recently bitten by rabid dogs, were sent to be cured by the kindly wizard. The children were surprised that the long journey should culminate in a few jabs which they hardly felt. They did not understand that behind each pin-prick was one of the greatest minds that ever blessed the human race. Instead of succumbing in agony and exhaustion, instead of being abandoned by terror-stricken parents, or being smothered between two mattresses as was frequently the fate of hydrophobic children in the pre-pasteurian era, these youngsters came back to their families in the best of condition. Time has passed, and it is no longer necessary to cross mountains and seas to reach a Pasteur Institute. That mother institute in Paris has offspring, not only throughout Europe and the Americas, but in Tunis, Indo-China, Morocco, and Cambodia.

The doctrine of the bacterial origin of infectious disease is

Medicine's greatest discovery. Man now looked at the microbe, and saw his immemorial foe. It was not the stars, but the "infinitely small" that brought the Black Death to overwhelm his cities. Invisible for centuries, he knew at last the witches that stole his children from the cradle. He had groped after strange causes, while the real cause lay hidden around him. Spread and stained on the slide, lay his terrible enemy. He saw the germs that tortured and deformed him, burned him with fever, filled him with pus, stabbed him with pain, deprived him of reason, drove him to the grave. His untutored brothers of the Stone Age were right—little demons were everywhere. They locked men's jaws, set him coughing, twisted him into inhuman shapes, got inside him, burst his skin, poisoned his blood. His ignorant brothers of the Stone Age were wrong in thinking these little demons—we call them *cocci* and *bacilli*—could be frightened away with noises and smells, or placated by gifts. In the ceaseless warfare of man and microbe, man needs keener weapons.

The bacterial theory shed light on many obscure conditions. The gall-bladder was intended to be a reservoir, but too often it becomes a quarry. That is why, although its average capacity is less than two ounces, its capacity for pain is infinite. When a calculus begins its passage down the cystic duct, it starts on one of the most painful journeys that a human being can experience. Gall-stones were observed in the fourteenth century by Gentile da Foligno, yet it was not until much later (1618) that the first gall-stone was taken from a living patient by the Father of German Surgery, and when Fabricius Hildanus removed that historic calculus perhaps he felt more trepidation than when he amputated the human thigh. But with Hildanus this was an accidental or sporadic procedure; for its popularization, mankind is indebted to the foremost French surgeon of the following century, Jean-Louis Petit, who had occasion to lament: "How many people have died because this disease was not recognized, or because no operator could be found who would undertake to rid them of their disease by means of an operation." The modern history of cholelithiasis commenced when Galippe found germs in biliary calculi (1886), thus suggesting the microbic origin of gall-stones, and preparing the way for the epigram: "Every gall-stone is a tombstone erected to the memory of the dead germs that lie within it."

The morbid history of leprosy stretches across humanity's trail for thousands of years. We may still read the futile prescriptions of the Egyptians for this affliction. Throughout medieval Christendom we hear the ringing of the leper-bell, and the warning cry, "Unclean, Unclean." Every large town had its leper-house—there were 19,000 of these houses of doom. The condition was hopeless—once a leper, always a leper. In the modern era, the disease was studied internationally, and by none more assiduously than the Norwegian physicians, Carl Wilhelm Boeck and Daniel Cornelius Danielssen whose collaborative investigation of anesthetic leprosy is known as Danielssen-Boeck disease; their pupil, Armauer Hansen, discovered the short and slender rod that has caused all the leprosy in the world (Bacillus leprae, 1871). Numerous remedies were tried and discarded, until it was found that the seed of an East Indian tree contained an oil which rendered lepers bacteriologically negative. Lepers, if they come in time, are now cleansed by chaulmoogra oil, and discharged safe and cured. It is a remarkable victory for man in his battle with the microbe.

Among the case-histories of Hippocrates is one which, from the clinical description, we recognize as diphtheria. Under the names of Egyptian disease and Syrian ulcer, Aretaeus drew a vivid picture of its essential features. It is thus an ancient disease, and its virulence did not decrease with time. Diphtheria was among the first and worst epidemics that ravaged the New England colonists, and legislatures decreed a day of thanksgiving at their cessation. Diphtheria has long been notorious for its fatality to attending physicians, for it is highly contagious. The murderous membrane, creeping from tonsils to the fauces, inexorably suffocating its victims, makes it one of the cruelest diseases of the nursery. In the throats of those dying from diphtheria, Klebs found a club-shaped bacillus, and Loeffler separated it from other bacteria.

If the Klebs-Loeffler bacilli are grown on a certain broth, they elaborate a powerful poison; if a horse is inoculated with small and increasing doses of this toxin, it produces in defense a counterpoison or antitoxin. An enormous amount of antitoxin can be recovered from the horse's jugular vein, and this fluid is one of the most beneficent triumphs of modern medicine. An immunized horse will manufacture enough antitoxin to protect over eight hundred horses against diphtheritic toxins that would otherwise have killed them all. In the human world, this antitoxin has saved countless children from an agonized death. Where once the physician stood helpless as the false membrane spread without hindrance, today if he is called early enough, he wards off disaster. The child in the Berlin clinic who was the first to be saved by diphtheria antitoxin (1891), lived in the new world of immunity. Mankind is indebted principally to the Prussian army surgeon, Emil von Behring, working in Koch's laboratory, for this discovery. The use of *toxin-antitoxin*—a mixture of diphtheria toxin with its antitoxin—as a prophylactic against the disease, was later suggested by von Behring, and developed in New York by William Hallock Park and Abraham Zingher. This marked a considerable advance, since the immunity conferred by diphtheria antitoxin is transitory, while the immunity from toxin-antitoxin is lasting. Bela Schick's test—injection into the skin of a minute quantity of diphtheria toxin, which produces inflammation in the unprotected—enables us to determine who is immune and who is susceptible. Thus step by step, in the bacteriologic age, man has attacked the *Bacillus diphtheriae*.

Back in the Renaissance, old Ambroise Paré, reviewing his life-work, wrote: "God is my witness, and men are not ignorant of it, that I have labored more than forty years to throw light on the art of surgery and to bring it to perfection. And in this labor I have striven so hard to attain my end, that the ancients have naught wherein to excel us, save the discovery of first principles: and posterity will not be able to surpass us (be it said without malice or offense) save by some additions, such as are easily made to things already discovered."

A bold prophecy, but for two hundred and fifty years after Paré's death, his words remained substantially true. Surgery was as painful on the day that Astley Cooper laid down his knife as in Paré's time. The thought of an operation was torture, and patients suffered agonies beforehand; finally tied to the table and held down by force, they tore madly at their straps, shrieking in uncontrolled terror—the one saving aspect of the whole ghastly affair was that no one understood the meaning of surgical shock. The soporific draughts of Dioscorides and the sleeping sponge of the Middle Ages were forgotten or discarded as unreliable. Haste was the great thing, and he was the best surgeon who operated fastest. Robert Liston amputated a thigh by compressing the artery with his left hand and cutting and sawing with his right—if he needed the use of both hands he held the saw between his teeth. Liston's knife flashed, and if the spectator sneezed or winked or turned his head, he missed the operation because it was over. In spite of his speed Liston had harrowing memories: a man who was to be cut for stone lost his courage on the operating-table, rushed down the long corridor and locked himself in the lavatory until Liston made a battering-ram of his powerful shoulder, broke down the door and carried the patient back.

Then came the wonderful news from America: Pain had been conquered at the Massachusetts General Hospital. Liston gave ether its first European trial, and on November 4, 1847, James Young Simpson of Edinburgh discovered the anesthetic properties of chloroform. The practical application of anesthesia closed forever one of the most terrible chapters in surgery, but the worst of all remained. In fact, the conquest of pain, by increasing the number and variety of operations, augmented the evil. Every hospital gloried in what was called "a good old surgical stink." Every surgeon was proud of his old operating coat, which he neither washed nor changed, for the accumulating incrustations of dried blood and pus attested to his experience. Operators and their assistants—as Semmelweis knew only too well—came from autopsies or the dissecting-room, and without cleaning their hands, examined patients and parturient women. Surgery was dangerous, because surgery was dirty. The following suggestion in the Visitors' Book of Radcliffe Infirmary is characteristic of hospital conditions in the first half of the nineteenth century: "There should be a positive order that sheets should be changed in ordinary cases at least once a month without waiting for special request." The nursing service, until the reforms of Florence Nightingale became effective, only added to hospital horrors.

Simpson left incomplete what must nevertheless be regarded as one of his greatest achievements—his protest against Hospitalism. That same humanity which led him to seek a method of assuaging pain, likewise drove him to attempt to lessen hospital mortality. Appalled at the frightful statistics he collected, he remarked that "a man laid on the operating table in one of our surgical hospitals is exposed to more chances of death than the English soldier on the field of Waterloo." Septic poisoning was an ever-present horror, often supervening the slightest operation; the stench of infection filled every ward, and phagedena was rarely absent; pestilence followed in the footsteps of the most careful surgeon, and often the number of coffins carried out of a hospital corresponded to the number of patients who had entered. So Simpson tried to abolish the hospital system altogether, or urged that hospitals be constructed of iron, that they might frequently be removed, rebuilt and renovated. The suggestion does credit to his warm heart, but it indicates how he and his generation worked in darkness.

The answer to the world's cry came from a young Quaker teaching in the Scotch universities, and it is sad to recall that even Simpson did not perceive the light and spoke in derision of "mythical fungi." He opposed his teachings, and when his colleague came down from Edinburgh to London to demonstrate the new principles, he found himself unwelcome to surgeons, students and nurses; resentful of a strange method, hating his carbolic spray, and shocked at his sacrilege of changing dressings on the Sabbath, the sisters of St. John lined up in solid opposition to this man, and it was in the midst of innumerable insults and stiff white caps held high in air, that Joseph Lister established antiseptic surgery.

Lister did not introduce the term antiseptic. Perhaps the first who used it was the wholly unknown Place, who wrote in his *Hypothetical Notion of the Plague* (1712): "As this phenomenon shows the motion of the pestilential poison to be putrefactive, it makes the use of *antisepticks* a reasonable way to oppose it, and whatever resists and is preservative against putrefaction, admits not of the generation of insects. If this hypothesis is proceeded upon, our proper and promising materials to yield medicine and for physical preparations against it, such as cedar, Irish oak, cinnamon, spices, and what was used by the ancients in their embalments of dead bodies; for the same virtues that preserved dead bodies from insects and putrefaction I know no reason why they should not preserve the same bodies living from the same thing." In the next generation, Sir John Pringle, father of military sanitation, published his important *Experiments upon Aseptic and Antiseptic Substances* (1750). By this time the word was evidently familiar to the public, for it occurs in the Gentleman's Magazine (1751): "Myrrh in a watery solution is twelve times more *antiseptic* than sea salt." Yet over a hundred years later, Lister had to begin at the beginning.

The subscribers to the Lancet, who turned the pages of their journal between March-July 1867, and skipped a difficult-looking article, signed Joseph Lister, bearing the title, *On a New Method of treating Compound Fractures, Abscess, etc., with Observations on the Conditions of Suppuration;* and the members of the British Medical Association who attended the session that August at Dublin, languid in the summer heat as Lister read his paper *On the Antiseptic Principle in the Practice of Surgery,* little realized that the long reign of "laudable pus" was at an end, and that the call for the most beneficent of surgical revolutions had been sounded. The battle extended to all countries and went on for many years, and when it was over, surgery was transformed and divided into two epochs—the pre-Listerian and the Listerian. As its originator announced, Listerism is simply applied Pasteurism. By his recognition of the rôle of pathogenic bacteria in wounds, and the necessity of keeping them out of wounds, Lister sterilized the practitioner, the nurse, the patient, and his surroundings. Joseph Lister's manifold labors may be read in the volumes of his *Collected Papers* (1909), but his life-work is summed up in a phrase: he made surgery clean.

Without the bacterial theory, it was impossible to understand gonorrhea and syphilis. We must now pick up the thread of venereal disease where we dropped it in the eighteenth century. Syphilis achieved in the name of science is as dangerous as that acquired in the quest of pleasure, and John Hunter's syphilis complicated his angina pectoris. In the very year that Hunter dropped dead in his hospital from angina pectoris and an insult, a new era dawned in venereal disease through the work of Benjamin Bell. With definite knowledge of the differences and similarities of the two diseases, Bell drew a line of demarcation between gonorrhea and syphilis, and sounded the death-knell of the identistic theory. This work was translated and promulgated in France in the early nineteenth century by Edouard Bosquillon (1802), who gave us the term urethritis, added valuable notes on congestion of the prostate, and energetically opposed the use of mercury in gonorrhea.

Jean-François Hernandez showed (1812) with his famous experiments on the convicts of Toulon that by the inoculation of gonorrhea, syphilis is not communicated. It was the era of inoculations, and gonorrhea was experimentally passed from urethra to urethra. At times medical students and physicians offered themselves as volunteers, but frequently hospital patients participated in these experiments without their knowledge. The profession finally learned that all urethral discharges are not gonorrheal, that gonorrhea is caused only by gonorrhea, and syphilis only by syphilis.

The chief venereologist of the period was Philippe Ricord, a typical Frenchman despite his Baltimore birth and Philadelphia education—in Paris he was known as "The great American doctor." Ricord's experience was enormous; unfortunately he was obstinate, and made inexcusable blunders. He claimed the secondary stage of syphilis cannot be transmitted and hence is not dangerous; physicians in various countries, accepting his authority, inoculated many patients with the secondary lesions, and of course the results were disastrous. Had Ricord been familiar with the history and jurisprudence of syphilis in the sixteenth century, he would not have made this mistake. Ricord summed up the results of his unparalleled experience in the epigram: "We know when a gonorrhea begins, but only God knows when it ends." Ricord kept an ivory-handled gold-plated vaginal speculum for the exclusive use of the Empress Eugenie. Considering how much venereal disease Ricord saw in his long life, he cannot be blamed for his mocking opinion of human chastity. Oliver Wendell Holmes in *Some of my Early Teachers* (1882), called him "the Voltaire of pelvic literature, a skeptic as to the morality of the race in general, who would have submitted Diana to treatment with his mineral specifics, and ordered a course of blue pills for the vestal virgins."

In the seventies, a Bonn graduate who lived nearly thirty years in New York, enraged the profession. Even physicians can be shocked, and it was not pleasant, in the Victorian era, to see that "inordinately lean, tall man of saturnine mien," the long-fingered, grim-thinking Emil Noeggerath, stand up at the first meeting of the American Gynecological Society, and say: "About ninety per cent of sterile women are married to husbands who have suffered from gonorrhea either previous to, or during, married life." Noeggerath maintained that most of the acute and chronic inflammations of the female genitalia came from gonorrheal infection, often contracted in the marriage-bed—honeymoon gonorrhea. He showed that not only florid gonorrhea and a chronic gleet on the part of the male, but an apparently disappeared, a really latent gonorrhea, could cause the infection. Physicians of all nations united in denouncing him. The tragedy of this affair is not that Noeggerath was abused, but that he was right. Years later, the foremost gynecologist of the time, Sir Spencer Wells, said sarcastically: "I have not seen these cases of gonorrhea, no doubt they all go to Birmingham." This of course was a thrust at his rival, Lawson Tait, who founded modern pelvic surgery largely upon the ravages of gonorrhea in the female. When Lawson Tait was challenged to a duel in Berlin by a fellow gynecologist, he answered: "I choose the deadliest of all weapons—the clamp of Spencer Wells."

An assistant in the Dermatological Clinic at Breslau, Albert Neisser, twenty-four years of age, following the recently-discovered bacteriological methods of Robert Koch, spread out gonorrheal pus on a slide, and after allowing it to dry, stained it by pouring over it a watery solution of methyl violet, then examined it under high power illumination with the least amount of diaphragming off of light. In this manner he was the first to see the coccus, shaped like a coffee-bean, occurring in pairs with the flat surfaces apposed—the sole cause of the most prevalent malady of adolescence. He described the result in a very brief communication entitled "On a form of Micrococcus characteristic of Gonorrhea" (1879). It is interesting to note that even in this preliminary paper Neisser gives warm thanks, for encouragement received, to Ferdinand Cohn. In his first paper, Neisser did not call his micrococcus the *gonococcus*, though he did so subsequently (1882). The young Neisser, by detecting the specific etiology of gonorrhea, solved the riddle of centuries.

The Leipzig obstetrician, Karl Siegmund Franz Credé, stimulated by the work of Noeggerath, had been wondering how to prevent the most frequent cause of blindness in the newborn—blindness due to the mother's gonorrhea. All the pens in the world could not begin to tell the extent and horrors of ophthalmia neonatorum. Credé was not the first who thought of this problem—Soranus, obstetrician of antiquity, poured oil in the child's eyes, and in the course of time seemingly everything else was employed, even corrosive sublimate and carbolic acid. At first Credé knew so little that he directed his efforts to the cleansing of the parturient canal: he soon learned that this would have baffled Hercules. He then began to instil various injections into the eyes of the newborn, and it was not until 1884 that he perfected his method. Immediately after the cutting of the umbilical cord, and before the infant was dressed, the secretions were wiped from its eyes, each eye was then opened by two fingers of an assistant, and a single drop of a two per cent solution of silver nitrate, hanging from a glass rod, was approached to the cornea and allowed to fall upon it. There was no further treatment of any sort, and the instillation was not to be repeated. As a result of this simple technique, blindness was abolished entirely in Credé's clinic. This prophylactic, applied in a moment, could wipe out all the purulent conjunctivitis of the newborn in the world, but because of its unlawful neglect, uncounted thousands still go through life in darkness.

The pale, thread-like, twisted parasite of syphilis lay coiled and concealed until the twentieth century. An innkeeper's son, Fritz Schaudinn, whose researches brought the protozoa within the domain of biology and medicine, exposed this scourge of mankind. Schaudinn's discovery of the organismal cause of syphilis (*Spirochaeta pallida,* 1905), is one of those ineffaceable landmarks which stand out clearer against the background of time. The following year, Schaudinn experimented upon himself with *Entamoeba histolytica,* and perished at thirty-five. It throws a sidelight on human nature to recall that Koch, who was an important Prussian official when Schaudinn was struggling for recognition, saw no merit in the young man's ideas—it reminds us of Galileo, who gave us a new heaven, but laughed when Kepler said the tide is influenced by the moon.

Paul Ehrlich, the despair of his teachers in his university days, was irregular in attendance, especially avoided the classes in chemistry, and after five years could not pass the required examinations. He remained another year, and was graduated to the great relief of the janitors. For Ehrlich was constantly playing with dye-stuffs, and never a neat worker, he squirted color-spots everywhere. Those who saw Ehrlich in later life with the ashes from his perpetual cigars falling unheeded all over his clothes, may imagine what ravages the young Ehrlich committed with basic aniline stains. Years later, one professor looked at his desk and wrote to another, "The traces of Ehrlich's industry are indeed indestructible." A favorite story, that Robert Koch told very often, was to the effect that when he came to Breslau to demonstrate the anthrax bacillus, he was taken on a tour of inspection through the laboratory: they pointed out Ehrlich's table to him with the remark, "This here belongs to little Ehrlich, he is a very good dyer, but his examination he will never pass."

In his early twenties, Ehrlich made significant discoveries with these stains, which are now used by all bacteriologists. His "vital staining" laid the foundation of chemotherapy, and created an epoch in immunity. Although Ehrlich, because of his seemingly haphazard "trial and error" methods, referred to his chemical researches as "play chemistry" (*Spiel-Chemie*), he realized that his "chemical imagination" was his chief asset. This imagination made him the greatest biochemical philosopher of all times. If his much-criticized "side-chain theory" has many weak links, yet it was by following this chain that August von Wassermann discovered the diagnostic test for syphilis which has since been a household word. Ehrlich became a savior of the race by his introduction of the arsenical derivative—the six hundred and sixth of the series—for the sterilization of syphilis. As a therapeutic achievement, the production of salvarsan (606) and neosalvarsan (914) has never been surpassed.

Paul Ehrlich and Elie Metchnikoff shared the Nobel Prize (1908) for their researches in immunity. Metchnikoff grew up in tsaristic Russia, where a gendarme sat astride the halls of learning, and the knout lay over the book; the crucifix and the gallows met on every crossroad, and the Romanoffs imprisoned the human spirit. After his second attempt at suicide Metchnikoff went to Messina, taking with him his wife and her five brothers and sisters. One day some clever apes arrived in town, and Madame Metchnikoff and all the children went to the circus.

Metchnikoff has told how he remained alone with his microscope, watching the moving cells of a transparent star-fish larva. The idea flashed across his brain that the mobilization of such cells might serve in the defense of the organism against the invaders of the body. Feeling himself on the trail of a great discovery, an intense excitement possessed Elie Metchnikoff. He began by striding up and down the room, but finally rushed to the seashore to collect his thoughts. In the Sicilian garden which he rented, grew a small tangerine tree which had been arranged as a Christmas tree for the children. Taking a few rose thorns from it, he introduced them within the skin of the star-fish larvae, and found that in spite of the larva's lack of vascular and nervous systems, its mesodermic cells accumulated around the intruding thorns, just as the white blood cells of man surrounded a splinter or germ that enters the body. Thus was born the theory of *phagocytosis*—the doctrine that when microbes or other deleterious substances attack the body, an army of phagocytes rush to the injured part, hurl themselves upon the enemy, attempting to engulf and devour the invaders. While his family was away at the circus, Metchnikoff had climbed to immortality. Upon their return, the children spoke of the wonderful tricks of the performing apes, and no one knew of the revolution which had taken place in Metchnikoff's life. His career as a zoölogist was over: he was transformed into a pathologist, and although he had no medical training, he became a leader in humanity's warfare against infectious diseases.

In his forty-fourth year, Metchnikoff entered the Pasteur Institute a misfit, but through the open door he carried his far-reaching discovery. Immediately a new life dawned for Elie Metchnikoff. He never again lived in Russia. This exile, who could not feel at home in his native country, found a haven among the Pasteurians. At first a small laboratory was placed at his disposal, and his wife served as his assistant; physicians overflowed this limited space, and an entire floor was given to him for his numerous pupils. Two rooms were set aside for his personal use, and Metchnikoff never gave up those rooms. In his latter years, working with Emile Roux, Metchnikoff was the first who definitely succeeded in inoculating anthropoid apes with syphilis. As man and monkey are the only animals capable of being systemically infected with this disease, a blood-relationship is thus established between them. Before this time (1903), physicians could study experimental syphilis only upon heroic volunteers—often themselves—or upon unsuspecting hospital-patients. The chapter dealing with the purposeful inoculation of human beings with veneral disease for scientific investigation, is one of the most mysterious and carefully-guarded in the annals of medicine. It was Metchnikoff also, again in conjunction with his friend Roux, who devised calomel ointment as a protection against syphilis. Thousands of homes, where perhaps the name of Metchnikoff has never been mentioned, have been saved from venereal disease by this prophylactic. As soon as it comes into general use we will cease to see new chancres every day. Both Metchnikoff and Ehrlich, who did so much to save mankind from syphilization, died broken-hearted victims of the World War.

It is remarkable how many paths in modern physiology and medicine start from the laboratory door of Claude Bernard. The secrets hidden in the internal secretions of the ductless glands are writing a new story of science, and Claude Bernard is the author of such chapters as Understanding the Pancreas, the Romance of the Liver, the Conversion of Glycogen, and the Puncture that Produces Diabetes. The very term, internal secretion (*sécrétion interne*), is of Claude Bernard's coinage.

One would like to believe that this master of experimental medicine passed the winter of his life in happy comfort amidst his devoted family. But whoever knocked at No. 40 Rue des Écoles, found that Claude Bernard lived alone with an old housekeeper who never let her duties to God interfere with her services to the physiologist. Claude Bernard sacrificed his home on the altar of his laboratory. Early in his career, this investigator made a bitter discovery—his wife was not interested in the experimental method. Hearing from his companions that he was clever, she demanded that he employ his talents to build up a large practice. That he should lock himself up in his laboratory, and after a long period of hard work emerge with nothing but the discovery of the vasomotor system, filled her with undisguised indignation. Claude Bernard knitted his ample brow, and realized he must choose between his spouse and science. But the rough call of Magendie, "I say, you there, I take you as my *préparateur* at the Collège de France," rang in his ears as a sacred passport to the temple of the experimental method, and Claude Bernard remained forever within its portals. The outraged Madame gathered together her belongings, took her daughters with her, and left the scientist homeless. A highly incensed police commissioner, who found in the belly of his missing dog, "the accusing cannula of a physiologist," later became the friend and protector of Claude Bernard, but his family remained unforgiving. His daughters grew up to hate their father, and one of them, who regarded him as a sinful vivisector, devoted her spare money to founding hospitals for cats and dogs.

Claude Bernard never had a son, but he had a spiritual heir who succeeded him as professor of experimental medicine at the College of France, and wore his mantle, if not with all the master's greatness, at least with a never-failing piquancy. We refer of course, to that enthusiastic, impulsive, roving, restless physiologist, Charles Édouard Brown-Séquard. Everything connected with this name is interesting. Brown-Séquard's nationality is a problem in ethics, ethnopsychology and anthropology, for he was born on the Island of Mauritius, the posthumous son of a Philadelphia-Irish sea-captain and a French girl, and yet regarded himself as a British subject, although he preferred to live in Paris. The mariner evidently found no fortune upon the waters, for after his death his widow found it necessary to support herself and child with the needle. Her family name was Séquard, and her son added this to his father's more prosaic patronymic of Brown.

Brown-Séquard's first passion was literature, and as his early efforts met with success, when he and his mother sailed for

France, during his twenty-first year, he carried with him the manuscript of a novel and a letter of introduction to one of the most romantic figures in French literature—Charles Nodier. Politician and entomologist, wanderer and booklover, newspaper editor and lexicographer, exile and Academician, prisoner and member of the legion of honor, bohemian and librarian, likewise historian, philologist, dramatist, poet, biographer, and patron of Victor Hugo, Alfred de Musset, Sainte-Beuve, and a host of lesser authors, Nodier drank deeply from the cup of life. The career of Nodier, without any embellishments, would make a drama of intense and ever-shifting scenes. Nodier, who had written dissertations on themes ranging from the antennae of insects to a diary of emotions of a love-sick heart, knew the uncertainty of literary rewards, and advised Brown-Séquard to become a doctor.

It is curious to recall that Claude Bernard, also at the age of twenty-one, had come down to Paris from his vine-covered cottage on the hill-slopes of Beaujolais, bringing the manuscript of a dramatic tragedy in five acts and a letter of introduction to the famous critic, Saint-Marc Girardin, professor at the Sorbonne. Claude Bernard's vaudeville sketch, La Rose du Rhône—composed during drug-store days—had already been produced with success, and Girardin acknowledged that his ambitious drama possessed considerable merit, but he put his hand on the young provincial's shoulder, and said kindly, "You already know something about pharmacy; now study medicine, and you will be more sure of making a living." Thus, to the advice of two eminent literary critics, endocrinology owes its chief founders, Claude Bernard and Brown-Séquard.

Brown-Séquard plunged into medicine with his usual ardor, but many years were to elapse before he obtained his doctorate, for a dissection-wound interrupted his studies for a time, and then the death of his mother darkened the world for him. Stunned with pain and incapable of work, he began a career of restless wandering that was Paracelsian.

Finally graduating at Paris with a thesis on "Researches and

Experiments on the Physiology of the Spinal Cord," he entered a military hospital, and in due time fought a cholera epidemic; opposing the imperialism of Louis Napoleon, he fled to America when the usurper was successful; upon returning to France, he decided to practise in Mauritius, and landed among the coral-reefs of the Indian ocean in the midst of another cholera outbreak; soon he was in America again, teaching medical jurisprudence at the Virginia Medical College; but Paris called, and here he made his mark by his lectures on the nervous system; when the National Hospital for the Paralyzed and Epileptic was opened in London, the physician-in-chief was no other than Brown-Séquard, and later he taught and practised in various cities of Scotland and Ireland; the news spread throughout the medical circles of the United States that Boston had a brilliant professor of neurology—it was Brown-Séquard; Harvard could not hold him, and he returned to Paris to teach comparative and experimental physiology, and to edit a medical journal; few men can leave the allurements of a combined professorial and editorial chair, but we next find Brown-Séquard an active practitioner in New York; our metropolis lost him, and London and Paris again knew his bronzed face and those long locks; in Geneva he became professor of physiology, and just as Switzerland was about to congratulate herself that she had acquired the international scientist, he stepped over the Alps into Claude Bernard's place at the College of France.

One would be justified in surmising that a physician who from youth to age had been driven across continents by travel fever, would be incapable of completing much scientific work, but this amazing individual, eternally traveling, lecturing, practising, experimenting, produced a bibliography so copious that it has never been compiled. The fame of Brown-Séquard is popularly associated with one spectacular experiment, but as a matter of fact he produced solid work of an enduring character, such as his pioneer investigations on the physiology of the spinal cord, his numerous researches in the nervous system, and his artificial production of epilepsy and its inheritance. After confirming by original experimentation, Claude Bernard's discovery of vasoconstrictor nerves, which has become "one of the keystones of modern physiology," Brown-Séquard followed the master into the realms of endocrinology, clearing new paths by his production of Addison's disease by excision of the suprarenal capsules, by his treatment of acromegaly by animal extracts, by his contention that the ovaries and kidneys possess an internal secretion, and by his pronouncement, "The internal secretions whether by direct favorable influence, or whether through the hindrances of deleterious processes, seem to be of great utility in maintaining the organism in its normal state."

The years passed, and Brown-Séquard grew old. Honors came to him, and in his sixty-third year he received the LL.D. from Cambridge. At that session, the highest honorary degree of the University was likewise bestowed upon the American surgeon, Samuel David Gross, then seventy-five years of age, and the elder man wrote in his Autobiography, "Dr. Brown-Séquard I had seen many years before, but I had not met him for a long time, and was sorry to find that he looked much older than is usual with one of his age."

Nine years later, Brown-Séquard, at seventy-two, was aged indeed. Beneath the dying flames of his ardor for science, only a few embers now flickered. The fire of Brown-Séquard had burnt out amidst the ashes of the years. He was irritable, impotent, suffered from gastrointestinal troubles and was plagued by urinary disturbances, and no longer cared to be surrounded by eager students in a laboratory. His career appeared over, and it seemed as if no new laurels would weigh down that wrinkled brow.

But Brown-Séquard's greatest day was yet to come: on June 1, 1889, he stood before the Société de Biologie and added a new thrill to science. The Brown-Séquard who addressed his colleagues on that historic day, looked twenty years younger than the Brown-Séquard they had known, and he reported that by testicular injections he had rejuvenated himself: his irritability, impotence, gastric and vesical infirmities had disappeared, and by means of the dynamometer and the ergograph he demonstrated his increased strength and energy. He rolled the clock of time backward for two decades, and mentally, physically, sexually, Brown-Séquard at seventy-two resembled the Brown-Séquard of fifty-two.

When his reports appeared in the Archives of Physiology, which Brown-Séquard edited in collaboration with Vulpian and Charcot, there arose an uproar of incredulity and wrath which has not yet entirely subsided. His alleged results were ascribed to his "senile-erotic imagination," and many physicians were either incensed or amused at what they considered the obscene folly of a scientist in his dotage. Brown-Séquard insisted that not chemical substances of the gland, but emulsions of the testicle were essential for success, yet he was discredited by men who did not even attempt to follow his technique. His self-experiment is now regarded as the "definite birthday" of the science of the internal secretions. We would celebrate this birthday with more happiness if we could duplicate his results, but we cannot. Nevertheless, we may regard his spectacular experiment as the origin of modern organotherapy.

Situated in the neck, saddled upon the windpipe, is a two-lobed organ without an excretory duct, pouring its internal secretion directly into the blood-stream; this ductless gland is shield-shaped, and hence known as the *thyroid*. If the thyroid does not function in early life, the result is a big-bellied, frog-like animal, a thick-tongued dwarfed idiot, hitherto existing in hopeless darkness—this is *cretinism,* and those affected are *cretins*. If the thyroid ceases to function in later life, the victim begins to speak in slow, monotonous tones, grows sluggish in movement, dull in intellect, and finally relapses into idiocy—the condition of *myxedema*. Deficient activity of the thyroid gland is spoken of as *hypothyroidism,* and excessive activity results in *hyperthyroidism*. Surgical removal of the thyroid is known as *thyroidectomy,* and produces the myxedematous condition of *cachexia thyropriva*. The thyroid is subject to a dangerous enlargement known as Derbyshire neck, bronchocele, struma, or *goiter;* if the goiter is marked by bulging eyeballs, it is referred to as *exophthalmic goiter*. In regions remote from the sea, in the so-called "goiter-belts," *goitrous cretinism* is especially common. The human thyroid weighs about one ounce (30-40 grams), and upon this ounce of glandular tissue, Medicine has gained some of its greatest victories. Let us trace the steps by which this has come about.

It is highly remarkable that in the prehistoric era, burnt sponges and sea-weed ashes were used by the Chinese in goiter, since these substances contain iodides. In the Roman era, Caesar speaks of big neck among the Gauls as one of their characteristics; and the Romans recognized that slaves with bulging eyes fatigue readily; the prevalence of goiter in Switzerland is apparent in the question of Juvenal: "Who marvels at goiter in the Alps?" Celsus described the technique for the removal of bronchocele (goiter), and Pliny said goiter is caused by impurities in water: "Only men and swine are subject to swellings in the throat, which are mostly caused by the noxious quality of the water they drink." There are vague allusions to the thyroid in Galen (*De voce*), and Paulus Aegineta refers to bronchocele, but there was no increase in knowledge of thyroid disease until the Renaissance.

Paracelsus was the first to establish the relationship between cretinism and endemic goiter. Vesalius referred to the thyroid (*Fabrica*, 1543), which was named by Thomas Wharton, who gave the first satisfactory description of its anatomy (*Adenographia*, 1656). T. Prosser wrote "An account and method of cure of the bronchocele, or Derby neck" (1769). Haller classified thyroid, thymus and spleen as glands without ducts, pouring a special fluid into the blood. Caleb Hillier Parry, of Bath, wrote the original account of exophthalmic goiter (Parry's disease, 1786). François-Emmanuel Fodere's "Essay on Goiter and Cretinism" (1792), was followed by his Treatise (1800), in which year Benjamin Smith Barton published his "Memoir concerning the disease of goiter, as it prevails in different parts of North America."

In the nineteenth century, Giuseppe Flajani described the goiter and cardiac palpitation of two cases of bronchocele or *gozzo* (Flajani's disease, 1802). Bernard Curtois, experimenting in extracting alkali from sea-weed, discovered iodine (1811). After Fyfe had isolated iodine from sponges, Jean-François Coindet, reasoning that iodine is the active constituent of burnt sponge, introduced it as a remedy for goiter—and thus were the Chinese vindicated. Carl Adolf Basedow, of Merseburg, who wrote the first monograph on exophthalmic goiter (Basedow's disease, 1840), called attention to the three cardinal symptoms: the swelling, exophthalmos, and tachycardia (Merseburg triad). Thomas Blizard Curling's "symmetric swellings of fat tissue at the sides of the neck connected with defective cerebral development" (1850), is the first reference to the condition now called myxedema. Moritz Schiff removed the thyroid of various animals, these being the first thyroidectomies (1856). Charcot described the fourth cardinal symptom of exophthalmic goiter, the tremor (1863). W. W. Gull in "On a cretenoid state supervening in adult life in women" (1873), described the condition later known as myxedema. P. H. Watson was the first to excise the thyroid for exophtlamic goiter (1874). W. M. Ord introduced the term myxedema, "On myxedema, a term proposed to be applied to the cretinoid affection occasionally observed in middle-aged women" (1878). J. L. Reverdin and Theodor Kocher, treating exophthalmic goiter by total thyroidectomy, discovered the thyroid to be a vital organ (1883). Victor Horsley was the first to investigate the thyroid of monkeys (1884). Moritz Schiff demonstrated that the symptoms of cachexia thyropriva following thyroidectomy could be prevented by a previous graft of thyroid substance, or by the administration of thyroid, hypodermically or by mouth (1884).

With this new information, Medicine was ready to raise dumb and dwarfish imbeciles to the status of normal mankind. George Redmayne Murray began to use hypodermic injections of the thyroid gland in the treatment of hypothyroidism (1891):

The symptoms of the disease having thus been traced to loss of the thyroid gland, the next advance was in the direction of supplying the deficiency. Schiff had already shown that the usual fatal result of thyroidectomy in the dog could be averted by a preliminary transplantation of another thyroid gland into the abdomen of the animal, and von Eiselsberg proved that the same result could be obtained in the cat, provided the graft was successful. Quite independently, 1890, thyroid grafting was suggested by Sir Victor Horsley as a method of arresting the disease in man. This suggestion was acted upon by several surgeons, especially by Bettencourt and Serrano, who noticed that in their case the operation was immediately followed by improvement, which they attributed to absorption of the juice of the transplanted thyroid gland. This observation appeared to me to be extremely important, as it indicated that the thyroid gland carried on its function by means of an internal secretion. I, therefore, concluded that if this was the case the regular use of the secretion, obtained in the form of an extract of the gland, would remove the symptoms of myxedema, and suggested this line of treatment at a meeting of the Northumberland and Durham Medical Society in February, 1891. In order to test this a glycerin extract of the sheep's thyroid gland was prepared, and injected at intervals beneath the skin so as to ensure its absorption by the lymphatics in the same manner as the normal secretion is conveyed into the circulation from the healthy gland. The symptoms of myxedema in the first case I treated in this manner rapidly disappeared, thus proving that the thyroid gland is a true internal secretory gland, and that the thyroid extract is a specific remedy for myxedema. The following year it was shown by Howitz, of Copenhagen, and by Dr. Hector Mackenzie and Dr. E. L. Fox, in England, that the same results could be obtained by the simple method of giving thyroid extract or the raw gland itself by the mouth.

In former times, the curse of cretinism was ended only by death; today this deformed and drivelling idiot, properly treated with thyroid, is turned into a normal specimen of childhood. It is one of the miracles of modern medicine, for the child that emerges is literally "born anew." For example, a cretin whom Hector Mackenzie had treated since the age of eleven, became a university student (1908). Just as the ideal of bacteriology is the discovery of pathogenic microbes and the preparation of antitoxins, so the object of endocrinology is the isolation of the hidden hormones and the production of organotherapy. Endocrinology is the obscurer science, and we stand today at the gates, and cannot pass beyond. Another generation shall enter, and much that is closed to our eyes, shall be open to those who succeed us. Where we stumble in uncertainty, they shall advance by the light of the new knowledge. Where we attempt to halt the monsters of disease with imperfect weapons, they shall conquer with swords dipped in a hundred discoveries. Yet some of the results already achieved justify us in repeating the paean of a representative endocrinologist: "When we see misshapen, stunted imbeciles transformed to normal, happy children, diabetics starving in the midst of plenty restored to health and strength, giants and dwarfs produced at will, sex manifestations engendered or reversed before our very eyes by control of endocrine factors, who can regard endocrinology as other than a most significant phase of modern biology?"

A peasant-monk strolled through his cloister-garden at Brünn, watching the common pea. Before it ripened, he removed the male element from the flower, which he fertilized later with ripe pollen from another breed. He crossed a tall with a dwarf, and the hybrids of the first generation were not intermediate, but all were tall; after self-fertilization of these hybrids, the next generation consisted of three talls and one dwarf; when the hybrid dwarfs were self-fertilized, they produced only dwarfs; one of the talls produced only talls; and the other talls produced three talls to one dwarf. He crossed a yellow-seeded with a green seeded pea, and the seeds of all the resulting hybrids were yellow; in the succeeding generation three of the seeds were yellow, and one was green; when the green seeds bred again, all the seeds were green; one of the yellow produced only yellows; and the other yellows produced the ratio of three yellows to one green. He crossed red-colored with white-colored flowers, and all the hybrids were red; after they fertilized themselves, three were red in the next generation, and one was white;

the offspring of the white were white, one of the red always remained red, and the other reds produced three reds to one white.

For several years this Augustinian monk watched his peas acting with mathematical precision. Gregor Mendel performed thousands of experiments in his monastery garden, and discovered the principle of alternative inheritance: The unit-characters do not blend. The sexual cells or gametes remain pure. In cross fertilization of plants, the resulting progeny exhibits the character of one parent only. The persisting character which is visibly inherited by the hybrids is *dominant*, the character which is undeveloped in the first filial generation is *recessive*. In the experiments above, the tall is dominant to the recessive dwarf, the yellow seed is dominant to the recessive green, the red flower is dominant to the recessive white. But the recessive is latent and is not lost, and will make its appearance in the next inbreeding of the hybrids, three-quarters of which will be dominants and one-quarter recessives. In inbreeding of these recessives, all will be recessives; in inbreeding of these dominants, one-third will remain dominants, the rest will breed as true hybrids in the ratio of three dominants to one recessive.

Mendel wrote out his *Experiments on Plant Hybrids* (1865) for the Proceedings of the Natural History Society of Brünn. No one read the amateur's monograph. Mendel corresponded with Karl Wilhelm von Naegeli, the great Swiss botanist and cytologist, who had coined "idioplasm" as the basic material of heredity. Naegeli had no idea what Mendel was talking about. In the nineteenth century, Mendel planted his peas on sterile soil. In the meantime he was appointed abbot of Brünn, and stormy years dawned for Moravia. Austria decided to tax the monasteries, and Mendel was too staunch a Catholic to submit. If the Austrian government had realized what Mendel accomplished in his monastery garden, it should have overlooked the disputed tax. But Mendel fell ill and died, and no one knew that the priest who passed away was the discoverer of the laws of heredity. Thirty-five years after the publication of Mendel's paper, it was read by a group of investigators interested in the problems of genetics. The effect was startling. They found the basis for all their researches in Mendel's peas. From that time, on Mendelism gave biology a new impetus. Mendel, as an observer of nature, now ranks with Darwin.

At the turn of the century, a middle-aged Moravian who was teaching in Vienna, committed the boldest act of modern times. Sigmund Freud, in his interpretation of dreams (*Die Traumdeutung*, 1900), developed a new method of diagnosis and treatment, which differed materially from the classic ideal of curing "quickly, safely, pleasantly." The auricular confession of the Church is child's play in comparison with the confessional established by this Jewish physician. From the subconscious depths of forgotten memories, Freud has dragged up the psychic traumata of early childhood. He exposed the origin of compulsion-neuroses, and reopened destructive wounds long buried in oblivion. Unheeding the opposition of his profession and society, he emphasized the dominance of sexuality and the neurotic diseases arising from its repression. Submerged mental processes, struggling to be born, were brought to light by the new obstetrician. To psychology he added depth-psychology, and to physical pathology the vaster realms of psychopathology.

Freud has covered so much unfamiliar ground that undoubtedly he has often gone astray; some of his chief disciples have forsaken him, and struck out into organic paths. Psychoanalysis, as originally propounded, may be largely revised in another generation. That does not detract from its value, nor from the merit of the founder. Freud has opened new territory for our investigation, and we will never again live in the narrower pre-Freudian era. Not only the medical sciences, but mythology, religion, history, biography, literature and art, have been influenced by the application of psychoanalytic methods. There is substantial truth in Freud's contention that the three cultural epochs of mankind are the Copernican revolution, Darwinism, and Freudism. Psychoanalysis, howsoever modified in the future, will continue to explore the hitherto uncharted regions of the mind, and Freud will be remembered as the great geographer who first mapped the Subconscious World.

In its dying years, the nineteenth century bequeathed to its successor three discoveries, infinitely romantic and of enduring importance. In October 1895, a teacher of physics, contemplating an exhausted vacuum tube in a black box, noticed that a paper screen covered with barium platinocyanide which accidentally lay near by, became fluorescent. His curiosity aroused, he soon found that the unknown radiations from the tube could pass through substances opaque to ordinary light, and possessed the power of developing a photographic plate. Two months later, Wilhelm Konrad Roentgen gave to mankind as a Christmas gift, the x-ray. At about the same time, a young Dane, the Hamlet of medicine, born among the fjords and fogs of the Faeroe Islands of the North Sea, reared in Iceland, hopelessly ill since youth, captured the sun for therapeutics. Niels Finsen was the first, consciously and scientifically, to employ artificial sunlight in the treatment of disease. The light from Finsen's lamp gave us phototherapy. While these experiments, blended with genius and pathos, went on in the north, a man and woman moved into an abandoned shed on the outskirts of Paris, and worked there for many hours during the day, boiling and stirring in a large cast-iron vessel tons of waste material—brown dust and pine-needles that had come from the forests of Bohemia. Sometimes the man wrote formulas on the blackboard, while his wife prepared the tea on the broken stove. Often they returned to the shack in the evening, for out of that basin had come strange products—luminous silhouettes, glowing like fairy lights in the dark. One night Pierre and Marie Curie looked longer than ever, for in their magic pot they found Radium. The relationship of radium and the x-ray to the living cell—the marriage of physics and biology in the realm of light—initiates problems which no single generation can hope to solve.

The most hopeful aspect of modern science is the victory of the Experimental Method over the assumptions of authority. Carl Voit said to his students: "You need not believe anything that I tell you in my lectures, you need believe only what I can demonstrate to you." The advent of this new spirit was of more importance to medicine than the discovery of many microbes and drugs. There is so much to be done, that we no longer have time for pompousness and pretense. Medicine is yet an impotent art. Of all the earth-born, the majority are prematurely returned to earth by disease. Will the time ever come when mortals will live the normal cycle of their years, free from infection, safe from organic disease, secure from mental blight?

In Life, as in Death, we cannot answer the main problems. As we stand before the veil that hides the Truth from men, we hear once more the voice of Ernest Renan: "An immense river of oblivion sweeps us onward into a gulf without a name. O abyss, thou art the only God! All here below is but symbol and dream. The gods pass away like men; it would not be well did they last forever. The faith which we have held ought never to be a chain. We have done our duty by it when we have carefully wrapped it round in the purple shroud wherein the dead gods sleep."

Life is a great experiment in physiology, in which we all take part: the unknown holds the protocols, and Death writes the conclusions. We do not know where the experiment is tending, nor can we control the outcome. There are gates we cannot open, and impassable roads without a guide-post. Yet we have pressed immeasurably forward; the sable curtain still shrouds us in darkness, but it is no longer so frightening. Often it has lifted, and where once most impenetrable, are seams through which we steal a glance at the mysteries beyond. We have mounted our present height over the accumulated discoveries of the centuries, but chiefly those of modern times. We linger still on the lower rungs, and the upward climb is uncertain, but never was the way so clear. In the eternal quest, Medicine and Biology are halted by a speck of protoplasm, within whose nucleated cell is locked the mystery of animated matter. With ever new, yet ever insufficient knowledge, we continue the never-to-be ended Journey.

XII

MEDICINE IN AMERICA

AMERICA is the youngest of the great nations, and if it seems strange that we know no more of the first English physicians in America than of the first Greek physicians in Rome, the same reason is operative in both instances. Eminent physicians remain at home, if for no other purpose than to annoy their rivals, and are not likely to be found on the first ship that touches a new shore. In the year that Jamestown was settled (1607), William Harvey was elected a Fellow of the Royal College of Physicians, and his prospects in London looked brighter than in Virginia; when the *Half-Moon* sailed up the river that we now call the Hudson (1609), Thomas Fryer, graduate of Cambridge and Padua, was enjoying the honors of Consiliarius; when the Pilgrims landed on Plymouth Rock (1620), the Oxonian Matthew Gwinne was appointed Tobacco Inspector by James I, the royal enemy of the weed. Such men, professionally or socially successful, had no incentive to follow fortune in a wilderness. The social standing that comes to first settlers is always posthumous.

The practitioners who first set foot on American soil have left us nothing except their names. Among the Jamestown pioneers were the physicians Thomas Wootton, whose possible knowledge of dietetics was of little avail, since he was compelled for a considerable time to subsist on crabs; and Walter Russell, who treated both Captain Smith and an Indian chief. The following year, Anthony Bagnall, surgeon to the fort, while visiting one of his patients, received an Indian arrow through his hat. It seems that young America did not agree with these medical adventurers, who soon disappear from the colony. In the fall of 1609, the valiant John Smith being wounded by the explosion of a bag of gunpowder, was compelled to return to England, "for there was neither chirurgeon nor chirurgery at the fort." Upon the arrival of Lawrence Bohun in Virginia, he was appointed physician-general of the colony, for he had no competition; in the spring (1611) he sailed with the sick Lord Delaware to the West Indies, and was killed by a Spanish warship. The next physician of the Virginia Company, John Pot, for a brief time held the office of governor.

The Bishop of London, official follower of the Carpenter, voiced the opinion of all well-bred Englishmen when he scornfully referred to the Pilgrims as "cobblers, tailors, feltmakers, and such-like trash": the Bishop of London did not foresee that their very numerous descendants would constitute the aristocracy of America. The *Mayflower* carried 102 passengers from the old to the new Plymouth; they landed in winter, and the snows covered half of them: a dozen men, and a small group of women and children, saw the first summer. Among the survivors was the butcher's son, Samuel Fuller, deacon and physician. He had been married thrice before coming to America, but of his medical education we know nothing. As the sole practitioner in the settlement, he was in considerable demand, and his death during a smallpox epidemic (1633) "was most deeply lamented by all the colonists." The combination of preacher-physician—called by Cotton Mather an "Angelic Conjunction"—or even preacher-physician-pedagogue, was common in early America, since one profession did not suffice for a livelihood. For example, John Wilson, who graduated at the first Commencement of Harvard College (1642), is described as "pastor, schoolmaster and physician." The practice of law was sometimes added, and almost invariably the physician was also a farmer.

The effective founder of puritanism in America, John Winthrop, governor of Massachusetts, felt the need of standardized medical practice; he appealed to an English physician for an authoritative text, and Ed. Stafford, of whom we know nothing else, sent him nine pages of manuscript (1643). Stafford took advantage of the occasion to advertise "my black powder against ye plague, smallpox." For pains in the breast, he recommended the wearing of the skin of a wildcat. For green wounds, "Clownes all-heal prescribed in Gerrits Herball"—John Gerard's *Herbal* is the extent of his quotations. For old sores, he suggests the charm known as St. John's Wort, pounded with quicklime, mixed with rain water, stirred every day in the sun for a month: "Wash ye soares with it; it cureth Wonderfully." For the King's evil, he prescribes two fasting toads, boiled in oil in a new pipkin, the oil to be expressed from the toads and combined with yellow wax, to be applied to the running sores, while the patient sweats upon his black powder: he concludes, truthfully enough, "By this course there is no doubt of the Cure by God's assistance."

Stafford's instructions did not help the colonials in diagnosis. The first outbreak of syphilis in Boston (1646) infected sixteen persons because it was unrecognized. "But see the providence of God," writes Winthrop, "at that very season there came by accident a young surgeon out of the West Indies, who had had experience of the right way of the cure of that disease. He took them in hand and through the Lord's blessing recovered them all in a short time." To cure syphilis in the seventeenth century in a short time certainly required the Lord's blessing.

If the colonists did not know venereal disease when they saw it, they had no difficulty in detecting witchcraft. A female physician named Margaret Jones, according to Winthrop (1648) possessed "such a malignant touch, as many persons were taken with deafness or vomiting, or other violent pains or sickness; her medicines, though harmless in themselves, yet had extraordinarily violent effects; such as refused her medicines she would tell that they would never be healed, and accordingly their diseases and hurts continued with relapses against the ordinary course, and beyond the apprehension of all physicians and surgeons." Winthrop thus proves she was a witch: "She had upon search an apparent teat in her secret parts as fresh as if it had been newly sucked, and after it had been scanned, upon a forced search, that was withered, and another began on the opposite side. In the prison in the clear daylight there was seen, she sitting on the floor, and her clothes up, a little child, which ran from her into another room, and the officer following it, it was vanished. . . . The same day and hour she was executed [the first execution in the colony] there was a very great tempest in Connecticut, which blew down many trees."

Kenelm Digby informed the younger John Winthrop, governor of Connecticut, that crabs' eyes, beaten to a subtle powder and placed in a glass of strong vinegar, perform miraculous cures in all sorts of ulcers and broken bones (1656). Sir Kenelm felt qualified to give medical advice, for his Powder of Sympathy made him internationally famous. The sympathetic powder was applied, not to the wound, but to the weapon which caused the injury, or to a portion of the sufferer's garment. For example, the Duke of Buckingham's secretary had been so severely stabbed that death from gangrene was the doctor's prognosis, but Kenelm Digby came to the rescue. Asking for the secretary's blood-stained garter, he bathed it in a basin containing a solution of his sympathetic powder, and within an hour the secretary felt "an agreeable coolness," and was soon completely cured. Credulity writes testimonials for every delusion. Among the numerous laudatory letters which were sent to Digby, was one about a carpenter who had cut himself with an axe, and attempted a sympathetic cure by annointing the axe and hanging it upon a hook. The wound was progressing favorably, until one day it reopened, because the axe had fallen from its hook. Since the sophisticated Madame de Sévigné pronounced the Powder of Sympathy "a perfectly divine remedy," we need not be surprised if the colonists found crabs' eyes in vinegar equally efficacious.

Thomas Thacher, preacher and physician, issued in Boston a broadside which he called "A Brief Rule to guide the Common

People of New-England how to order themselves and theirs in the Small Pocks, or Measles" (1677). It is apparent from the title that the "well wisher to the sick," as Thacher styled himself, did not make a differential diagnosis between the two diseases. This single sheet—a double-columned poster, printed on one side of the paper, fifteen and one-half inches long and ten inches across—was the first and only medical publication in the colonies during the seventeenth century. The inventory (1680) of Samuel Seabury, surgeon of Duxbury, revealed the following books: Nicholas Culpepper's Practice of Physic, Nicholas Culpepper's Anatomy, Reed's Practice of Surgery, Physician's Practice, Latin Herbal, John French's Art of Distillation. Many medical libraries of the time were less extensive. Science had not a single votary in the old colonial days, and statements to the contrary are due to patriotism. The medicine of Massachusetts Bay was all folklore. New England medicine in the seventeenth century is as dreary as its literature and as repellent as its theology.

Early in the eighteenth century, in this seemingly sterile soil, opposite the old South Church of Boston, was born the most richly endowed of all Americans. Hatched in the same nest with a large brood of mediocrities, removed from school at ten to follow his father's trade of tallow-chandler and soap-boiler, entering Philadelphia as a runaway printer of seventeen eating buns, laughed at for his ridiculous appearance by the girl he married later, reëntering the city as a world-famous freethinking philosopher, there is no explaining Benjamin Franklin. An unaffected provincial and chief cosmopolite of his age, he sighed for the privacy of his laboratory while amusing himself in the center of history. Living in America, England and France, equally celebrated in each country, he knew personally, in addition to the diplomats, the foremost scientists, philosophers and physicians.

In scientific as well as in political matters, the colonies asked: "Have you consulted Franklin on this business? And what does he think of it?" Franklin had his finger, and it was usually the index finger, in the founding of our first philosophical society, first circulating library, first hospital and first medical school. He was one of our earliest medical printers and booksellers; his letters on hygiene are masterpieces; his dialogue with the gout is classic; his counsel to a young man on the advantages of choosing an elderly mistress, is a landmark in sexology. His inventions include bifocal spectacles, a flexible catheter, and the "Pennsylvania fireplace," which marked so great an improvement in domestic ventilation. Franklin, preaching the gospel of fresh air, opened the windows of America. That his theory of "catching colds" was modern, is apparent from this passage in the autobiography of John Adams:

At Brunswick [1776], but one bed could be procured for Dr. Franklin and me, in a chamber little larger than the bed, without a chimney, and with only one small window. The window was open, and I who was an invalid and afraid of the air of night, shut it close. "Oh!" says Franklin, "don't shut the window, we shall be suffocated." I answered I was afraid of the evening air. Dr. Franklin replied, "The air within this chamber will soon be, and indeed is now, worse than that without doors. Come, open the window and come to bed, and I will convince you. I believe you are not acquainted with my theory of colds?"

Opening the window, and leaping into bed, I said I had read his letters to Dr. Cooper, in which he had advanced, that nobody ever got cold by going into a cold church or any other cold air, but the theory was so little consistent with my experience, that I thought it a paradox. However, I had so much curiosity to hear his reasons that I would run the risk of a cold. The Dr. then began a harangue upon air and cold, and respiration and perspiration, with which I was so much amused that I soon fell asleep, and left him and his philosophy together, but I believe they were equally sound and insensible within a few minutes after me, for the last words I heard were pronounced as he was more than half asleep. I remember little of the lecture, except that the human body, by respiration and perspiration, destroys a gallon of air in a minute; that two such persons as were now in that chamber, would consume all the air in it in an hour or two; that by breathing over again the matter thrown off by the lungs and the skin, we should imbibe the real cause of colds, not from abroad, but from within.

The outstanding event in eighteenth-century electricity was the experimental demonstration of the identity of lightning and the electric spark. This discovery was accomplished in a thunderstorm, by means of a silk handkerchief, a key and a kite—but it was the hand of Benjamin Franklin that held the kite. The practical-minded Franklin was not content merely to draw the electric fire from the heavens; he provided himself with a static generator, opened a clinic on Green Street, Philadelphia, and inaugurated medical electricity in America. Franklin's final comment on the electrotherapy of his day was remarkable for its candor, sagacity, and lack of laudatory testimonials. His work in this field survives in various eponyms: we still speak of the Franklin plate, Franklinic reaction of degeneration, franklinism and franklinization.

Franklin's influence did much to make Philadelphia the medical cradle of early America. In this city Thomas Cadwalader was the first in the colonies to teach practical anatomy (1730); William Shippen first lectured on midwifery (1765) and established a small lying-in hospital; and John Morgan published the first work on medical education in America (1765), memorable for its argument to separate medicine and pharmacy as independent professions. The Revolution transformed the colonies into a nation; as late as the summer of 1792, Philadelphia was the largest city in the Union, and its medical, cultural and commercial center. In the summer of 1793, the twilight mosquito conquered the city: every road leading from Philadelphia was crowded with human beings flying in panic, children expired alone in empty houses, and all day resounded the cry of negro grave-diggers, "Bring out your dead, bring out your dead." It was the hour of trial of Benjamin Rush, and we must now pause to look at the most conspicuous figure in American medicine.

"When I was a boy of twelve years old," wrote Charles Delucena Meigs, "the name of Dr. Rush was a sort of myth in my young ears, and was known by all the people of yon sequestered village on the Creek Frontier; and when in the autumn of 1812 I first entered his lecture-room in the old university building on Ninth Street, I was enrapt; his voice, sweeter than any flute, fell on my ears like droppings from a sanctuary, and the spectacle of his beautiful radiant countenance, with his earnest, most sincere, most persuasive accents, sunk so deep into my heart that neither time nor change could eradicate them from where they are at this hour freshly remembered. Oh! but he was a most charming gentleman!" The bitter Charles Caldwell, who of course included Rush within the circle of his hatred, has nevertheless testified, "the resources of his amenity and courtesy were all but boundless." These tributes to Rush's urbanity—and they could be multiplied indefinitely—simply confirm Claude Bernard's contention: "But medicine is still in the shades of empiricism and suffers the consequences of its backward condition. We see it still more or less mingled with religion and the supernatural. . . . Medical personality is placed above science by physicians themselves; they seek their authority in tradition, in doctrines or in medical tact. This state of affairs is the clearest of proofs that the experimental method has by no means come into its own in medicine."

The career of Rush proves that having a fine personality, being a perfect gentleman, signing the Declaration of Independence, founding various important societies and taking an active part in public affairs, do not necessarily make a scientist; it proves that a physician with a facile pen may leave behind him several volumes entitled "Medical Inquiries and Observations" —and not one page of scientific value; it proves too, that the influence of the foremost physician of his age, hailed as the father of his country's medicine, as the American Sydenham, and even as the Hippocrates of Pennsylvania, may be distinctly mischievous. It is probably known that physicians are apt to be dogmatic in therapeutics—else the history of medicine would have had a different development! Benjamin Rush was more than dogmatic: he considered himself infallible, and unfortunately for American medicine, he succeeded in impressing this conviction upon his contemporaries.

The fame of Rush was at its zenith in 1793 when Philadelphia was decimated by an epidemic that ranks with the historic plagues—and all eyes turned to the oracle who occupied the chair of the Institutes and Practice of Medicine. Rush accepted the challenge and acted characteristically: instead of investigating the abundant clinical material at his disposal, he retired to his desk—how old Paracelsus would have railed at him!—and began to look through his books and documents. "See," said Ambroise Paré, after making his first discovery on the battlefield, "how I learned to treat gunshot wounds; not by books." Rush paused over every sentence, sometimes every word, of an old manuscript, which Franklin had given him, written more than fifty years previously by the botanist John Mitchell of Virginia; when Rush issued from his library, he felt himself the conqueror of yellow fever. The hard-hitting Cobbett was justified in describing what followed as a "reign of blood." Rush bled and purged without mercy, and although the majority of the physicians followed his precepts, and although every apothecary in town overworked himself to fulfil his calomel-and-jalap prescriptions, Philadelphia then lost its supremacy over American cities.

In his lengthy account of the epidemic, Rush wrote: "A meteor was seen at two o'clock in the morning, on or about the twelfth of September. It fell between Third-street and the hospital, nearly in a line with Pine-street. Moschetoes (the usual attendants of a sickly autumn) were uncommonly numerous. Here and there a dead cat added to the impurity of the air of the streets." Had Rush been able to forget Mitchell's manuscript, had he disregarded the meteor and the dead cat, and had he paid some attention to these "moschetoes" that buzzed around him, he would have advanced medicine by over a century. But Rush, in spite of ample opportunities, never discovered anything.

In many respects Rush did not reach the best medical thought of his own time. His conception of fever was more confused than that of Nathan Smith; while Rush finally asserted that the sole cause of the yellow fever epidemic in Philadelphia was the damaged coffee on a wharf, John Crawford (1790) maintained that such diseases as yellow fever, malaria and dysentery were due to tiny insects; while Rush whetted his lancet to shed ever more streams of human blood, Johann Gottlieb Wolstein, in a truly remarkable work (1791), based on observations of animals, demonstrated the evils of venesection; while Pinel struck the chains from the mentally afflicted, Rush prepared for them a "tranquilising chair," wherein the patient was strapped at the ankles and wrists, and across the abdomen and chest, while his head was confined in a wooden box. Nothing more gruesome was ever contributed to medicine.

Rush knew less about diabetes than Aretaeus, and less about pulmonary consumption than Galen. He declared the latter disease was not contagious, and he invariably prescribed exercise for the consumptive; as for the treatment, he gives us this specific: "The pulmonary consumption . . . even when tending rapidly to its last stage has been cured by bleedings, digitalis and mercurial salivation." In fact, this heroic doctor did not fear any disease; concerning scarlatina, he wrote: "Whenever I have been called to a patient where the scarlatina appeared to be in a forming state, a vomit of ipecacuanha or tartar emetic, mixed with a few grains of calomel, has never failed of completely checking the disease. . . . When the matter which produces this disease has been received into the body, a purge has prevented its being excited into action, or rendered it mild, throughout a whole family." Even lock-jaw held no terrors for him: "Tetanus is prevented by inflaming the injured parts . . . and often cured by opium, bark and wine." He admitted hydrophobia was a formidable disease, but he added that he could prevent the manifestations by giving mercury, and cure the malady itself by copious bloodletting.

Rush was our pioneer prohibitionist, and his "Inquiry into

the Effects of Ardent Spirits" went into several editions; Rush, who had a flair for publicity, himself sent a thousand copies to the Presbyterian Church for distribution. Its scientific value may be judged from this typical passage: "A noted drunkard was once followed by a favorite goat, to a tavern, into which he was invited by his master, and drenched with some of his liquor. The poor animal staggered home with his master, a good deal intoxicated. The next day he followed him to his accustomed tavern. When the goat came to the door, he paused: his master made signs to him to follow him into the house. The goat stood still. An attempt was made to thrust him into the tavern. He resisted, as if struck with the recollection of what he suffered from being intoxicated the night before. His master was so much affected by a sense of shame, in observing the conduct of his goat to be so much more rational than his own, that he ceased from that time to drink spirituous liquors."

Even in the sixteenth century, Michael Servetus was progressive enough to write a treatise in favor of palatable therapeutics. Rush, reactionary in most things medical, maintained: "The Author of Nature seems to have had a design, in rendering medicines unpalatable. Had they been more agreeable to the taste, they would probably have yielded long ago to the unbounded appetite of man, and by becoming articles of diet, or condiments, have lost their efficacy in diseases." There are few medical writers, and certainly none of celebrity, whose works are less worthy of perusal today than those of Rush. The books of our forefathers often amaze us by their knowledge and insight, but Rush is equally surprising by his paucity of thought. Endless trivial and unverified anecdotes, dictatorial but incorrect assertions, a total absence of humor and eternal preaching and moralizing in inflated rhetoric—these are the characteristics of the voluminous writings which Rush has bequeathed to a posterity which honors his memory and does not read his productions.

Among the first to prick the Rush legend was the inimitable Oliver Wendell Holmes. In reply to Rush's pompous epigram, "Medicine is my wife and Science is my mistress," Holmes answered: "I do not think that the breach of the seventh commandment can be shown to have been of advantage to the legitimate owner of his affections. Read what Dr. Elisha Bartlett says of him as a practitioner, or ask one of our own honored ex-professors, who studied under him, whether Dr. Rush had ever learned the meaning of that saying of Lord Bacon, that man is the minister and interpreter of Nature, or whether he did not speak habitually of Nature, as an intruder in the sick room, from which his art was to expel her as an incompetent and a meddler."

In the Centennial Year, that mighty man, John S. Billings, gave the reputation of Rush a thrust from which it will never recover. He quoted from David Ramsay's tribute to Rush, in which the eulogist affirmed that upon the correctness of Rush's universal employment of the lancet his fame as an improver of medicine in a great degree must eventually rest. Billings added this comment: "And to the correctness of this judgment we entirely assent"—thus demonstrating that at times the pen is sharper than the scalpel.

In every age, opposition to the cardinal doctrine of the healing power of nature, promulgated by Hippocrates, has been a sign of the obstructionist in medicine. Rush was conspicuous among those who sought to overthrow the Hippocratic maxim that nature heals and the physician is only nature's assistant. Everywhere he attempted to cast out nature by unlimited bloodletting and overdrugging—the famous physician was really a menace in the sick-room. Rush erred in joining the Conway Cabal against the father of his country, and he erred equally by denying the father of his profession. Due largely to Rush's influence, our art lay in bondage to drugs until the Apollonian Osler liberated us from the medicine-spoon. Rush expressed his attitude plainly enough: "It is impossible to calculate the mischief which Hippocrates has done, by first marking Nature with his name and afterwards letting her loose upon sick people. Millions have perished by her hands in all ages and countries." No other evidence is needed of the status of Benjamin Rush in modern medicine.

This is written, not in detraction, but in evaluation, of Rush. He was a man of many sterling merits. He was the most prominent figure at the cradle of American medicine. But he fussed over the baby until he spoiled it. If he had only known enough medical grammar to be able to differentiate between a conjecture and a conclusion—if he had only inquired more, and sermonized less! The history of medicine has no room for myths, and to say today that the work of Benjamin Rush belongs to the classics of medicine is to be guilty of myth-making. The ancient Hippocrates (460-370 B. C.) is modern; the modern Rush (1745-1813 A. D.) is antiquated.

In the days when New York was a cross between a Dutch-English trading village and a rising American metropolis—when the water from the De Voor mill-stream went splashing beneath the Kissing Bridge while the cornerstone of the first Park Theater was being laid—three doctors strolled along the leafy lanes of Broadway, discussing a daring project. They were young, unmarried, and idealistic, and they talked about starting the first medical journal in America.

They felt the time was ripe for such a periodical, for terrifying and highly destructive epidemics, especially of yellow fever, aroused the apprehensions of the public and quickened the zeal of the physicians. They decided to devote their journal to the following departments: the diseases of localities; veterinary medicine; insects noxious to men, beasts, plants; the condition of vegetation; the state of the atmosphere, including the direction and force of winds, and the sensible quantity of electricity. Feeling that these topics did not adequately cover the ground, the enthusiasts added other subjects to their prospectus: diseases which formerly prevailed in any part of the United States; useful histories of particular cases; occupational diseases; new methods of curing diseases; new remedies; extracts from rare works or manuscripts dealing with diseases that exist in the United States; interesting information relative to the minerals, plants and animals of our country; American medical biography; accounts of former American medical pamphlets and books; reviews of new American medical publications; medical news. Above all, their journal was to demonstrate that systems of medicine, whether ancient or contemporaneous, were preposterous, and that though conjecture may precede experiment, facts are the only rational basis of theory. One of the main points of discussion was whether the journal should be an annual or a quarterly, and with some trepidation the editors agreed upon the more frequent form of publication. Their Circular Address —with its curious blending of old-fashioned farm-medicine and the modern experimental method—was dated November 15, 1796, and signed by Samuel L. Mitchill, Columbia College; Edward Miller, 158 Broadway; and E. H. Smith, 45 Pine Street.

Delays, inevitable and excusable in a pioneer publishing venture, occurred and recurred, but on July 26, 1797, American medical journalism was born; on that day, there came from the press of T. & J. Swords, the first issue of the first American medical journal—the *Medical Repository*. When the call went forth for subscribers, the doctors could not claim that they already subscribed to more journals than they had time to read, and there was an immediate and gratifying response from the leading physicians in all parts of the Union, while such eminent laymen as Noah Webster, James Kent, and De Witt Clinton, likewise supported the undertaking. Not only were Benjamin Rush and Philip Syng Physick among the original subscribers, but one of the first subscriptions came from Elisha Perkins, whose wonderful Metallic Tractors were to render the medical profession superfluous. Thus, in at least one instance, the Father of American Medicine, and the Father of American Surgery, found themselves in the same boat with the Father of American Quackery. When we peruse the New York list, finding there the names of Stephen Van Rensselaer, Cornelius C. Van Allen, Arondt Van Hook, James L. Van Kleeck, and Peter Vander Lyn, windmills seem to turn along canals, again we see the silver bands around the wooden leg of the doughty Peter Stuyvesant, and we are reminded that New York was once New Amsterdam.

Not only was American medical journalism inaugurated by the *Medical Repository*, but this quarterly was the sole representative of our periodical professional literature during the eighteenth century. As late as 1803, when John Conrad Otto, of Philadelphia, wrote the first modern description of hemophilia, he sent it to the *Medical Repository* for the simple reason that there was then no other journal in the country. Previous to the appearance of the *Medical Repository*, our physicians either kept their observations in their heads or in manuscript, or sent them abroad for publication—as did John Bard, in reporting the first case of an extra-uterine fetus in America. The *Medical Repository* changed this situation, and published numerous original investigations of importance: for example, in its pages, Richard Bayley pointed out the difference between angina trachealis and putrid sore throat (membranous croup and diphtheria), founded upon autopsies; Wright Post explained the technic of his ligation of the primitive carotid; and John Stearns introduced the use of ergot in childbirth. Since the *Medical Repository* is of such historic significance in American medicine, let us look again at the names of the three editors, as perhaps the first time we passed them by without any particular interest.

We need not be surprised to find among them the name of Samuel Latham Mitchill, for in those days he was everywhere. A pamphlet published during his lifetime, entitled "Some of the Memorable Events in the Life of Samuel L. Mitchill," lists 192 of these memorabilia! He had an aversion to practice, but a craving for everything else. At public functions, in literary circles, at philosophical discussions, at faculty conclaves, in Congress—he was both a representative and a senator—in botanical gardens, at reunions and on grandstands, Mitchill could be found, frequently the orator of the occasion. Whether in laborer's attire, or in powdered cue and buckled shoes, or in the dress of the Fiji Islanders, or in the scholastic robes of the LL.D., or in Indian costume, he was usually the center of admiration and conversation. When a mammoth was dug up, Mitchill was there, bubbling with excitement, thinking of the treatise he was going to write; when that immortal engineer rode up the Hudson on the world's first steamboat, changing Fulton's folly to Fulton's wonder, Mitchill was the beaming guest of honor; when De Witt Clinton opened the great canal, wedding the waters of Lake Erie and the Hudson River, Mitchill was present, spilling much laudatory eloquence.

He was prolix, pedantic, bombastic and dogmatic; his assertion that the Garden of Eden was located in Onondaga Hollow in New York State, his determination to alter the nursery rhymes with verses of his own devising, and his attempt to change the name of America to Fredonia, and to call our people Fredes instead of Americans, indicate that Samuel Latham Mitchill was a busybody. Mitchill, because of his versatility, has been designated the prototype of Holmes but we can hardly let his comparison pass unchallenged: both of these doctors wrote of The Nautilus, and the poem of Holmes is among the treasures of literature, while Mitchill's tribute begins as follows:

> I saw thee, beauteous form,
> As late I walked the oceanic strand,
> And as my curiosity was warm,
> I took thee in my hand.
> Soon I discovered, a terrific storm,
> Which nothing human could command,
> Had robbed thee of thy life and cast thee on the sand.

It is difficult to understand how a man who revelled in the perfect decasyllables of Pope, could have sent to the printer hosts of such lines limping on crippled metrical feet, but in those days all doctors wrote atrocious poetry—even the sulphureous Charles Caldwell. Mitchill's pomposity, his credulity—he maintained in court that a white woman gave birth to a black child because her husband accidentally upset a bottle of ink in her shoe—the seriousness with which he took himself, and his complacent belief that he was an oracle, made him a conspicuous target for the barbed shafts of ridicule which were aimed at him in the New York Evening Post by the youthful physician-poet, Joseph Rodman Drake. The laughing satire was clever, and it wounded Mitchill deeply, but in reading it today, our sympathy goes out rather to its perpetrator than to its victim, for in parenthesis Drake reminded Mitchill that life is brief—and at the age of twenty-five, the brilliant and beloved Drake, "the handsomest man in New York," perished of tuberculosis.

Mitchill went on accumulating honors, and had so many diplomas and decorations that a cart was required to remove them, and he was called the nestor of American science, the human dictionary, the Congressional Library—and also a Chaos of Knowledge. His memory was phenomenal, and his repertoire encyclopedic: "Tap the Doctor at any time, and he will flow." A colleague pointed out that Mitchill "could discourse in turn, on a Babylonian brick, meteoric stones, the theory of chemical combination, the construction of a windmill, the fishes of North America, or the geology of Niagara Falls," but to this eulogium we must add, that men of such heterogenous attainments, howsoever much they may dazzle their contemporaries, usually leave little to posterity.

Mitchill was still in his twenties when he became professor, in Columbia College, of botany, natural history, chemistry and agriculture, but he easily devoted himself to zoölogy, geology, and anthropology in addition; he was among the first to investigate the American aborigines, and the condition of the deaf and dumb in this country; his finding of the resemblance between symptoms of poisoning by snake venom and infective fever, served as a starting-point for the later researches of Weir Mitchell; while his work on the fishes of New York, entitles him to be considered the father of American ichthyology.

Of vast learning, of splendid physique, and of benevolent disposition, we may gratefully remember him as one of the makers of American science and one of our pioneer medical editors, and if we do recall that the first time Samuel David Gross met Samuel Latham Mitchill, the latter was in a horizontal position because he was too drunk to walk, we may interpret the incident as illustrating that Mitchill was incapable of drinking skilfully from any source except the founts of knowledge.

Edward Miller was Mitchill's co-editor on the *Medical Repository*, his fellow-professor at Columbia College, and his affectionate friend in general. Miller did not possess Mitchill's many-sidedness—or his overweeningness. Edward Miller was an earnest practitioner of medicine, and although he enjoyed a classical education, his writings are exclusively clinical, dealing mainly with the most baffling and formidable American disease of the period —yellow fever. Not only at the bedsides of strangers, but in his own family, Edward Miller witnessed the limitations of the Hippocratic art. There were once seven Miller brothers, but two died in infancy; his eldest brother, John, a physician and army surgeon in 1776, died at twenty-five; his next eldest brother, Joseph, a counselor at law and a member of the legislature, was killed by yellow fever, a few weeks after his marriage, at thirty-four; his youngest brother James, also an attorney, succumbed to pulmonary consumption at twenty-three.

The Millers came from Delaware, and Edward practised in his native state, in New Jersey, and in Maryland, but his professional life was more intimately associated with Philadelphia where he graduated, and New York where he spent his mature years. His eminent talents as a physician, and the unblemished integrity of his conduct, have been put on record by his friend, David Hosack, the foremost New York physician of the day; while the foremost physician of Philadelphia suggested—and the suggestions of Benjamin Rush were royal commands—that the writings of Edward Miller, which lie scattered through the *Medical Repository*, be collected and published in a volume, to which he would prefix a memoir of the author.

The most piquant of that editorial triumvirate, was the youngest of the group, Elihu Hubbard Smith. The idea of the journal really originated with Smith; first he won over Miller, and together they called upon Mitchill, naturally finding in this lover of the quill an enthusiastic ally. Smith was a Connecticut man—he entered Yale at eleven—but he settled in New York for the same reason that Galen came from Pergamum to Rome. The youthful Smith rapidly became conspicuous in the medical and literary circles of the growing city: his diagnoses were respected, and his poems applauded. He was appointed physician to the New York Hospital, and produced the prologue for the opening of the Park Theatre. He annotated the American edition of Erasmus Darwin's Botanic Garden—with a poetic epistle of his own—and with equal facility wrote essays on the Athenian plague, yellow fever, the natural history of the American elk, and a three-act opera entitled Edwin and Angelina, or the Banditti.

He lived about a block from Trinity Church, on Pine Street, "the prettiest street in all the town," and entertained most of the interesting people in New York. With him lived his bosom friend, Charles Brockden Brown, the first American novelist, remembered by physicians for his graphic descriptions of yellow fever and smallpox. In this home Smith set aside a room for the young Italian physician, I. B. Scandella—"the accomplished and elegant Scandella," as Mitchell called him. It happened in this way: Dr. Scandella was a member of an ancient Venetian family, had been secretary to the Venetian Embassy in London, and then traveled in America to study the rise of a new nation. After a sojourn of two years in our country, he embarked for Europe, but as his vessel was found unfit for the voyage he returned to Philadelphia, and then came to New York. A ship lay waiting for him in the harbor; his baggage, however, had not arrived from Philadelphia, and he tarried. But it was the summer of 1798, and the ever-dreaded yellow fever again overwhelmed Philadelphia, and Scandella hastened there to aid a family in distress. On coming back to New York, he found it likewise in the grip of the yellow terror, and so great was the confusion that it was impossible for him to obtain lodgings. Then the hospitable doors of Number 45 Pine Street swung open, and the lovable Scandella became Smith's guest—alas! his last guest. Scandella was stricken with the prevailing epidemic, and Mitchill was sent for; he did all that was possible, but on the sixth day Scandella was no longer Smith's guest. Mitchill now entered Smith's chamber, and unlocked the inner shutters. Smith was in a stuporous sleep, and unaware that in the next room his friend lay dead. Mitchill aroused him, and asked him how he felt. He said not very unwell, and would be better by and by. His handsome face was suffused, and the once noble eyes were inflamed and glassy. It was early morning, and Smith asked Mitchill if it was not almost sundown.

Thoroughly alarmed by these symptoms, Mitchill called for Miller, and it was decided to try the mercurial treatment upon Smith. A nurse from the hospital begged permission to apply the strongest ointment with her own hands. The nurse salivated herself, and without avail. It was 1798, and all worked in darkness. These editors had written about noxious insects, and no one knew that a mosquito was sending Smith to his grave. The nurse wept and rubbed, and Mitchill and Miller bowed their heads, and the black vomit came, and Smith's body turned yellow.

That jaundiced hue seemed to encircle the city, and so high was the mortality and so widespread the consternation, that only Miller and Mitchill and a very few others, followed the hearse of Elihu Hubbard Smith to the yard of the Presbyterian Church in Wall Street. He was in the twenty-seventh year of his age, and his journal in its second volume, when they buried the young father of American medical journalism.

In the autumn of 1811 there appeared in Philadelphia the first issue of the *Eclectic Repertory and Analytical Review*. This was long before Wooster Beach had founded Eclecticism, and as the journal went out of existence before there was an American eclectic school of medicine, it obviously had no sectarian affiliations, and employed the word "eclectic" in the sense of "selective." The reason for the name is apparent enough when we examine the journal, for it opened with reprints of essays by such English scientists as William Heberden, Edward Jenner, Astley Cooper, Humphry Davy, Benjamin Brodie and William Clift. To this useful publication, Philip Syng Physick and John

Syng Dorsey contributed papers of importance in the development of American surgical literature, but the editors—they were Thomas Tickell Hewson, Joseph Parrish, John Conrad Otto, Thomas Chalkley James—seemed especially proud of the quality of their reprints, and at one time thought of changing the name of their review to the Journal of Foreign Medical Science and Literature.

While their editorial eyes were scanning the European horizon for copy, there arrived from the backwoods of America a manuscript so brief that when published in the seventh volume (1817), it occupied only pages 242, 243, 244. It was entitled, *Three Cases of Extirpation of Diseased Ovaria*, it was signed Ephraim M'Dowell, M.D., of Danville, Kentucky, and it began, "In December 1809, I was called to see a Mrs. Crawford." Eight years had thus passed since that historic visit, but this was McDowell's first communication on the subject.

The case is one of the most celebrated in the story of diseases of women. Jane Todd Crawford was enormously distended; although beyond term, she thought she was in labor, and two physicians requested McDowell's aid in delivering her. Upon vaginal examination, McDowell found the womb empty, and thus realized that the enlarged abdomen was not due to a fetus but to an ovarian tumor. McDowell, with the frankness of a frontiersman, explained that never had he seen so large a substance extracted, nor heard of an attempt; he informed her that the situation was dangerous, and the experiment uncertain, but he promised to perform it if she would come to his home in Danville. The tall, powerfully-built McDowell was neither a talker nor a writer, but there must have been something about him that inspired confidence. The doomed Mrs. Crawford looked into his "piercing black eyes" and made her decision.

The waters of Motley's Glen, where Mrs. Crawford lived, did not run to Danville, sixty miles away; mounting a horse, resting her tumor on the horn of the saddle, she arrived after a journey of a few days in McDowell's village. Without trained assistants, anesthetics or a precedent, McDowell placed her on a table and made a long incision. Immediately her intestines rushed out upon the table, and remained there during the twenty-five minutes of the operation. Cutting open the tumor, he took out fifteen pounds of gelatinous material, and extracted the sack which weighed seven pounds and a half. He turned her upon her left side, stitched and plastered her, and put her to bed. McDowell did not know how to write a case-report, and he skips the first four days: "In five days I visited her, and much to my astonishment found her engaged in making up her bed. I gave her particular caution for the future; and in twenty-five days, she returned home as she came, in good health, which she continues to enjoy." Jane Todd Crawford's heroic confidence in her doctor was not misplaced; she reached the age of seventy-eight, outliving for several years the man whom she made the "Father of Ovariotomy." Their combined courage opened the abdomen to surgery. We wish that her portrait had been preserved for posterity.

In the early nineteenth century, the wilderness of Sackett's Harbor, in the extreme north of the State of New York near the Canadian border, was young and beautiful, but already stained with human blood. The harbor was a battlefield in the War of 1812—here the British attacked the former colonists, and from this port the Americans sailed to Toronto: the British evacuated the garrison, but left some of their men to explode three hundred barrels of gunpowder in the midst of the advancing and victorious Americans, and the carnage that resulted was described in his diary by a young doctor from Connecticut who had just quit his preceptor:

A most distressing scene ensues in the Hospital—nothing but the groans of the wounded and agonies of the dying are to be heard. The Surgeons wading in blood, cutting off arms, legs, and trepanning heads to rescue their fellow creatures from untimely deaths. To hear the poor creatures crying . . . "Do, Doctor, Doctor! Do cut off my leg, my arm, my head . . . I can't live, I can't live!" would have rent the heart of steel, and shocked the insensibility of the most hardened assassin and the cruelest savage. It awoke my liveliest sympathy, and

I cut and slashed for 48 hours without food or sleep. My God! Who can think of the shocking scene when his fellow-creatures lie mashed and mangled in every part with a leg, an arm, a head, or a body ground in pieces, without having his very heart pained with the acutest sensibility and his blood chill in his veins. Then, who can behold it without agonizing sympathy!

William Beaumont, the surgeon who wrote these words, never attended medical school. By this time there were already famous medical faculties in America, which included John Morgan and Benjamin Rush of the university of Pennsylvania, Valentine Mott and David Hosack of the New York schools, the Warrens and James Jackson of Harvard, while Nathan Smith at Darmouth constituted "its entire Faculty, and a very able Faculty at that." But pioneer conditions were still upon us, and medical college was regarded as a luxury beyond the dreams of many students of medicine. Thousands of youths became physicians and surgeons by entering the office of a busy practitioner. It is scornfully asserted that they studied medicine by sweeping out the office, running the doctor's errands, polishing his instruments, and holding his horses. If this is true—and it is to some extent —it is all the more odd that these youths who never saw a sheepskin except with the sheep inside of it, should compare so favorably with highly-trained graduates of today. Perhaps there was more merit in the preceptor system—which taught medicine by actual cases as master and pupil jogged over rough country roads from patient to patient—than we realize, or perhaps too much group-diagnosis, too much reliance on case-reports taken by internes and too many laboratory aids and registered nurses, have made us clinically lazy. A century ago, many an ungainly disciple of Aesculapius took his equipment out of his much-traveled saddle-bags, entered the patient's house (chewing tobacco), spat the juice over the carpet, rolled up his sleeves over his hairy arms, sat down by the patient's bedside, and while shifting the quid to the other cheek, diagnosed the disease without syndicating it to the medical journals and prescribed effective treatment.

After the war, Beaumont practised medicine and surgery, and opened a store. He and his partner believed in advertising, and inserted in the *Plattsburgh Republican* (September 6, 1816) an announcement intended to be irresistible:

> Beaumont & Wheelock have just received and offer for sale at the lowest prices a large and well-selected assortment of GROCERIES, consisting of Madeira, Port, London Particular, and Sherry Wines, Cognac and French Brandy, Jamaica, St. Croix and New England Rum, Pierpont Gin, Molasses, Tea, Lump and Loaf Sugar, Rice, Coffee, Salt, Pepper, Allspice, Ginger, Plug and Paper Tobacco, Pipes, Codfish, Shad, Mackerel, Chocolate, Spanish Segars, Window Glass, Snuff, Starch, Powder, Shot, Almonds, &c. Also in addition to their former stock a large assortment of Drugs & Medicines, Dye Woods, &c., &c.

That Beaumont was a keen observer is obvious from his maxim: "Trust not to man's honesty, whether Christian, Jew or Gentile. Deal with all as though they were rogues and villains; it will never injure an honest person, and it will always protect you from being cheated by friend or foe. Selfishness or villainy, or both combined, govern the world, with a very few exceptions." Nevertheless, he could not sell groceries, or what he thought were groceries. Before long he was in uniform again, and the first steamboat of the west, *Walk-in-the-Water*, carried him to the outposts of civilization.

Michilimackinac in primitive Michigan was then a fur-post and a fort. Voyageurs, Indians, half-breeds, trappers, traders, adventurers, crowded the store of the American Fur Company. A shotgun was accidentally discharged, and a young French-Canadian, standing a few feet from the muzzle, dropped to the floor. His shirt caught fire, and wadding, pieces of clothing, powder and duck shot entered his body. Beaumont came from the fort, and bending over the insensible Alexis St. Martin, smelled the burnt flesh; he noted the torn muscles and fractured ribs; through the frightful wound, which admitted a man's fist, the lungs and the punctured stomach protruded. No one was surprised when Beaumont declared the youth could not recover, and no one could have guessed how much time this physician and patient were destined to spend together.

Alexis St. Martin displayed astounding vitality and began to mend. He lived but could not work, and the Mackinac authorities, impatient of supporting an alien pauper, insisted that he return in a batteau to his Canadian home, two thousand miles away. It is extremely doubtful if Alexis could have survived this second ordeal; the indignant Beaumont, on his monthly salary of forty dollars and rations, took the injured woodsman into his own home, and kept him for two years. "During this time," says Beaumont, "I nursed him, fed him, clothed him, lodged him and furnished him with every comfort, and dressed his wounds daily and for the most part twice a day." Alexis grew strong again, and could chop logs as well as any man in Mackinac. He was normal, except that below his left nipple an opening remained, communicating with an opening in the stomach. Thus when Alexis required a cathartic, Beaumont administered it, "as never medicine was before administered to man since the creation of the world—to wit, by pouring it in through the ribs at the puncture of the stomach." Beaumont was able to look directly into the cavity of St. Martin's stomach, and practically witness the process of digestion.

About three years after the accident, Beaumont realized that St. Martin's gastric fistula offered a unique opportunity for experiments in the physiology of digestion: "I can pour in water with a funnel, or put in food with a spoon, and draw them out again with a syphon. I have frequently suspended flesh, raw and wasted, and other substances into the perforation to ascertain the length of time required to digest each; and at one time used a tent of raw beef, instead of lint, to stop the orifice, and found that in less than five hours it was completely digested off, as smooth and even as if it had been cut with a knife." Beaumont began to make the most of his opportunities. He introduced all sorts of foods into St. Martin's aperture, withdrew them, reintroduced them, and learned what the gastric juice did to each. He was the first who was able to collect, directly from the human stomach, gastric juice either pure or mixed with bright yellow bile.

Suddenly Alexis St. Martin disappeared. Not until four years later did Beaumont learn that his former patient had returned to Canada, had married Marie Jolly, and was working for the Hudson Bay Fur Company as a voyageur to the Indian country. Beaumont was so anxious to get hold of Alexis again, that he paid for his transportation, and that of his wife and two children. Altogether, Beaumont performed four series of experiments upon Alexis: at Fort Mackinac, Michigan Territory (1825), Fort Crawford, Upper Mississippi (1828), Washington, District of Columbia (1832), and Plattsburgh Barracks, New York (1833). He published at Plattsburgh the first edition of *Experiments and Observations on the Gastric Juice and the Physiology of Digestion* (1833); a second edition, edited by his cousin Samuel Beaumont, was published at Burlington, Vermont (1847). For several years, Beaumont and Alexis played a grim game of hide-and-seek across a continent; after 1833, Beaumont could not get his hands upon the elusive Alexis; he offered to support him and his entire family, and give him a large sum of money in addition, but in vain. The wife of Alexis wanted her man on their little Canadian farm, and Beaumont's 238th published experiment was his last. These experiments to a marked degree advanced our knowledge of the digestive processes.

As the years passed, and Beaumont found it impossible to procure his subject to continue the experiments, he spoke in anger of "that old, fistulous Alexis." It is easy to understand the physiologist's irritation, but it is impossible to blame Alexis St. Martin. He was tired of eating for scientific observation, tired of having his food taken from him in various stages of digestion, tired of the thermometers that registered his gastric temperature, tired of being exhibited to doctors and students, tired of the bottles that collected his juice, tired of being treated as a stomach with a window. He was a human being, not only a "human test tube." Alexis was illiterate: his contracts with

Beaumont are marked with a cross, for he could not sign his name. It meant nothing to him that children in the schools were beginning to study his case in the elementary texts of Physiology, or that Claude Bernard, master of physiology, inquired about him. Alexis belonged to the woods and waters. He put his family in an open canoe, and without mishap ascended the rivers and crossed great lakes as large as seas. He liked his wife and naked children, he liked to get drunk on his neglected farm. He did not know what physiology meant, but he knew it was good to lie on the earth beneath the tall pines. He would take all the money he could wheedle out of Beaumont, but he would keep miles away from those stirring rods and thermometers. An ungrateful savage, growled Beaumont, and both were right. It is true that Beaumont saved the life of St. Martin—the woodsman reached the age of eighty-three, outliving the surgeon twenty-eight years—but it is equally true that St. Martin made Beaumont the pioneer physiologist of America. William Beaumont's experiments were not surpassed until the close of the century, when there appeared at St. Petersburg the researches of Pavloff and his pupils on *The Digestive Glands* (1897).

John Lambert Richmond, farm-boy and coal-miner, studied Greek and Latin in the fields, and became a Baptist minister. Later he served as janitor in the Medical College of Ohio, where Daniel Drake, the builder of the medical west, helped him to graduate as a physician. Five years later (1827), Richmond was preaching an evening sermon at Newtown, outside Cincinnati. He was informed that a woman across the river, in labor for thirty hours, was succumbing to repeated convulsions. Night and distance and the Little Miami River in flood did not stay him. Rowing in a skiff, he reached the patient, a fat colored primipara with a deformed pelvis. Only the knife could save her from inevitable death, and Richmond made the incision. In five weeks the woman walked a mile and back the same day. The pioneer breed did not rush into print, and Richmond waited three years before reporting (1830), in the journal edited by Drake, the first Cesarean section in America:

With only a case of common pocket instruments, about one o'clock at night, I commenced the Cesarean section. Here I must take the liberty to digress from my subject, and relate the condition of the house, which was made of logs that were green, and put together not more than a week before. The crevices were not chinked, there was no chimney, nor chamber floor. The night was stormy and windy, insomuch that the assistants had to hold blankets to keep the candles from being blown out. Under these circumstances it is hard to conceive the state of my feelings, when I was convinced that the patient must die, or the operation be performed.

Samuel Guthrie, who had no diploma, was obviously of the true pioneer breed, for after his brief contact with the two principal cities of America, he felt that even Chenango County was too civilized; with his wife Sybil he sought the seclusion of Sackett's Harbor (1817). Patients were few, and Guthrie did not long continue in practice, for many engrossing matters soon required his full energy and attention. His lancet rusted, while pick and axe cleared the wilderness away; virgin clay from the nearby bank made a comfortable dwelling, and pure water was conducted to the new home. Gardens, orchards and vineyards spread throughout the forest; stone-walls enclosed well-cultivated fields, and barns and other buildings arose on both sides of the creek. The blacksmith shop had its forge, bellows, anvil; on the shelves were tools, spelter and borax, solder and rosin; in the corners were found sheet copper, crucibles, melting ladles. His vinegar house was patronized by farmers' wives for miles around, and he distilled a famous brand of alcohol.

In the midst of the newly-conquered ground was erected a mysterious structure—a chemical laboratory. Odors mingled with apparatus, a dome-shaped charcoal-oven was conspicuous, and a still with its condensing worm immersed in a barrel of water was destined to make medical history. Numerous explosions occurred, which so scarred the physiognomy of Guthrie that he permitted only one daguerreotype of himself to be taken, and he destroyed that one with an expletive. Not his features, but his deeds have come down to us, for at Sackett's Harbor this backwoods chemist discovered chloroform (1831).

Guthrie called his chloroform "sweet whiskey," and Silliman of Yale hoped it was not another "intoxicating spirit." Guthrie did not realize that he had prepared the waters of the modern Lethe. In the evening of Guthrie's life, the medical world rang with a new name. A Scotch teacher of midwifery had risen to greatness on the fumes of chloroform. James Young Simpson uncorked a bottle of the heavy fluid, and at the same time opened a new era in anesthesia. The power of chloroform to conquer pain, assuaging the pangs of parturition, spreading the mantle of oblivion over operative tortures, was finally revealed (1847).

Before this, however, the anesthetic properties of other vapors had been demonstrated in America, and anesthesia may be regarded as America's greatest gift to the world. Yet this boon could have been picked up by anyone, and as a matter of fact not one of the discoverers of anesthesia was a distinguished physician. For several years, wandering lecturers and amateur chemists, passing through our southern towns, entertained their auditors by making them drunk on various gases. Nitrous oxide or "laughing gas" parties became a popular form of amusement, and sometimes young men would seize a Negro and press an ether-saturated handkerchief against his nose until he became unconscious. Among those who indulged in these "ether frolics" was Crawford Williamson Long, a recent graduate of the university of Pennsylvania, practising in his native state of Georgia. In some of the parties held in his office, he noted that he and others who inhaled ether, staggered and fell, but felt no pain from their bruises.

One of his acquaintances, James M. Venables, attending the village academy, frequently inhaled ether for its exhilarating effects, and declared under oath that he was very fond of its use. Venables had two tumors on the back of his neck, and wanted Long to cut them off. The operation was postponed from time to time, but one evening (March 30, 1842) after school was dismissed, Venables sat in Long's office; the doctor poured some ether on a towel, and the patient inhaled it; Long operated, and when Venables awoke he did not believe that the tumor had been removed until it was shown to him. Long wrote in his ledger: "James Venables, 1842. Ether and excising tumor, $2.00." Long went to bed that night without knowing there was anything remarkable in his ledger; he used ether on a few other occasions, but never in a major operation; he did not concern himself with the principles of anesthesia; he did not write out his experiences, and the subject which he had learned in jest he abandoned without further thought.

Up north, at Hartford, Connecticut, the dentist Horace Wells attended a popular scientific lecture; as part of the performance, the effects of nitrous oxide were exhibited. Wells tried it, and his wife reproached him for making a fool of himself in public. Another member of the audience ran and jumped all over the room, striking against various objects, and not until the influence of the gas had worn off did he realize he had injured his legs. Wells asked the lecturer if teeth could not be drawn painlessly under the influence of this gas, but the lecturer was not a dentist and said he had never considered the matter. Wells was suffering from a troublesome tooth, and asked his friend J. M. Riggs to extract it after he had become insensible from inhaling the gas. Riggs took out an upper molar, and Wells did not feel so much as the prick of a pin. "A new era in tooth-pulling!" he exclaimed (December 11, 1844) upon awakening.

Wells now began to extract teeth without pain, proving the value of the suggestion that Humphry Davy had published (1800) in his *Researches, Chemical and Philosophical*: "As nitrous oxide in its extensive operation seems capable of destroying physical pain, it may probably be used with advantage during surgical operations in which no great effuson of blood takes place." Wells arranged for a public demonstration of his method at the Massachusetts General Hospital, under the leading New England surgeon, the venerated John Collins Warren. On this occasion the gas-bag was removed too soon, and as Wells drew out the tooth, the patient howled, and the medical students shouted "Humbug!" That cry was the doom of Horace Wells.

At this fiasco, Wells was assisted by his former student and brief-time partner, William Thomas Green Morton of Massachusetts. Wells introduced Morton to Boston's versatile scientist, Charles Thomas Jackson. Morton, who had always wanted to be a doctor, and had compromised on dentistry because his shopkeeping father could not send him to medical school, now enrolled as a medical student under Jackson. Morton, who was manufacturing artificial teeth, was anxious to remove the stumps of old teeth without pain. He learned from Horace Wells whatever he knew about nitrous oxide, and then began to question Jackson. "Try ether," said Jackson the chemist. Morton acted as if he had never heard of ether, and Jackson explained its properties, showed him ether and the apparatus in which it was administered, and told him where it could be procured. Jackson's interest in ether was theoretical: about this time his wife and aunt had some of their teeth extracted by Morton without anesthesia. Jackson knew enough about ether to be afraid of it.

Morton was bolder, shrewder, and more practical. Fearing to be forestalled, keeping his teacher in the dark about his intentions, he consulted apothecaries and instrument-makers about their methods of preparing and administering ether; he learned how to handle this volatile liquid, produced insensibility in various animals, and employed it in his dental practice. He was thinking of a patent, but as hundreds of college boys and factory girls had already inhaled ether with gayety, and medical men were familiar with its peculiar and pleasant odor, Morton disguised his ether with aromatic oils—Jackson had told him how —and further disguised it with the name of *letheon*. Thus protected, he appealed to Warren for a surgical test. The old Warren consented, and Morton arrived at the Massachusetts General Hospital with his letheon in a tube connected to a glass globe. Warren's ever-repeated exclamation at the end of this first public operation under ether, "Gentlemen, this is no humbug!" was matched by Bigelow's solemn words: "I have seen something today that will go round the world." Ether Day—October 16, 1846—is a blessed day in the history of humanity.

Oliver Wendell Holmes, in a letter to Morton (November 21, 1846), suggested the terms *anesthetic* and *anesthesia*, which were adopted at once. The word *anesthesia* occurs originally in Plato and Dioscorides, and the conception is older than the second chapter in Genesis. The word and deed were forgotten during the centuries that failed, and the abolition of operative tortures appeared impossible. At the University Hospital College of London, anesthesia had its first European trial. Among the students in the crowded amphitheater sat a handsome Quaker youth, but that day Joseph Lister was only a spectator in surgery. Robert Liston was the surgeon, and as he entered the arena, he addressed his audience: "We are going to try a Yankee dodge today, gentleman, for making men insensible." At the conclusion of that amputation of the thigh, Liston saw the conquest of pain. Previously, all surgeons subscribed to the opinion of Velpeau, the great surgeon of France: "To avoid pain, in surgical operations, is a chimera, which it is not permitted to follow at this day. Knife and pain, in operative surgery, are two words, which never suggest themselves the one without the other to the mind of the patient, and it is necessary to admit the connection" (1839). Within a few years of this hopeless prognostication, American enterprise severed the melancholy connection.

It is America's epoch of glory and shame, for on the trail of this revelation strode tragedy, suicide, scandal, greed and lawsuits. Warren and Bigelow were above suspicion, and their disinterested advocacy of etherization made it known in all countries—then human selfishness came to the surface. Long, who had remained silent for seven years, wrote his first article on the subject (December 1849); Wells claimed to be the sole discoverer of the principle of anesthesia; his mind unhinged by failing where Morton succeeded, he was caught throwing vitriol at the Broadway prostitutes, and committed to prison; Jackson insisted that he had told Morton everything, and he wrote to Humboldt of America's ingratitude; Morton quarreled over his patent-rights, and said he would sue every physician who used ether without his permission. Of the four principal claimants, Long died in obscurity; Wells died by his own hand in jail; Jackson died in a lunatic-asylum; Morton died in poverty. On the question of their priority, volumes will continue to be written, but the best summary is that of Holmes: when asked to whom the credit belongs, he answered: "To e(i)ther."

Ambitious men have pursued both Physic and Poetry; the tradition dates back to Apollo, god alike of the Muses and of Medicine. For mortals this is a fatal combination, since the double laurels are reserved for few brows. The outstanding exception is Oliver Wendell Holmes, lyricist and medical philosopher. Had Holmes been able to suppress his wit, he would have been a successful practitioner. When he announced, "Small fevers thankfully received," the Bostonians smiled, and consulted other doctors. After teaching at Dartmouth, Holmes occupied the chair of anatomy at Harvard for thirty-five years; his students never forgot his description of the female pelvis as the triumphal arch under which we must all pass in entering life, but they may have concluded that less poetical obstetricians were safer.

The humor of Holmes, permanently enriching English literature, was often carried over to his medical labors. Humor did not prevent him from being in deadly earnest when occasion demanded, and few Harvard men have received as much abuse as the genial Holmes. It must be remembered that he was not always famous; in fact, there was a time when he was "a very young gentleman," and his ideas were characterized as belonging to the "jejune and fizenless dreamings of sophomore writers." Wishing to illustrate that prevention is better than treatment, Holmes quoted the words of the mother to her child who had a poisonous berry in its mouth—"Spit it out!" To such an extent did this simple statement annoy a well-known practitioner in New York, that he advised the Massachusetts Medical Society to spit out the offending speaker. No man knew the medical classics better than Holmes—"These books were very dear to me as they stood upon my shelves. A twig from some one of my nerves ran to every one of them"—yet at a time when scholasticism still reigned in medicine, he made his magnificent plea for bedside teaching.

Small, smiling, asthmatic, Holmes did not consider himself a fighting type of man, but the same pen which saved "Old Ironsides," was ready to battle for science. Homeopathy, whose mystic vagaries once confused many physicians, found its keenest antagonist in Holmes: no subsequent exposure of medical sectarianism can compare with his *Homeopathy and its Kindred Delusions* (1842). The intelligence which caused him to explode the infinitesimal globules, likewise made him the foremost critic of overdrugging—in those days, orthodox practitioners had some harsh epithets for Oliver Wendell Holmes. It is frequently asserted that Holmes said: "If all the drugs in the Pharmacopeia were thrown into the sea, it would be all the better for mankind and all the worse for the fishes." This is a misquotation and a decided misrepresentation. The fact is, he desired to rescue certain drugs from the fatal ship-load which was to incommode the fishes. What he actually said—he used the words first at the annual meeting of the Massachusetts Medical Society (May 30, 1860)—was something quite different, and even his italics are significant:

Throw out opium, which the Creator himself seems to prescribe, for we often see the scarlet poppy growing in the cornfields, as if it were foreseen that wherever there is hunger to be fed there must also be pain to be soothed; throw out a few specifics which our art did not discover, and is hardly needed to apply; throw out wine, which is a food, and the vapors which produce the miracle of anesthesia, and I firmly believe that if the whole materia medica, *as now used*, could be sunk to the bottom of the sea, it would be all the better for mankind—and all the worse for the fishes.

One year after his homeopathic onslaught, Holmes published the essay which made him the most useful physician in America. During the first half of the nineteenth century, motherhood was unsafe. Countless thousands died in childbed fever. There were hospital-wards which needed a coffin for every parturient woman that entered, there were obstetricians whose visits were invariably followed by funerals. This had been going on for a long time, and the profession called it an act of God. Attempts to investigate the cause of this tragedy of birth, were met with impatience. A few men, Charles White of Manchester (1773), Thomas Kirkland of Leicestershire (1774), and Gordon of Aberdeen (1795), in the years indicated, went over the fatal road that led from the lying-in chamber to the dead-house, and their books gathered dust. Oliver Wendell Holmes was unable to let the matter rest.

It is remarkable that one whose clinical experience was not extensive, should have been able to advance the proposition: "The disease known as Puerperal Fever is so far contagious as to be frequently carried from patient to patient by physicians and nurses." Holmes thus transferred the blame from God to man. Years later, Meigs maintained: "I prefer to attribute them to accident, or Providence, of which I can form a conception, rather than to a contagion of which I cannot form any clear idea, at least as to this particular malady." Later still, Meigs declared that in the propagation of childbed fever, the attendants are no more responsible than "with the propagation of cholera from Jessore to San Francisco, and from Mauritius to St. Petersburg." Such was the attitude of Charles Delucena Meigs, professor of obstetrics at Jefferson Medical College, and accounted the most eminent American obstetrician of his time. Meigs denounced Holmes with the same virulence that he later opposed Simpson's use of chloroform in labor.

Holmes was so chicken-hearted that he ran from his lecture-room whenever a rabbit was chloroformed, but he was not afraid of Meigs. In connection with his work on childbed fever, Holmes wrote: "No man makes a quarrel with me over the counterpane that covers a mother, with her new-born infant at her breast. There is no epithet in the vocabulary of slight and sarcasm that can reach my personal sensibilities in such a controversy. . . .

Let it be remembered that persons are nothing in this matter; better that twenty pamphleteers should be silenced, or as many professors unseated, than that one mother's life should be taken. There is no quarrel here between men, but there is deadly incompatibility and exterminating warfare between doctrines."

The concluding appeal of Holmes' essay, *The Contagiousness of Puerperal Fever* (1843), is unforgettable: "The woman about to become a mother, or with new-born infant upon her bosom, should be the object of trembling care and sympathy wherever she bears her tender burden, or stretches her aching limbs. The very outcast of the streets has pity upon her sister in degradation, when the seal of promised maternity is impressed upon her. The remorseless vengeance of the law, brought down upon its victims by a machinery as sure as destiny, is arrested in its fall at a word which reveals her transient claim for mercy. The solemn prayer of the liturgy singles out her sorrows from the multiplied trials of life, to plead for her in the hour of peril. God forbid that any member of the profession to which she trusts her life, doubly precious at that eventful period, should hazard it negligently, unadvisedly, or selfishly."

Holmes, academic physician, vaguely perceived the nature of puerperal sepsis, but was unable to reveal its etiology and prophylaxis. This discovery belongs wholly to a young Hungarian, serving as an assistant in obstetrics. The emotional Semmelweis, obsessed with his one great idea, was not as well-poised as Holmes. Driven from Vienna by the obstetrical leaders of Europe, goaded to desperation by the Motherhood he saw unceasingly massacred in childbed because men would not wash their hands with chloride of lime, he was brought back to Vienna to die a lunatic's death in an asylum. His grave had hardly closed when Pasteur in the laboratory and Lister in the clinics reckoned with the microbe, and then all the world saw that Semmelweis had been right ever since he promulgated his doctrine in Vienna (1847). So they raised a monument to his memory in his native Budapest; the obstetrician is seen in full, holding his book under his arm; on the step of the pedestal sits a woman, with her infant in her arms, gazing reverently at her benefactor; it is very beautiful and is kept green by a special watchman. Yet the words of Fritsch remain true: "There is a dark chapter in the history of midwifery, and it is headed—Semmelweis." At the conclusion of his splendid career, Oliver Wendell Holmes knew that the early paper which he had written "in a great heat and with passionate indignation," was the best thing he ever did.

In the summer of 1835, a young doctor in South Carolina tore the tin sign from his office-door, and dropped it in an abandoned well. His practice had consisted of two patients, both babies, and both had died. The recent graduate ceased to be a doctor in his native town. He fled in despair, and only poverty chained him to his profession. He settled in the forests of Alabama, and rode his horse through Indian camps and howling wolves. Everywhere he saw patients literally murdered by bloodletting. He was sick at heart, and wished he could sell clothes or cobble shoes for a living. We cannot know what destiny has in store for us. Ten years later this man thought, "If there is anything I hate, it is investigating the organs of the female pelvis." He invariably informed gynecological cases, "This is out of my line." So little did James Marion Sims know himself.

Sometimes in a difficult labor, the pressure of the fetal head produces an opening from the bladder into the vagina—the dreaded *vesico-vaginal fistula*. Few conditions were more appalling, and the prognosis was practically hopeless. Drip, drip, drip, never as long as the woman lived did the urine cease its eternal drip, drip, drip. Standing or sitting, awake or asleep, whether the hole in the bladder was large or very small, the urine kept up its everlasting dribble. The victims lay in isolated places, hidden from the sight of all. Here Paré had failed, and his successors could do nothing. In the mid-nineteenth century, Jobert de Lamballe of Paris grappled with the problem, operating innumerable times on the same women, adding the tortures of surgery to the blunders of nature. Oddly enough, now and then an American surgeon achieved success; such cases were reported by John Peter Mettauer of Virginia (1838), George Hayward of Boston (1839), and Joseph Pancoast of Philadelphia (1847). These cases were incidental, and exercised little influence upon the general calamity.

Entirely against his will, cases of vesico-vaginal fistula were sent to Marion Sims. He refused to attend these young colored mothers, saying over and over again that nothing could be done for them, and threatening to send them back at once. We often do what we swear we will never do. Sims built a little hospital for six of these slave-girls, and kept them for four years at his own expense. He found that when he placed a woman in the knee-chest position, the admission of air expanded the vagina. With a pewter spoon he originated the duckbill vaginal speculum: "Introducing the bent angle of the spoon I saw everything, as no man had ever seen it before." Walking from his house to the office, he picked up in his yard a piece of brass wire that was used in suspenders before the days of India rubber; this fine brass wire gave him the idea for his silver-wire suture. From an onrush of air, a bent spoon and a torn suspender, Marion Sims learned how to revolutionize gynecology. The first colored girl that was sent to him was named Anarcha, and Sims thus describes her condition:

> She had not only an enormous fistula in the base of the bladder, but there was an extensive destruction of the posterior wall of the vagina, opening into the rectum. This woman had the very worst form of vesico-vaginal fistula. The urine was running day and night, saturating the bedding and clothing, and producing an inflammation of the external parts. The odor from this saturation permeated everything, and every corner of the room; and, of course, her life was one of suffering and disgust. Death would have been preferable. But patients of this kind never die; they must live and suffer. Anarcha had added to the fistula an opening which extended into the rectum, by which gas—intestinal gas—escaped involuntarily, and was passing off continually, so that her person was not only loathsome and disgusting to herself, but to every one who came near her.

Twenty-nine times Marion Sims operated upon Anarcha, and the thirtieth operation was a success (1849). One after the other,

Sims healed his colored girls. "Then," he says, "I realized the fact that, at last my efforts had been blessed with success, and that I had made, perhaps, one of the most important discoveries of the age for the relief of suffering humanity." He published, with illustrations, his paper *On the Treatment of Vesico-Vaginal Fistula* (1852); this was followed by "A Case of Vesico-Vaginal Fistula resisting the Actual Cautery for more than Seven Years; Cured in Thirteen Days by the Author's Process" (1854). Sims was a bit superstitious; he always claimed 13 was his lucky number.

The malarias and chronic diarrheas of the South often brought Sims to within a hairbreadth of the grave; few have survived such prolonged and frightful illnesses; although above middle height, he frequently weighed less than ninety pounds; he insists that in one extremity his life was saved by drinking the iron waters at Cooper's Well, Mississippi, and thereafter he carried demijohns of the water with him, and ate pickled salt pork. In time he realized he could not remain in the South in which he was born: "I was always a little better in New York and Philadelphia than in any other place." In 1853 he left his Alabama home, and settled in New York. After some preliminary skirmishes with the foremost physicians, Sims organized the Woman's Hospital. Long afterwards he wrote: "The Woman's Hospital from the day it was opened had no friends among the leaders—among hospital men. I was called a quack and a humbug, and the hospital pronounced a fraud." The sweet-tempered Sims was unusually bitter about his early New York experiences; in time, he dominated the gynecological practice of the metropolis.

At the age of forty-eight, Sims arrived in Paris (1861) with a letter of introduction from Valentine Mott to Velpeau. Sims' friend, Phineas T. Barnum, was the American best known to Europe, and it was thought that every American had a touch of Barnum in him. Especially did this seem to be the case when Sims announced he had discovered a method of curing vesico-vaginal fistula. The French knew that no one in the world cured this condition except Jobert de Lamballe, and he succeeded only in the rarest instances. Sims could not speak a word of French, but a man who could smile like Sims spoke an international language. His personal charm, more than their faith in his skill, induced the French to let him operate in the amphitheater where Jobert de Lamballe had failed seventeen times on the same woman. Before long, reports reached America that a savior of womanhood, named J. Marion Sims, was accomplishing wonders in the hospitals of Paris.

The most hopeless cases were now brought to him. There was a woman of forty who had a vesico-vaginal fistula for more than twenty years. No man in France had been able to help her; the mouths of the ureters were visible, and Sims saw the urine passing in spurts; the base of the bladder was destroyed, and the remainder "hung outside her body in a little hernial mass as large as a child's fist." Mungenier could not obtain a bed for her in any hospital; Sims said he would operate in his hotel. The peeved Jobert de Lamballe would not come, but every one else was there—Nélaton, Velpeau, Civiale, Larrey, Olliffe, Campbell, and Huguier. In one week's time, when the sutures were removed, the patient was found perfectly cured.

Then there was the little Countess of twenty-one, who had been delivered of an enormous-headed child (hydrocephalus) which tore her bladder. Sims has described her: "She was young, beautiful, rich, accomplished; and, as Dr. Nélaton had told her six months before that she was absolutely incurable, she was praying for death, but in vain, for patients seldom die of afflictions of this kind. In all my experience I have never seen a case of this kind which was attended by such extreme suffering." Sims wrote about her to his wife in New York: "Although it has been but forty-eight hours since the operation, I am able to pronounce the verdict of a perfect cure. If you could only see her, you could not help loving her. As she lies in bed her happiness is manifest to all. She warbles as innocently as a little bird." In a subsequent letter, Sims wrote: "I have been the guest of the countess four weeks, and it is the pleasantest time I have had since I left my happy home. I am quite domesticated and hate to leave."

It was customary for Americans to come to Europe to study, but few had come to teach. Sims was urged to settle in London; he was decorated by the governments of France, Portugal, Spain, Belgium and Italy. No American breast had ever been covered with so many ribbons. He dearly loved his medals and his contacts with royalty, but through it all he remained boyish and unspoiled, the same kind-hearted and fun-loving doctor that he had been down in Alabama. He and his countess acted like two children. "Come, doctor," she would say, "you must put on the dignity now"—but would never allow him to remain dignified long. His autobiography is evidence of his simplicity: he tells of the pin which he stuck in his teacher's chair, how he attended the theater in women's clothes, and how he ripped his breeches in the presence of two charming girls. As a steadfast lover, Sims has never been surpassed: he fell in love with Theresa Jones when he was eleven; was engaged secretly—her family objected to him—at twenty; married her at twenty-two; and wooed her when he was seventy. It is written in J. Marion Sims' *Story of my Life* (1884): "She gave me the bud through the garden fence; and now, my dear readers, whenever you may call to see me, I will show you that rose-bud. This was just fifty years ago."

America, in its colonial period and statehood, learned its medical alphabet in Europe. In time the student-nation began to read lessons which the older eyes did not discern. American medicine has no antiquity, but in the young story are bold deeds. By candle-light in a New Hampshire town, a surgeon saw a lad bleeding to death from a wounded artery in the neck; it was too late to seek trained assistants, and aided only by the patient's mother, he saved the fast-ebbing life; he rode off on horseback without plaudits—he had been rejected by Harvard because he lacked preliminary education—but he was the first in history who tied the common carotid. In America the ligature was first placed around such important arteries as the innominate, subclavian and common iliac. In the backwoods of Kentucky woman was first relieved of ovarian tumor, and among the wilds of Michilimackinac the human stomach was first seen and studied in situ. An American pen wrote the first burning protest against the slaughter of mothers in childbed, and an American knife removed the vesico-vaginal fistula from the hopeless afflictions of the female sex.

A primitive forest on our northern border surrounded the laboratory where chloroform was discovered. Not from the Asklepion at Epidaurus, not from St. Bartholomew's Hospital at London, but from the Massachusetts General Hospital first arose the vapor of ether that has spread like a benediction over the earth. The injection of cocaine into nerves, the production of spinal analgesia, and the localization of surgical shock, are of American origin. The rubber glove, devised by a surgeon in Baltimore to protect the hands of the nurse he loved, is now used everywhere. Those pathological shadows, undiagnosed abscesses in the right iliac fossa, were finally classified as an entity and named appendicitis; it was found that pressure of the finger on a certain spot detects a diseased appendix; these American achievements permitted the surgical invasion of the peritoneum, which opened up a hitherto dark continent to the lifesaving scalpel. Europe gave to America tracheotomy—bloody and horrible; America gave back to Europe intubation—a procedure so simple that it cannot be classed as surgical. Here, amid general incredulity, the medicated probang was applied to the organ of the voice, and here the larynx was first completely photographed.

The paleontologists who gathered fossils in the western half of our country have made important contributions to the science of extinct life, and hence to the ancestry of present forms. American researches in sex-chromosomes, and in the life-history of the fruit-fly, investigated by the million, are fundamental in the cytology of heredity, and throw light on inheritable physical and mental disease. Other nations have watched us suture bloodvessels, grow tumors, transplant organs, rejuvenate tissue, cultivate nerve-cells outside the organism, and produce normal larvae by chemical means from the unfertilized eggs of the sea-urchin. The fatherless frog was born in America.

First differentiating the two widespread fevers, America demonstrated typhoid is transmitted by the house-fly and typhus by the head-louse. The hookworm, menace of the warm lands since the days of the Egyptians, has unfastened its teeth in our southern states. American investigators have been among the foremost in the preventive treatment of goiter, pellagra, beri-beri, rickets and pernicious anemia. Nowhere have the bacterial diseases of plants and the infected ticks of cattle been studied with such constancy as in this country. An army doctor from Virginia, tracking pestilence in Cuba, proved that only an impregnated mosquito, striking before night, carries the unknown parasite of yellow fever.

The coconut palms of Panama waved over the White Man's Grave. Five hundred young engineers came gayly out of France to dig the Canal, and the mosquito of yellow fever dug their last resting-places; twenty thousand corpses rapidly filled the pest-hole, until France abandoned the task, heeding the warning that there were not trees enough on the Isthmus to make crosses for all her laborers. A surgeon in the United States Army, handicapped for years by uncomprehending officials, hunted the wriggling larvae on that narrow strip of jungle; he transformed the death-trap of the tropics into a health-resort; the United States was able to break the barrier between the Atlantic and Pacific, because this Theseus slew the devouring Minotaur of yellow fever.

An alien from Japan, whose medical life was passed in America, hunted the parasite of yellow fever in Ecuador, and sacrificed himself to the disease in Africa—there are no frontiers in medicine. In that international brotherhood, hearing the voice of the father of preventive medicine, "It is in the power of man to cause all infectious diseases to disappear from the world," all the true children of Hippocrates work together for the Disease-less Future.

XIII

SOCIOLOGY IN AMERICA

COLONIAL HOME.—John Bartram, the botanist who never attended an academy, attended a sheriff's sale: he bought land on the banks of the Schuylkill River, and on this land he built a house. At first the house was one room deep, but as his family increased, room after room was added. The attic was enlarged, the peak of the roof lifted, and the whole house extended toward the river. He built an honest house, which did not cheat on space, air and sunlight. John Bartram, aside from acting as herbalist and physician to his neighbors who could not afford the fashionable practitioners of Philadelphia, was his own mason, carpenter, tool-maker and blacksmith. As he explained to a kindred spirit, the physician-preacher Jared Eliot, who introduced the white mulberry tree into Connecticut: "I have split rocks, seventeen feet long, and built four houses of hewn stone split out of the rock with my own hands." With his own hands, and later with the helping hands of his growing sons, he made steps, door-sills, large window-cases, pig troughs and water troughs, all of stone. Life was good to John Bartram, and even Death came as a gentle friend: the day the aged man felt tired, he lay down in his house and passed away. The year was 1777: Year One of these United States of America.

The date-stone on the south side of the house is plain: John Ann Bartram 1731. Weathering the centuries, the house is as substantial as the day it came from the hand of the builder. In the garden by the river, the windows of the house have looked out upon much American history. When young John Bartram dug its foundations, Washington and Jefferson were yet unborn: when John Bartram was an old man, Washington and Jefferson often rested in his garden by the house. The rock-hewn cider mill on the soothing Schuylkill has long been silent, but daily the knocker on John Bartram's door resounds through his house. The strength and harmony of the whole house; the carvings on the east windows; the original Franklin stove near the entrance (the gift of the inventor himself); the cupboard within a cupboard (the wife of Benjamin Franklin presented to wife Ann Bartram a blue china tea-set); the spacious closets, with wooden pegs serving as hooks; the massive doors with their ingenious locks; the wide and solid flooring of age-defying wood; the splendid open fireplaces where mighty logs can burn; the room of looms and spinning-wheels; the study where the self-taught master wrote his letters by candlelight to Linnaeus and to Dillenius of Oxford and to Gronovius of Holland; the broad stairways extending their welcome throughout the house—all bring back the spirit of America's first native botanist.

Tenement House.—There is a gracious charm about a surviving colonial house which is part of the heritage of America. Yet before the eighteenth century had run its course, the slum invaded America, and the evil grew with the passing years. Spacious private homes in New York were partitioned into windowless cubby-holes devoid of light and ventilation. As unceasing tidal waves of poverty, famine and persecution carried millions of immigrants—hopefully burning with "America fever" —to the uncleanable Augean stables of the East Side, speculators learned that an unlimited number of human beings can be crowded into a limited area. The term "tenement-house" became a symbol of reproach. Such fundamentals as air and water were neither expected nor offered in a district which had become the most densely populated on earth. The gardens where the Knickerbockers had planted their tulips were cut up into backyards, and as rear-tenements enroached upon rear-tenements even the backyards disappeared. New York began to produce slum-children who imagined open sewers were playgrounds, and regarded fire-escapes as the best of beds. There were little natives of Mulberry Bend who never sat under a tree, and never inhaled a flower. Wedge-shaped bells once tinkled along this very street, when the cows came home from pasture, but that was before the slum-children were created.

The Code of Hammurabi, known as the oldest code of laws in the world, contains the following regulation: "If a builder build a house for a man and do not make the construction firm, and the house which he has built collapse and cause the death of the owner of the house, that builder shall be put to death." There were times when citizens of the nineteenth century wished that even this primitive principle had been inserted into the building code of Manhattan Island, for when our houses tumbled to the ground, no one was punished except the victims. Fire-traps and fever-nests were always overcrowded, for poverty closes the gates of choice. The sanitary inspector Gerrit Forbes wrote the first report (1834) connecting the slums of New York with the origin and spread of its epidemics, but he spoke a language that his contemporaries did not understand. The physician John Haskins Griscom, a fighting Quaker who battled all his life against corrupt politicians, exposing the ordeals of aliens on incoming vessels, including ship fever to which he himself nearly succumbed during one of his seven thousand examinations, wrote a more detailed report on the housing horrors of New York (1842), but this was likewise pushed aside by indifference and swamped by the ever-swelling streams of immigration.

New York passed through an era when its mayors were corrupt, its judges bartered justice, and its boss grafted millions to the tune of "As long as I count the votes, what are you going to do about it?" It was the era when members of exclusive clubs and of the best churches collected rents from the worst tenements. It was the era when health wardens were usually saloon-keepers, and one of them thought he was giving the right answer when he defined Hygiene as "the vapor which rises from stagnant water." A new era dawned with the creation of the city's Board of Health (1866), which administered the first Tenement House Law (1867), enacted by the legislature at the behest of a distinguished voluntary group known as the Council of Hygiene. No longer could the owner cover 100 percent of his lot with a tenement-house, for it was necessary to leave a 10-foot yard in the rear; no longer could apartments which were entirely underground be rented—thousands of tenants had lived in cellars below tide-water—for in the new dispensation the ceiling had to be a foot above the level of the curb; no longer could premises be offered if they lacked running water, though a backyard spigot was sufficient. To certain New Yorkers it seemed like a revolution in real estate, but there was no cause for alarm: within a few years, most of the provisions for light and air were revoked (1872), and those that were not repealed were unenforced.

Aside from the inevitable names of Robert M. Hartley, Robert Weeks de Forest, Robert Fulton Cutting, Josephine Shaw Lowell and Lillian D. Wald, reformers attempting to uproot the superstition that the slums of New York were due to the shape of the city, included the surgeon Stephen Smith, who undertook a sanitary survey of the city when an epidemic of typhus overwhelmed Bellevue Hospital (1864), tracing upwards of one hundred cases to a single tenement occupied by Irish immigrants; the Brooklyn merchant Alfred Tredway White, who arranged the first seaside home for the summer relief of poor children and erected the first successful improved tenements in the nation (1876); the ethical culture leader Felix Adler, founder of the first free kindergarten in the city and the first American society for child study, whose revelations of the vile conditions in our tenements resulted in legislative investigation (1884); the editor-poet Richard Watson Gilder, who served as the angry and active chairman of the New York Tenement House Commission (1894); the Canadian-born Elgin Ralston Lovell Gould, who formed the

City and Suburban Homes Company of New York (1896) to prove that sanitary dwellings could be built for the laboring classes at moderate rentals.

There was considerable hard work on the part of the reformers, there was much talk with many fine resolutions: and the outcome was practically nothing. Oh yes, a law was passed (1879) prohibiting the building of rooms without windows, but it was either overlooked—the discovery was made that inspectors could be bribed—or it gave rise to the dreary dumb-bell tenement. The indictment by Ernest Flagg, pioneer of house planning, architect of the United States Naval Academy at Annapolis and of Saint Luke's Hospital of New York, remained throughout the nineties: "The greatest evil which ever befell New York City was the division of blocks into lots of 25 x 100 feet. So true is this, that no other disaster can for a moment be compared with it. Fires, pestilence, and financial troubles are as nothing in comparison; for from this division has arisen the New York system of tenement-houses, the worst curse which ever afflicted any great community." With the coming of the new century, the passage of the model New York Tenement House Law (1901) awoke new hope in the stout hearts of social workers, but multitudes of "old law tenements" still held their ground, and New York still retained the undisputed title of the world's greatest slum. Yet such is the social cleavage, even in a democratic country, that the million-peopled slum acreage of the city was unknown foreign territory to an astonishing number of New Yorkers.

At the close of the first decade of the twentieth century, Lawrence Veiller issued his handbook on Housing Reform (1910), in which he stated: "The conditions in New York are without parallel in the civilized world. In no city of Europe, not in Naples nor in Rome, neither in London nor in Paris, neither in Berlin, Vienna nor Buda Pesth, not in Constantinople nor in St. Petersburg, not in ancient Edinburgh nor modern Glasgow, not in heathen Canton nor Bombay, are to be found such conditions as prevail in modern, enlightened, twentieth century, Christian New York. In no other city are there the same appalling conditions with regard to lack of light and air in the homes of the poor. In no other city is there so great congestion and overcrowding. In no other city do the poor so suffer from excessive rents; in no city are the conditions of city life so complex. Nowhere are the evils of modern life so varied, nowhere are the problems so difficult of solution."

After the elapse of another decade, Lawrence Veiller, invited to express his views on housing as a factor in health, declared: "The bad conditions of housing which prevailed fifty years ago were limited to a few cities and to a few spots in those cities. In such great centers of population as New York were slums chiefly to be found. To-day the slum has spread all over the United States and its menace has increased a thousandfold. No part of the country is free from this blight—East, West, North, South; in the great city and the small one; in the town, village and suburb—even on the prairies this evil is to be found." The detractors of Lawrence Veiller called him a visionary Ruskinite, but he knew the old tenement better than any man in America, knew it from blueprint to completed building, from yard privies to the little black rooms, from sewage-filled cellars and damp walls up to falling ceilings and leaking roofs. Devoting his entire career to the subject, he realized that the tenement disease is preventable—but to cure it after it has intrenched itself in a community, requires the most drastic of social surgery.

One who came from a Russian village was born anew in the slums of Boston, when she wandered into Hale House named after her friend Edward Everett Hale, or when she passed beyond the colonnade of Bates Hall of the public library imagining herself a Greek of the classic days treading on sandalled feet through the marbled porticoes of Athens: "Here is where I liked to remind myself of Polotzk, the better to bring out the wonder of my life. That I who was born in the prison of the Pale should roam at will in the land of freedom was a marvel that it did me good to realize. That I who was brought up to my teens almost without a book should be set down in the midst of all the books that ever were written was a miracle as great as any on record. That an outcast should become a privileged citizen, that a beggar should dwell in a palace—this was a romance more thrilling than poet ever sung." So she found her salvation in the slums, and stood on tip-toe to pluck a star from the American sky. But to do this, it is first necessary to be a Mary Antin, capable of turning Dover Street and the muck of Applepie Alley and Letterbox Lane into The Promised Land (1912). For the vast army of nameless ones, the slum remains a morass without sunrise.

BATH-ROOM.—Clio was in a careless mood when she failed to preserve the name of the first American plumber. Colonial America scrubbed itself in wooden troughs which were also used for other household purposes: the water, heated in the fireplace, was poured in and taken out with dipper or pail. The alert Benjamin Franklin brought over from France the slipper bath, which was a large shoe-shaped copper tub with a seat for the bather: a fire under the heel warmed the water which could later be drained off at the toe. The bathtubs introduced by the Stephen Girard Estate into new homes in Philadelphia (1832-37) were regarded with suspicion; and Boston (1845) declared their use illegal unless prescribed by a physician. The White House did not have hot and cold running water for its kitchen and shower baths until the administration of Andrew Jackson. The first bathtub was installed in the White House for Millard Fillmore, and it had no successor until the outspoken Grover Cleveland demanded two bathtubs in the executive mansion. Perhaps the President with two bathtubs in his house felt undemocratic when he was informed (1894) by a leading statistician that only 2.33 percent of the families of New York lived in homes possessing bathtubs with water connection.

For many years the outdoor privy was as characteristic of American scenery as fields of waving corn. Its ubiquity led a sanitary engineer to predict (1885): "Out-of-door privies, those temples of defame and graves of decency, that disfigure almost every country home in America, and raise their suggestive heads above the garden-walls of elegant town-houses, are, I believe, doomed to disappear from off the face of the earth." This prophecy has not been fulfilled in its entirety, but in our cities at least, privies and close-stools and sick-chairs have given way to the water-closet. The rural South which goes barefoot and still uses Mother Earth as its privy, pays homage to the hookworm, Necator americanus. Unfortunately, our early water-closets were untrustworthy affairs often out-of-order—frequently they lacked water. Many fine houses were built around well-covered but defective plumbing, like a hidden ulcer on the body of a beautiful woman.

Years ago, there was a finishing-school for young ladies in Pittsfield, Massachusetts—in view of what happened, "finishing" acquired a sinister meaning. The spacious school, surrounded by trees (and cess-pools), went by the pretty name of Maplewood. One hundred and twelve individuals lived in the school, seventy-four being resident pupils. Their education and morals received careful attention—everything received careful attention except the drainage. So these nice American girls, with their clean faces and starched dresses, drank sewage. Most of them became violently ill, many of them died, and the rest scattered. The Maplewood fever, which was typhoid, broke up the school. Pious lips spoke of "the act of a mysterious Providence, to whose rulings all must submit." It was neither the first nor the last time that the blame was put on Providence when the fault was with the Plumbing.

A poet, declaiming against useful things, clinched his argument by stating, "The most useful thing in the house is the water-closet." Eliminating the scorn behind Théophile Gautier's words, the words themselves may be saved as a sanitary maxim, or appended to the axiom: "The house is the unit of sanitary administration." Public comfort-stations in our country are exceedingly scarce and cleverly concealed—a disagreeable surprise to the visiting European—but the private American bath-room has become world-famous. The loving care which Americans lavish on their bath-rooms has been a decided factor in the well-being of the nation. The evolution of the American bath-room is not only a triumph of modern ingenuity, but one of the outstanding victories of public health.

STREET-CLEANING.—In 1893, the City Club took a series of filthy photographs. The pictures were not contributions to pornography, they were exposures of the streets of New York. Unremoved ash-cans littered the streets, garbage overflowed the sidewalks and gutters. Tin cans and oyster shells were everywhere, and sewer inlets were clogged with tons of discarded paper. Those were the days when a street-cleaner was a political henchman, and he could not be dismissed when he gave the password, "I didn't come here to work." A jungle of unharnessed trucks and wagons darkened the streets—over sixty thousand on Sundays and holidays—and many of them remained in the streets for days at a time. Passers-by used them as toilets, homeless boys used them as hideouts, toughs and thieves used them as dens, whores used them as rent-free rooms. The wagons in the streets appeared as irremovable as the droppings from the horses.

In 1894, a Brazilian visitor wrote the following letter to a friend in Rio de Janeiro: "New York seems to be the dirtiest wealthy city that I have seen. There are portions of the city that are so packed with empty vehicles of every size and shape that one is apt to think, from a view of the filthy state of all their surroundings, that after eight o'clock at night the commercial portion of the city is converted into a huge dirty public stable, unsightly and disgustingly hideous, viewed from whatever point it may be looked at." Certain New Yorkers who heard of this letter proved that even New Yorkers can be sensitive.

In 1895, a bespectacled, bald-headed gentleman with an elongated waxed mustachio, was driving with his wife through the down-town streets of New York. The photographs of the City Club and the letter of J. S. Da Costa had accomplished nothing. The dirt had not been removed from the face of the city. Officials declared that New York could not be cleaned because of its peculiar construction, as there were no alleys through which the rear of lots could be reached. The carts of the Street-Cleaning

Department evidently remained in the stables, since they did not remove the accumulating garbage that was dumped in front of stores and houses. In many places the pavements could not be seen, for they were covered with slimy mud and coated with grease from wagon-axles. The city was a mess, and even in the clear air of January it stank. The lady endured it as long as she could, but when they passed through Elizabeth Street she turned and spoke to her husband, "Please let us go back to Newport. This is hopeless." The lady did not know her husband if she expected him to run away from dirt. His intellectual features relaxed into a grim smile. "Darling," he said, "I am going to clean up this town."

The speaker of these words was George Edwin Waring. Something unpredictable had occurred: cutting across political corruption, a reform ticket had routed Tammany Hall and elected as mayor of the city, William Lafayette Strong. To the old merchant's surprise and disgust, these friends now clamored for political prizes, which caused Strong to swear he would never accept public office again. Nothing that Strong accomplished in his single term was more memorable than his appointment of Waring as commissioner of street-cleaning. Waring was definitely wolf's-bane to politicians. They simply disappeared in the presence of the man who had been a major of the Garibaldi Guards and colonel of a regiment of Missouri cavalry in the Civil War, and had drained Central Park, and had recently reconstructed the plumbing of the United States Capitol at Washington. He created a sensation when he announced he wanted a man instead of a voter at the other end of the broom-handle. Waring, author of numerous volumes, wrote an important book on Street-Cleaning (1897), dedicated to Mayor Strong.

During the brief war with Spain (1898), there was yellow fever at Siboney. William Crawford Gorgas and Victor Clarence Vaughan, two of our foremost sanitarians, recommended the burning of the camp. So the little town, with all its medical equipment and quartermaster's supply, was given to the flames, to prevent the spread of yellow fever. The procedure was utterly senseless—unless by accident an indolent infected mosquito happened to have its proboscis singed. (Walter Reed had not yet spoken, and we still lived in the dark ages of the black vomit.) When the war with Spain was over, the United States Government requested Waring to clean up Havana as he had cleaned up New York. Waring, at sixty-five, entered upon his new duties with undiminished zeal: his preliminary report contained many useful suggestions. In the midst of his work, a mosquito bit him, and Waring was numbered among the millions who died of yellow fever without knowing its cause. His name survives in an eponym (Waring's system), and his epitaph may be written: Waring, with his White Wings, was the first who scrubbed New York behind the ears.

AMBULANCE.—Edward Barry Dalton was one of the Bellevue men who enlisted in the Civil War as regimental surgeon; in the Battles of the Wilderness he was in charge of the hospitals of the Army of the Potomac. In the early days of the war there had been little provision for the transportation of the wounded—the effective ambulance-wagons and tents projected by the military surgeon, Israel Moses, although recommended by a Board had not been built—and Dalton saw persons wandering for days over the battlefields, searching for missing relatives. As the war went on, he likewise saw the ambulance corps, instituted by Jonathan Letterman, rescue large numbers of soldiers who would otherwise have perished where they had fallen. At the conclusion of the fratricidal strife, Dalton was young in years and sad with experience.

After the war, Dalton became the first Sanitary Superintendent of the Metropolitan Board of Health of the City of New York (1866-69). In the midst of the city streets, the Army of the Potomac again passed before him: he held conferences with carriage-makers and dreamed of ambulances. Colonel Dalton would translate the military ambulance service into the terms of a growing metropolis, he would increase the usefulness of hospitals in large cities. He convinced the Commissioners of Public Charities and Correction of the feasibility of his plan, and at his suggestion the Medical Board of Bellevue held its first examination for ambulance surgeons (June 30, 1869). That summer, when two horse-drawn vehicles dashed out of the Bellevue gate, they rode into history.

Bellevue was the first hospital in the world to establish a municipal hospital service. The bell-clanging wagon, scattering everything in its path; the youthful and all-knowing Doc, riding the bus; the splendid horses, sensing an emergency; the never-failing cooperation of the Police Department; the Black Bottle of Bellevue; the racy-tongued drivers, with their remarkable knowledge of the shortest distance between any two points in the city, rejoicing in their right of way, rushing at break-neck speed around elevator-posts and through crowded streets—all became a part of life-and-death in New York. For ages the open doors of hospitals had awaited the entry of the sick and the injured. But the hospital was static, and rendered service only to those who could come within its walls. The hospital did not possess the arms of compassion to pick up those who had fallen by the wayside, nor the swift feet of mercy to race with death. It was Dalton who made the hospital mobile.

"Physician, heal thyself!" is the epitome of medical satire, and Dalton was one of those physicians who brought healing to others, but not to himself. Soon after the accomplishment of his beneficent work, he went off to California to die at an early age of pulmonary tuberculosis. Thousands of families who have been saved from tragedy by his foresight have never heard of this Dalton: a name appropriately carved on the north façade of the new building of the Department of Health of New York. Throughout the cities of America to-day, fleets of swift-moving automobile-ambulances, by day and by night, answer the Call—this is the true monument of Edward Barry Dalton.

CHILD CARE.—Child labor, in a period of adult unemployment, is a social sin, and though it cannot be condoned, at least it can be explained as one of the grave defects of the industrial system. The infantile death-rate in asylums and hospitals was a gruesome chapter of the past—Samuel Gridley Howe of Massachusetts revealed that in one year from 80 to 90 percent of all foundlings in the state infirmary were turned into corpses, and later Abraham Jacobi of New York was expelled by a wrathful lady manager from a certain institution because he objected to a 100 percent mortality among its babies—yet even this can be explained as part of the medical ignorance of the time. But what the present generation finds difficult to understand is why our pious forbears—and indeed they were pious—never heard the cry of homeless children. Long before Charles Loring Brace established the Children's Aid Society of New York (1853) and the first lodging-house for newsboys (1854), a visitor who consulted the city directory could not have located any institution for the welfare of the gutter children, but would have found the name and address of the American Society for the Promotion of Education in Africa.

In the spring of 1874, the strangest thing happened: a settlement worker, Etta Angell Wheeler, prowling through the slums of New York, stumbled upon a male and female sadist whom the Marquis de Sade would have disowned with disdain. This couple had taken little Mary Ellen from a charitable institution, and kept her alive for the purpose of torturing her. Mrs. Wheeler wanted to get her out of their hands, but found—and this is the part that makes the story so strange—there was no legal machinery to remove an ill-treated child from its guardians. In her perplexity she appealed to the protector of the animal world, Henry Bergh, founder of the American Society for the Prevention of Cruelty to Animals. A colorful figure of the town, a forceful personality with a touch of the fanatic, Bergh was the man who made it dangerous to kick a yellow puppy around, or to whip an underfed and overworked horse. When Bergh appeared on the scene, wearing the badge of his society, with the famous tie-clasp of a greyhound, culprits trembled.

After listening to Mrs. Wheeler, Bergh calls for the advice of the society's lawyer, bearer of a magic name, Elbridge Thomas Gerry, whose grandfather was one of the signers of the Declaration of Independence. Bergh and Mrs. Wheeler now learn that children have no status. A child is being beaten, but nothing can be done. Such elaborate legal phraseology, such a wealth of whereases, and not a single hereby has crept in for the protection of childhood: so many laws, but none for Mary Ellen. The cruel marks of the scissors are deep on her thin, bare legs, and there is no statute in the land to rescue her from her tormentors. The bonnet of Mrs. Wheeler moves up and down on her excited head, as she looks helplessly around the room. The lips of Henry Bergh are tightly drawn, for he is primed for battle. The dignified Gerry smooths his Prince Albert to hide his indignation. Suddenly an inspiration—a child is an animal! and therefore the animal society can act—it will prosecute the adults—and take Mary Ellen away, just as if she were a starved and flogged horse. A loophole is found in the law: an American child is saved by the biologic fact that it belongs to the same kingdom as cats and dogs.

At this period, thousands of homeless young vagabonds haunted the old docks of the city, and slept anywhere except in beds; other thousands led a precarious existence in homes that defiled the name of home. The case of Mary Ellen set a precedent. As soon as it became known that an institution would investigate cases of abused children, numerous complaints and appeals poured in, interfering with the regular work of the animal society. Henry Bergh and his collaborators thereupon brought into being—as the legitimate offspring of the American Society for the Prevention of Cruelty to Animals—the New York Society for the Prevention of Cruelty to Children (1875). The earliest organization of its kind, it was the origin of the movement for the protection of minors in the United States, and for the first time in history special laws were enacted for the defense of neglected children and for the punishment of wrongs against them. Gerry was counsel to the children's society, later its president, directing its policies in so masterful a manner that the Gerry Society, as everyone called it, was feared even by those it was designed to protect. Child welfare of the twentieth century has gone far beyond the planning of Bergh and the vision of Gerry, but their pioneering and uncompromising work should not be forgotten.

SOCIAL SETTLEMENTS.—In his twenties, Arnold Toynbee delivered lectures on industrial history at Balliol College, which virtually created that subject at Oxford and penetrated far beyond its ivy-covered walls. He then stepped out of the classic shades of Oxford to the submerged population in East London. One of his acquaintances (Alfred Milner) has left us this vignette of Arnold Toynbee: "His striking appearance, winning manners, and great power of expression, above all his transparent sincerity and high-mindedness, won the respect and affection of all with whom he came into contact, whether as pupil, teacher, or fellow worker in social causes. His intellectual and moral gifts made themselves equally felt in the academic world of Oxford and among the manufacturers and workmen of the great industrial centers where he delivered his popular addresses. He believed earnestly in the power of free corporative effort, such as that of cooperative and friendly societies and trade unions, to raise the standard of life among the mass of the people, and in the duty of the state to assist such effort by free education, by the regulation of the conditions of labor, and by contributing to voluntary insurance funds intended to provide for the laborer in sickness and old age."

There never was an old age for Arnold Toynbee himself. Absorbed in his work, he overtaxed his own delicate health, and passed away before his thirty-first birthday. A collection of his fragments, first published by his widow under the title of The Industrial Revolution, has frequently been reissued, and is known to all students of economics. In that year, Balliol College erected a monument to Arnold Toynbee in London's immeasurable slum —Toynbee Hall (1884). Canon Barnett, who with his young wife and active co-worker, Henrietta Octavia Rowland, had settled as vicar of St. Jude's in Whitechapel, was the principal founder and first warden of Toynbee Hall. In Toynbee Hall, the favored sons of Oxford, fresh from their luxurious surroundings, met the people of the depths. The spirit of Arnold Toynbee lived on in Toynbee Hall: the earliest university settlement, the first of all social settlements, Toynbee Hall in Whitechapel was the mother-house and the training-field of the social workers of England and America.

After residence in Toynbee Hall, Stanton Coit of Ohio took up residence in a tenement on Forsyth Street, on the lower East Side of New York. Here he established Neighborhood Guild (1886), later called University Settlement, the pioneer social settlement in America. Its announced purpose was "to bring men and women of education into closer relations with the laboring classes in this city, for their mutual benefit." Stanton Coit, the first head resident, was succeeded by Charles Bunstein Stover, who described the Neighborhood Guild in a volume in memory of Arnold Toynbee (Johns Hopkins University, 1889). Stover, a beloved figure in the midst of the immigrants of New York, constituted himself the sponsor of play spaces and protector of parks: there was much rejoicing among social workers when he was appointed park commissioner. At a later day, the name of Stover was carved on a rock in Central Park for posterity.

Jane Addams of Cedarville, Illinois, a graduate of Rockford Female Seminary, studied economic and sociological questions in her own country and abroad: she was a young pilgrim, and her church was Toynbee Hall. Back in Chicago, among enormous colonies of aliens, crowded between networks of narrow streets and the river, in the midst of hovels that had long ceased to deserve the name of homes, Jane Addams and her friend Ellen Gates Starr found a large old homestead. This was Hull House, at 800 South Halsted Street, and the two women opened it as a social settlement (September 18, 1889). So Jane Addams lived near the river, and made the address of the Toynbee Hall of Chicago one of the most famous in America. After Hull House had grown into a great settlement with numerous buildings and an international reputation, everything still revolved around Jane Addams. It was observed that when Miss Addams had a headache, the whole staff felt sick and needed medicine; when Miss Addams recovered, the whole staff was healthy and happy.

It must be a satisfying experience to aid sweat-shop workers organize labor unions for bearable conditions, to bring comfort to women who have washed public lavatories for a generation to hold a shiftless family together, to help the worthy offspring of poverty climb out of the bottomless abyss. It is different when one must record a case-history like the following: "You might say it's a disgrace to have your son beat you up for the sake of a bit of money you've earned by scrubbing, but I haven't the heart to blame the boy for doing what he's seen all his life, his father forever went wild when the drink was in him and struck me to the very day of his death." A quenchless social fire must be kindled in a soul to decide to spend life with the morally twisted, the mentally diseased, the physically deformed; feeble-minded girl-mothers producing nameless imbeciles; human trash that will not work, drunken wife-beaters, gun-carrying toughs; the jail-bird, the prostitute and the pimp; and always the unwanted old women whose broken hearts are open doors, "Set wide to every wind of pain." Jane Addams was the potter who moulded this clay, and with the spoiled material she became the foremost woman citizen of America.

In the rented rooms of a private family, Graham Taylor and three of his students founded Chicago Commons (1894), from which stemmed the Chicago School of Civics and Philanthropy, the alma mater of thousands of social workers. Since its inception, Chicago Commons was in the vanguard of the battle for the health and welfare of this vast melting-pot of a city. It was a receiving-station of the racial transformation from the northern to the southern Europeans: "In the place of every German, Scandinavian and Irish family removing, immigrant families still stranger to our American life and conditions arrive. Like the surf upon the sand, each new wave of immigration from southern Italy, Sicily, Poland, Armenia and Greece breaks over us here." A resident of Chicago Commons, John Palmer Gavit, founded the monthly magazine The Commons (1897), which combined with the periodical Charities under the title Charities and The Commons (1905), and then adopted the more convenient name of The Survey (1909), the best-known journal for the social workers of America.

In a section of Philadelphia that appeared disinherited, Theodore Starr bought an ash-heap: in that crowded alley Susan Wharton founded a library for colored children, Helen Parrish supervised an industrial school encircled by human wreckage, Hannah Fox and Sally Fox moved into the street of shame, and now that there were four girls who did not belong to the street, they formed a committee—then the ash-heap blossomed into a garden, and the committee widened into a settlement (1892), later the celebrated Starr Center. In space so small that visitors smiled when it was called an office, located among Jersey City's migrant laborers in factories and on the docks—in a quarter sordidly poor and in constant flux, with none of the picturesque and intellectual qualities which make poverty so interesting to authors and artists—Cornelia Bradford began the social work which developed into Whittier House (1894), whose manifold achievements included the city's first free kindergarten, first district nurse, and first public playground.

In the midst of 30,000 plantation Negroes of Alabama, Mabel Dillingham and Charlotte Thorpe established the Calhoun Settlement (1892), which maintained a graded school for the community, medical mission work by the school physician, and aimed to change the crop-mortgage renter into a small farmer with land and home of his own. Outside of Asheville, before the trolley linked the rural districts to the town, Susan Chester, a Vassar graduate, established the Log Cabin Settlement (1894) for the mountain people of North Carolina. In one of Louisville's old saloon buildings, Archibald Hill and Lucy Belknap established Neighborhood House (1897), which helped to secure a new tenement law, and Kentucky's excellent child labor legislation. In a former fashionable section of New Orleans, which had run down into an appalling slum, the teacher Catherine Hardy established Kingsley House (1899), which gave the city its earliest public playground, and conducted a detailed health survey of the neighborhood.

The first quarter-century (1886-1911) of social settlements in America showed a rapid development: in 1886, there was one settlement; in 1897, there were more than seventy; in 1900, more than one hundred; in 1905, more than two hundred; and in 1911, the year that Robert A. Woods and Albert J. Kennedy edited Handbook of Settlements, there were more than four hundred. They noted in the preface: "The typical settlement, under American conditions, is one which provides neutral territory traversing all the lines of racial and religious cleavage. The house which is wholly unsectarian not only from the point of view of its staff, but as judged by the various elements in its neighborhood, represents the main action of the kind of social enterprise here set forth. For the first time in any publication, the growing tendency toward joint action among settlements is expressed in the statements about settlement federations and other forms of organization. It is an interesting fact, also, that the appearance of this Handbook coincides in time with the creation in large outline of a common program on the part of the settlements of the whole country."

The social settlement of America is a table spread for the immigrants of all the nations. Here they bring their feuds and factions, their old racial hatreds and the dividing beliefs that preach the doctrine of exclusive salvation. The social settlement must draw a circle so inclusive that no one is shut out. Settlements have maintained day nurseries, kindergartens, schools, reading-rooms and libraries; inaugurated health surveys and provided milk stations, penny lunches, clinical services and visiting nurses; established clubs and classes in cooking, sewing, dancing, singing, dramatics, athletics; founded departments of carpentry, etching, photography, hammered copper and brass, rugweaving, printing and bookbinding; organized roof-gardens for the sick, summer camps, picnics, outings, vacations and nature studies; fostered interest in handicrafts, languages, art, music, literature and science; arranged concerts, lectures, entertainments, plays, pageants, festivals; opened a new world to the illiterates of the old world by courses in English, hygiene, citizenship, democracy; denounced child labor and sponsored employment bureaus for adults; exposed corrupt politics and fought for social legislation. The tasks of the settlements are varied, for each has problems peculiar to its neighborhood, but all their activities are contributory streams to their main work, which is Americanization.

PLAYGROUNDS.—Gypsy-Polish-German blood coursed in the veins of Marie Elisabeth Zakrzewska, who emigrated to America at twenty-four. Here she was to taste the bitterness of poverty, to endure social ostracism, and to weep over the hopeless chaos of the English language, yet she lived to write her name—which she thought should be easy for Americans to pronounce—among the educational pioneers of New England. A Berlin midwife by training and graduate of the Cleveland Medical College, she was the first resident physician of the New York Infirmary for Women and Children, founder of the clinical department of the New England Female Medical College of Boston, founder and first attending physician of the New England Hospital for Women and Children, and had her hand in the organization of the New England Hospital Training School for Nurses, from which institution Linda Richards received her diploma (1873) as "America's first trained nurse."

In the 1880s Marie went to Europe on vacation. Rest was imperative, for in her efforts to open the medical facilities of New England to her sex, she had walked for years in the paths of prejudice. Even victory was tinged with bias, as when the Boston Medical and Surgical Journal (October 9, 1879) editorially declared: "We regret to be obliged to announce that at a meeting of the councilors, held on October 1, it was voted to admit women to the Massachusetts Medical Society." We can, however, sympathize with that reactionary periodical when it complained, some years later, that the females of Boston were taught too much bad piano playing and too little good cooking. During her excursion abroad, Marie revisited her native Berlin and in a public park saw children playing on a sand pile. In the full-length biography of this woman, so crowded with battles for equality in education of the sexes, there was no room for this seemingly trivial incident. Yet nothing that she ever did in her life was more important than observing and remembering that sand pile.

Doc Zak, as she was familiarly called, opened a sand garden in Boston (1885), and this was the origin of the playground movement in America. Hull House transformed a vacant lot into Chicago's first playground (1893), and the Henry Street Settlement in New York turned its back yard into a neighborhood playground (1895), introducing various novelties (The Bunker Hill of Playgrounds). Every grain of sand of that original pile increased and multiplied, and at the turn of the century municipal playgrounds were in operation from New York to San Francisco. With the enormous increase of motor traffic which made city streets as dangerous as battlefields, the need for playgrounds grew in proportion, and thousands of volunteer and paid recreation leaders appeared on the American scene. The National Recreation Association, established as the Playground and Recreation Association of America (1906), expanded playgrounds on corner lots and back yards into the community recreation movement covering the whole country. Thus a sand pile grew into a great American institution. Considering how much our children love to play—they are the hardest and noisiest players in the world—it is startling to recall the recentness of our playground movement. We waited for a foreign woman who had no children of her own.

SOCIAL WORK.—The solitary horseman and the lone ranger appealed to early America. This independent spirit was apparent in the volunteer relief workers who sought to help destitute individuals or stricken families without attempting to change their community environment. Social work was private work, augmented by the number of separate persons or groups visited by charity workers. Undoubtedly there were excellent hearts among the organizers and associates of the Scots Charitable Society of Boston (1657), New York Society for the Prevention of Pauperism (1817), and in the later National Conference of Charities and Corrections (1873), and National Association of Societies for Organizing Charities (1888), but experience demonstrated that almsgiving, besprinkled with moral maxims and religious propaganda, was not social work. The word "Charity" grated on the American ear. When certain charity workers proved to be arrogant and aloof, it was wondered why such sour-faced, unimaginative and unsympathetic creatures should insist upon devoting themselves to the uplift of others (their descendants are found among some modern social workers).

The American attitude toward organized charity was expressed in the biting lines of the Irish-American poet, John Boyle O'Reilly: "The organized charity, scrimped and iced, In the name of a cautious, statistical Christ" (1891). The Hoosier author of Fables in Slang (1899) told the story of a high-toned charity worker who came into a poor home, with her lorgnette up to her eyes, inquiring of the woman bending over the washboard whether her husband worked and whether he drank. She was so grand and put on such airs, that the underprivileged child of the poor home resented the intrusion. As this "good fairy lady with the lorgnette" left the alleyway, she was followed by an overripe tomato, which landed just where the boy wanted it to land. "When uplifting, get underneath," is the moral not only of this tale, but of the entire social work movement. Largely on the strength of this story, George Ade was called "a great sociologist" by Lee Kaufer Frankel, himself one of the foremost figures in the organization of charity.

Social work is social sympathy translated into action for social welfare. One of its best representatives was Robert Weeks de Forest. To be called into de Forest's office was an exciting adventure. The leader of social service when the term meant philanthropy, de Forest remained the leader when the term denoted professional social work. He was the sort of man of whom it was said that if the best-known social workers of America came together for whatsoever purpose, by common consent de Forest would be chosen chairman of the committee. Corporation counsel and capitalist, he not only gave much to social causes himself, but he touched the purse strings of the wealthy, and millions came tumbling out. A hint from his lips originated the Russell Sage Foundation of which he was the president as long as he lived. A pioneer of housing reform, he was New York City's first tenement-house commissioner. Lawyer for a railroad and director of jute mills, de Forest looked like an artist, and worked like an apostle for a better America.

Abraham Flexner set unceasing debates in motion when he decided social work was not a profession (1915). This educator, who had gone from coast to coast literally kicking medical colleges to death, was a caustic scholar, though it should be remembered that most of the professional aspects of social work postdated his statement: formation of the Association of Training Schools for Professional Social Work (1919), later named the American Association of Schools of Social Work; the organization of the American Association of Social Workers (1921), which subsequently adopted high standards for full membership; and the official recognition of the United States Census (1930), which for the first time listed social workers as members of a distinct profession—31,241 of them. A decade later our government recognized sociology as a science when it issued a series of postage-stamps in honor of five American scientists: the ornithologist John James Audubon, the physicians Crawford Williamson Long and Walter Reed, the plant breeder Luther Burbank, and the social worker Jane Addams.

SOCIAL CASE WORK.—Scarlet fever attacked a little child, taking away her sight, her hearing, her speech, and depriving her of the sense of smell and taste. Only the sense of touch remained to Laura Bridgman, but the hand of Samuel Gridley Howe was laid upon her: he released her imprisoned spirit, and for the first time a blind deaf-mute was educated. Charles Dickens, passing through this country, found Laura Bridgman a fair young creature, her face radiant with intelligence and pleasure. In the Perkins Institution of Boston which Doctor Howe established, in the same cottage with Laura Bridgman, lived Anne Mansfield Sullivan. Almost totally blind since early childhood, though later her sight was partially restored, Miss Sullivan had entered the Perkins Institution at fourteen: in that year, in Tuscumbia, Alabama, was born a gifted child upon whom the darkness and the silence were soon to descend, for illness made her blind and deaf and mute and wild. At twenty, Miss Sullivan journeyed south to take charge of this pupil, then aged six. It was the meeting of two of the most remarkable women of the century. (As the pupil matured, she became the champion of so many social causes that her books were among the first to be cast into the flames in the unclean debauch of the Burning of the Books in Germany.)

The work of Samuel Gridley Howe with Laura Bridgman, and of Anne Mansfield Sullivan with Helen Keller, are the classic examples of social case work in America. They are, however, exceptional cases, and one does not need to be a social case worker to recognize the following experience as far more typical: "One case worker found her ingenuity taxed to reconcile an Italian father's social conventions with American ways of restoring a dangerously ill girl to health. An operation was needed and the hospital in which it could be performed had been found. But no entreaties moved the father, determined that his child should not leave her home. At last the case worker discovered that he regarded a young unmarried woman as permanently disgraced who spent a night away from the protection of the parental roof. The adaptation made was an arrangement by which father could accompany daughter to the hospital and stay there long enough to assure her restoration to health without blasting her reputation."

The most prominent name in social case work is that of Mary Ellen Richmond, of Belleville, Illinois, general secretary of the charity organization societies of Baltimore and of Philadelphia, and later director of the charity organization department of the Russell Sage Foundation, an institution of outstanding importance in social welfare, though it commemorates an antisocial individual who did not have a grain of charity in his multimillionaire soul. Miss Richmond was the author of Social Diagnosis (1917), the earliest authoritative text on social case work, and of What

Is Social Case Work? (1922); in addition she edited the Social Work Series which contained, among other volumes, Ada Eliot Sheffield's The Social Case History, a discussion of social case recording, and Joanna Carver Colcord's Broken Homes, an interpretation of the attitude of social case workers toward family maladjustments.

It is interesting to note that between the writing of Miss Richmond's two books, psychology had encroached on the field of sociology, with the result that social case workers began to insist on the development of personality. Within another decade, the invader was itself invaded by psychiatry. As summed up by Philip Klein: "Still more recently social case treatment along lines defined by psychiatric theory has tended to displace not only treatment in the older conception but also emphasis on social or psychological study." When psychiatry entered social case work, it was obvious that psychoanalysis could not be far behind. Leading studies of the latter aspects of social case work are Virginia Pollard Robinson's A Changing Psychology in Social Case Work (1930) and Jessie Taft's The Dynamics of Therapy in a Controlled Relationship (1933).

HOSPITAL SOCIAL SERVICE.—A baby suffering from stomach trouble was carried to the Massachusetts General Hospital by its frantic mother. In a few weeks the baby was "discharged-cured," and the overjoyed mother took it home. Baby was soon sick again, and the frantic mother carried it to the hospital. For the second time the baby was "discharged-cured," and the overjoyed mother took it home. Baby was soon sick again, and the frantic mother carried it to the hospital. For the third time the baby was "discharged-cured," and the overjoyed mother took it home. Richard Clarke Cabot, the physician who treated the baby, thus described the vicious circle: "Baby goes out, baby gets sick, baby comes back, baby goes out and so on forever." In this description can be detected an overtone of impatience.

The hospital could cure baby, but could not keep baby cured outside the hospital. Well in the hospital and sick at home—something must be wrong in the home. Physician and nurse did their duty when they cured baby in the hospital: it was not their function to supervise baby at home. It so happened that this particular baby was being overfed on a complicated and variegated diet that would have upset the digestion of a hardened Rocky Mountain goat. Cabot, unorthodox in method and fertile in ideas, clearly saw the need of the medical social worker. A hospitalized malaria patient does not need social service, he needs quinine; a child with a diphtheritic membrane does not require social service, he requires anatoxin injections. But a house-painter who recovers in a hospital-bed from lead-poisoning and plans to return to his former occupation because he knows no other trade is in need of social service; an unmarried mother who leaves the hospital with her infant and has neither support nor shelter is in need of social service.

Cabot figured that about two-fifths of the cases in public hospitals can be helped sufficiently by medicine alone, while medical social work is necessary for the remaining three-fifths. Thinking of that gastric baby, multiplied by sixty percent of the hospital population of America, Cabot originated hospital social service. His first hospital social worker was Garnet Isabel Pelton, a nurse who was succeeded by another nurse, Ida M. Cannon. Nurses do not necessarily make the most successful hospital social workers, for specific training is essential for social diagnosis. Both these nurses, however, were prominently identified with the movement: Miss Pelton related its history and status at the Conference of Charities and Correction (St. Louis, 1910), and Miss Cannon wrote the standard volume on Social Work in Hospitals (1913).

With advancing reputation, Cabot was appointed professor of clinical medicine at Harvard Medical School, but he fed his soul by serving as professor of social ethics at Harvard University. Cabot, who won the admiration of his colleagues when he published texts on physical diagnosis, and introduced the method of teaching medicine by case-histories, aroused their enmity by dangling irritating rows of figures showing that the clinician's diagnosis often bears no relationship to the pathologist's autopsy, and by his championship of the socialization of medicine. Had Cabot's position not been so secure in the Harvard milieu, he would have been expelled from professional societies on various occasions. Cabot was the author of several books on social service, for his social conscience would not let him rest. He possessed the initiator's touch: within a comparatively few years after he started medical social service at the Massachusetts General Hospital with a single worker (1905), there were enough followers to form at Kansas City the national organization, American Association of Medical Social Workers (1918); hundreds of hospitals inaugurated social service departments; and it was recognized that the best-staffed hospital remains incomplete until it becomes socially interested in sickness.

HYGIENE.—A generation ago, the main function of our manuals on hygiene was to emphasize the evils of tobacco and alcohol, while treatises on sexual hygiene, usually written by indignant clergymen, concentrated on the dangers of masturbation. Hygiene was a personal matter, concerned with exercise, proper food, plenty of sleep, and the correction of faulty habits in adolescence; the conception of hygiene as community hygiene was a quiet dawn witnessed by few. To-day, the term hygiene, extended from antenatal care to old-age pensions, has evolved into preventive medicine and public health. Only minor texts are devoted to personal hygiene, and teachers who formerly taught individual hygiene (really elementary physiology) now find themselves in the wider fields of preventive medicine and public health. Our early periodicals bore such names as The Hygeian Record and Family Adviser, The Hygieist, The Herald of Health, The Doctor of Hygiene, Hygienic Family Almanac, Hygienic Monitor, The Hygienic Teacher and Water-Cure Journal. Edited as a rule by faddists, they succumbed to editorial malnutrition or to financial marasmus. All the current periodicals in the field were established well within the twentieth century.

The first important document in American hygiene was the Report of the Massachusetts Sanitary Commission (1850), a complete blue print for public health organization, drafted by

Lemuel Shattuck. Like his forerunners in the public health movement in England, Shattuck was a social-minded statistician and not a physician. The epochal Report "fell stillborn from the hands of the printer," and the governor who signed it did not remember his name was there. Shattuck's suggestions were adopted posthumously. In the year of the Report, a farm boy came to the city of New York to complete his medical course. Stephen Smith saw New York as a perpetual fever-nest, with half a million members of the human race living in quarters unfit for swine. He remembered these conditions when he fathered the Metropolitan Board of Health (1866), and founded the American Public Health Association (1871), at whose jubilee (1921) he eagerly pointed out—he was then close to the century mark—that in the previous January the commissioner of health of the city of New York had made the following remarkable entry in the official records of his department: "Generally speaking, where two persons died fifty years ago, out of every 1000 population, only one died last year (1920)."

With the advent of the microbial doctrine that each infectious disease is caused by a specific microörganism, hygiene moved into the new house of science. The American pioneers in the demonstration of the relationship of bacteria to public health, were George Miller Sternberg, who made his reputation by his work on disinfection (1886), and wrote a manual of bacteriology (1892), standard in its day; Theophil Mitchell Prudden, who investigated the dangers of dust (1890), drinking-water and ice supplies (1891); William Henry Welch, who pointed out the invading Escherichia coli (colon bacillus) in numerous lesions of the human body (1891), and found the coccus of stitch-abscess and the bacillus of gas gangrene (1892). Prior to the European investigators, Theobold Smith and the veterinarian Daniel Elmer Salmon discovered the method of producing immunity from contagious diseases (1886).

William Thompson Sedgwick, director of the Massachusetts Institute of Technology, traced typhoid epidemics to contaminated brooks, and placed his index finger on the fly as the criminal. At the Lawrence Experiment Station (1887) a filter was "the first in America to stand between a water both highly polluted and highly infected, and a large industrial population." Between the filter and the people stood Sedgwick, undertaking the fundamental investigation of water supply and sewage disposal (1887) which remains a landmark in American sanitation. The name of a sanitarian, like that of a poet, may be "writ in water." Hermann Michael Biggs, whose watchfulness kept an epidemic of cholera out of America (1892), established in New York (1893) the first municipal bacteriological laboratories in the world; although rebuked by the New York Academy of Medicine, he was resolute in maintaining (1897), what we all know now, that pulmonary tuberculosis is an infectious and communicable disease which must be reported by physicians; again he showed his pioneer qualities by organizing the first municipal campaign against the venereal diseases (1912).

The biologist Herbert William Conn, of Fitchburg, was the first in this country to study the bacteriology of milk (1889). The liquid secreted by the mammary gland is Nature's perfect food, for it is the only single food containing a balanced diet; man's heedlessness and greed often made it the most dangerous food, for milk may swarm with more bacteria than sewage. Countless infants, alleged to have perished in the first year of life from constitutional weakness or from climatic conditions, actually sucked death from the milk of the cow. Aside from tuberculosis and cholera infantum, contaminated milk has carried many epidemics of typhoid, scarlet fever, diphtheria, and septic sore throat. In the pump-handle era, prior to sanitary control, polluted water was often added to milk. For years, New York drank its milk from diseased cows that never saw the sunlight, but were imprisoned in Long Island stables, feeding on brewer's swill. The merchant Nathan Straus, who lost his own child from milk-borne diphtheria, began to save thousands of lives annually by establishing sterilized milk depots (1893). Behind every bottle of Straus's safe milk, stood his medical mentor, Abraham Jacobi, the father of pediatrics in America. Henry Leber Coit, of New Jersey, who could not find a quart of clean milk for a dying son, originated the term and conception of certified milk (1892). Hervey D. Thatcher, of Potsdam, New York, the town's druggist, physician, and local inventor, devised the world's first milk bottle (1884). Now 30,000,000 bottles of milk are delivered to American doorsteps every morning—and there has been no milk-borne outbreak since the period of scientific inspection and pasteurization.

Industrial hygiene in America had an uneasy childhood. The American Medical Association, progressive in pharmacology, but shortsighted in sociology, attempted to strangle industrial hygiene in its cradle. The manager of a white lead factory expressed the bewilderment of his group when he asked in honest indignation, "Do you mean to imply that if my men get lead poisoning, I am to be held responsible?" The answer is Yes, but it took years to prove it. Case-reports on the menace of using white phosphorus in lucifer matches were published in the United States as early as 1851, but our workers continued to exhibit the terrible affliction of phossy jaw until John Bertram Andrews, a young economist in the service of the government, sounded the alarm (1910) which caused this condition to disappear from the American scene. Alice Hamilton, one of the memorable women who lived at Hull House, investigated poisonous trades for the Illinois Commission, the hygiene of the lead industry and high explosives for the United States Department of Labor, taught industrial medicine at Harvard, and wrote the authoritative texts, Industrial Poisons in the United States (1925) and Industrial Toxicology (1934). The bibliographies by the John Crerar librarian, Ella M. Salmonsen, on vitamins (1932) and silicosis (1934-7), are valuable as starting-points for future research.

The pioneer of naval hygiene was Albert Leary Gihon, author of the standard book on the subject (1871). Edward Lyman Munson wrote the main treatises on military hygiene (1902), sanitary tactics (1911), and the military shoe (1912). Clifford Whittingham Beers, of New Haven, who emerged from strait jacket and asylum to write A Mind That Found Itself (1908), created the mental hygiene movement. Milton Joseph Rosenau, of Philadelphia, for a decade the director of the United States Public Health Service, and for over a quarter of a century the professor of preventive medicine and hygiene at Harvard, wrote many useful papers based on his research, and was the author of Preventive Medicine and Hygiene (1913), the leading textbook covering the whole field. The names of William Freeman Snow and Maurice Alpheus Bigelow have long been associated with social hygiene, which received a new impetus when Thomas Parran, of St. Leonard, Maryland, the vigorous surgeon-general of the United States Public Health Service, succeeded in driving syphilis and gonorrhea into the light of open discussion (1936).

Lemuel Shattuck, our first sanitary statesman, noted the paradox of an abundant America, a modern land flowing with milk and honey, inhabited by an ailing population of frail physique. Present-day America has outgrown this reproach. During the quarter-century (1911-35), as the vital statisticians Louis Israel Dublin and Alfred James Lotka, have convincingly shown, we participated in a World War, passed through the most fatal pandemic of influenza in history, and suffered from a prolonged economic depression, yet during this period the national environment was so modified in the light of the new hygiene, that there was a marked decline in infant mortality and a corresponding increase in the average duration of human life. The American attitude toward health is expressed in Emerson's exultant cry: "Give me health and a day, and I will make the pomp of emperors ridiculous."

ACCIDENTS.—More employees have been maimed in the accidents of industry than soldiers have fallen on fields of battle: the casualties of work exceed those of war. It is therefore startling to recall that Maryland's cooperative insurance law (1902)—America's first effort to compensate injured workmen—was declared illegal. Since men who work in mines are constantly exposed to danger, Montana introduced a fund for miners (1910), but this attempt was likewise stranded on the rock of unconstitutionality. New York's earliest legislation (1910) for compulsory insurance in a selected list of hazardous occupations, was also blocked by constitutional lawyers until the State amended its constitution (1914). By this time several States had workmen's compensation laws on their statute-books, and it was obvious that the movement would become national. One of the most shocking aspects of the whole matter was the long and obstinate struggle to include occupational diseases in labor legislation. Much argument was needed before it was finally realized that a man at work, forced to inhale dangerous dusts until he contracts silicosis, the prelude to tuberculosis, is as much entitled to compensation as the man who is suddenly hit by a flying bolt.

Carelessness is one of the most fatal of American diseases. With the single exception of heart disease, more American males are killed by accident than by any other cause. Preventive medicine has saved countless lives which were later sacrificed to a moment's forgetfulness. The National Safety Council for Industrial Safety (1913) soon changed its name to the National Safety Council (1915), to include public as well as industrial protection. Death waits for life from the instant of birth: not long ago (1939), five newborn infants in a hospital were asphyxiated by steam because a radiator valve blew out, and this occurred because the defective valve had been carelessly repaired with adhesive tape.

The never-ceasing toll of automobile accidents in the United States is a national catastrophe. In a single year (1940), of the 35,000 persons killed, infants numbered 1,190; children, 2,870; youths and grown-ups, 25,410; old people, 5,530. Of the 1,320,000 persons injured that year, many of them disfigured and permanently crippled and disabled, infants totaled 47,520; children, 183,480; youths and grown-ups, 1,025,640; old people, 63,360. Figures are impersonal, and do not disclose the personal and family tragedies covered by these numbers which rise higher year by year. We have conquered pestilence, and are eliminating the life-destroying infectious diseases of the past, but we permit the automobile to erase our victories. The automobile is the modern plague which has turned our highways into roads of disaster and death. The automobile is in truth the devouring Minotaur of our Motor Age.

Home, which should be the safest place in the world for all of us, is in the aggregate the most dangerous of all. In one recent year (1941), accidents in American homes killed 31,500 persons, and injured 4,650,000 more. In time of war, accidents are not only individual misfortunes, but national wastage. Yet on unforgettable Pearl Harbor's first anniversary (1942), the National Safety Council revealed that in one year of war, America had lost through accidents in her homes and offices, in the factories and on her highways, sufficient man-power to have built 10 battleships, 50 destroyers, 10,000 heavy bombers, 20,000 fighter planes, and 50,000 light tanks. It is a terrible record, and it becomes all the more depressing when we remember the estimate of the Travelers Insurance Company: 98 percent of all accidents can be prevented. It is a challenge for America.

VITAL STATISTICS.—Actuarial science in America was born when the theologian, Edward Wigglesworth, analysing sixty-two bills of mortality, published A Table Shewing the Probability of the Duration, the Decrement, and the Expectation of Life, in the States of Massachusetts and New Hampshire (1789). This contribution was America's earliest life-table, and its author is the father of vital statistics in this country. The following year, as ordered by the Constitution, saw the taking of our first decennial Census (1790), inaugurating the modern era in the statistics of a nation. American contributions of the nineteenth century include Ezekiel Brown Elliott's logarithm of the probabilities of life (1856); James Wynne's important monograph on the vital statistics of the United States (1857); Sheppard Homan's classic survey of American mortality (1859); John Shaw Billing's introduction of mechanical aids in counting statistical data (1880), adopted by the United States Census; and Samuel Warren Abbott's model registration reports of births, marriages and deaths in Massachusetts (1886-96). More recent contributions to biometrics include Charles Benedict Davenport's applications of statistical methods in biological variations, and Raymond

Pearl's logistic curve of population-growth. It is now recognized that vital statistics comprise the alphabet of sanitary science, and that book-keeping is as essential in modern hygiene as in the industrial world.

THE NEW WORLD.—In the Rhenish valleys, Neanderthal Man stirs again, darkening our day with unspeakable crimes in the name of racism. Armed with terrible weapons, the eternal Hun demands the surrender of mankind. The Unclean Nation, self-styled the master-race, expresses his superiority by enslaving and butchering other nations. To lull with false security and strike in the back is his policy; to burn libraries and bomb hospitals is his method; to convert the women of vanquished people into prostitutes for soldiers is his ethics. More fatal than any plague of the past has been this demon of destruction, fattening on the pillage and murder of a continent. The fecolith of fascism has polluted our age with incredible foulness. The Unclean Nation, the chancre of civilization, has corrupted the blood of Mother Earth. The world-wreckage of centuries lies around us: Democracy, beguiled by appeasers and drugged by isolationists, has finally awakened from its perilous sleep. The Unclean Nation whose touch is death must be purified by fire. A new world is to be built on the ruins of the old: there are conquered nations to be unchained, there are human rights to be restored, and there are new values to be established.

In the upbuilding of the new world, science will be the chief architect. As the curative medicine of the past evolves into preventive medicine, the preservation of health becomes a problem of national scope. Social forces from all directions are taking the physician from his private office and placing him on the stage of socialized medicine. His domain is enlarged to the public health, and as he concerns himself with the prevention and control of disease, the rehabilitation of the crippled and handicapped, maternal and child care, the construction of required hospitals and maintenance of health centers, medical service to the unemployed and to the low-income population, disability insurance and other aspects of social security, and removal of the factors which predispose such large numbers to mental illness, he enters upon a career of increased usefulness as medical sociologist. To know what food people eat, what clothes they wear, in what sort of houses they live, and under what conditions they labor and take their recreation, has become the physician's business. Preventive medicine, vastly extending the physician's horizon, is destined to change him from private practitioner to the nobler occupation of a worker for the public health and welfare.

BIBLIOGRAPHICAL NOTES

I—MEDICINE IN THE STONE AGE

Origin of Man—Lucretius (*c.* 98-55 B.C.) wrote the first important account of the origin of man (De rerum natura, bk. v, 925-1157); no subsequent age has equaled its poetry and philosophy, and its anthropology cannot be surpassed even today. Translations by H. A. J. Munro (Bohn's Classical Library), Cyril Bailey (Oxford), W. H. D. Rouse (Loeb Classical Library), metrical version by William Ellery Leonard (Everyman's Library). We have used the edition of Cyril Bailey (1910).

Anthropology—The standard works of Edward Burnett Tylor (Early History of Mankind, 1865, Primitive Culture, 1871) and John Lubbock (Prehistoric Times, 1865, Origin of Civilization, 1870) have few direct references to medicine, but are valuable for background.—James George Frazer: The Golden Bough (12 vols.), abridged edition (1922).—Arthur Keith: New Discoveries Relating to the Antiquity of Man (1931).—Works of Franz Boas (1858-1942).

Primitive Medicine and Folklore—William George Black: Folk Medicine (1883).—Max Bartels: Die Medizin der Naturvölker (1893).—Oskar Hovorka and Adolf Kronfeld: Vergleichende Volksmedizin (1908-9, 2 vols., introduction by Max Neuburger).—Jonathan Wright: Demonology and Bacteriology in Medicine (Scientific Monthly, 1917, 494-508); Medicine of Primitive Man (Medical Life, beginning 1924, passim).—Leo Kanner: Folklore and Cultural History of Epilepsy (ibid., 1930, 167-214).

Fractures—Karl Jäger: Beiträge zur prähistorischen Chirurgie (Deutsche Zeitschrift für Chirurgie, 1909, 109-40) estimates that 53.8 per cent of prehistoric fractures were splinted and restored.

Trepanation—When Boucher de Perthes, the customs official who loved the Stone Age, picked up hand-chipped flints (1830) from the gravel-pits of the Somme valley, he carried back man's ancestry through geologic time to the Pleistocene period. The first prehistoric trepanned skull was found by Prunières (1865) in France, whose soil has yielded more neolithic specimens than the rest of Europe. The chief contributions to neolithic trepanation are French, as witness also the work of Broca, Cartailhac, Manouvrier (discoverer of the sincipital-T), Marcel Baudouin, and Lucas-Championnière (Trépanation néolithique, 1912).—In English, Robert Fletcher: On Prehistoric Trephining and Cranial Amulets (Contributions to North American Ethnology, 1882, 1-32).—Wilson Parry: Collective Evidence of Trephination of the Human Skull in Great Britain during Prehistoric Times (International Congress of History of Medicine, 1922, Proceedings, 1923, 135-41).—Victor Robinson: Trepanation After Lister (Ciba Symposia, Trepanation Number, 1939, i, 187-93).

II—MEDICINE IN ANCIENT EGYPT

General Survey—Well-selected bibliography of history, language, science and art, in Karl Baedeker: Egypt, A Handbook for Travellers (1878[1], based on manuscript of Georg Ebers; 1929[8]).

Egyptian Literature—Adolf Erman: Literature of the Ancient Egyptians (tr. by A. M. Blackman, 1927, 318 pp., containing "The Dispute with his Soul of One who is Tired of Life," 86-92).

Egyptian Healing Gods—Walter Addison Jayne: The Healing Gods of Ancient Civilizations (1925, Egyptian Deities, 3-86, bibliography, 523-7).—Jamieson Boyd Hurry: Imhotep (1926).—Seldom do scholars become so uncritical as when dealing with the Egyptian God of Medicine. In spite of William Osler's testimonial ("Imhotep, the first figure of a physician to stand out clearly from the mists of antiquity," Evolution of Modern Medicine, 1921, p. 10), we know little about the semi-mythical Imhotep, and not a line of his writings has survived. Richard Caton (Harveian Oration, 1904, p. 8) makes the unwarranted and irresponsible statement, "I-em-hotep rises before us as one of those intellectual giants who take all knowledge for their province. In his comprehensiveness he surpasses Leonardo da Vinci or our Linacre"; Caton (p. 9) suggests that Imhotep wrote the Papyrus Ebers, and even Breasted (infra) wishes us to believe that Imhotep is the author of the Edwin Smith Surgical Papyrus; as these papyri are dated a century apart, Imhotep could not have written both, and there is no evidence that he had his hand in any of the extant papyri.

Mummy—Herodotus (ii, 85-90; A. D. Godley, 4 vols.); our quotations from the ancient writers, as in this instance, are frequently from the Loeb Classical Library, which embodies the latest researches and is invariably bilingual.—Not to be placed by the side of Herodotus, is Diodorus Siculus, who however traveled in Egypt (60-57 B.C.), and whose history (bk. i) contains valuable information about Egyptian customs.—Thomas Joseph Pettigrew: A History of Egyptian Mummies (1834); for the most extensive life of Pettigrew (1791-1865), explaining his connection with antiquities, see Warren R. Dawson: Memoir of Pettigrew (Medical Life, 1931, 1-136).—Ernest Alfred Wallis Budge: The Mummy, A Handbook of Egyptian Funerary Archaeology (1925).

Palæopathology—Marc Armand Ruffer: Studies in the Palaeopathology of Egypt (1921); the work of Ruffer (1859-1917), with that of William Matthew Flinders Petrie, Grafton Elliot Smith, Frederick Wood Jones, and others, inaugurated the scientific method of studying the diseases of ancient mummies, for which Ruffer devised the term palaeopathology. His collected papers, with numerous plates, constitute an important contribution to which we are much indebted.

Surgical Instruments—John Dixon Comrie: Die ältesten chirurgischen Instrumente (Archiv für Geschichte der Medizin, 1909, 269-72), and by the same author: Medicine among the Assyrians and Egyptians in 1500 B.C. (Edinburgh Medical Journal, 1909, reprint of 32 pp.).

Papyrus Ebers—The Therapeutic Papyrus of Thebes (1552 B.C.) was found by Georg Ebers (1837-98), who announced his discovery to scholars in these words (Zeitschrift für Aegyptologie, May-June 1873): "I was successful on my last journey in finding a medical papyrus of extraordinary size and beauty which promises in many directions to bring rich fruit to our science." This roll, which created an epoch in medical Egyptology, has since been known as the Papyrus Ebers. See his autobiography, Die Geschichte meines Lebens (Stuttgart, 1893). Ebers was docent of Egyptology at Jena, and professor of the Egyptian language and antiquities at Leipzig. Ebers' historical novel, An Egyptian Princess (Eine ägyptische Königstochter, 1864), was the first of several in which he combined his archaeological knowledge with fiction; these novels were successful and undoubtedly helped to popularize Egyptology, but they belong rather to the follies of scholarship. His "Gesammelte Werke" appeared in 25 vols. (1893-5). —Bayard Holmes and Peter Gad Kitterman: Medicine in Ancient Egypt (The Hieratic Material, A Review of Carl H. von Klein's Manuscript Translation of the Papyrus Ebers, 1914)—Carl H. von Klein: The Medical Aspects of the Papyrus Ebers (Journal American Medical Association, 1905, 1928-35).

Edwin Smith Papyrus—Bayard Holmes' survey of Egyptian medicine is not limited, despite its title (supra), to the Papyrus Ebers; however, he wrote when little was known about Edwin Smith, whom he inaccurately describes as "an American farmer." The Surgical Papyrus of the Seventeenth Century B.C., is named the Edwin Smith Papyrus, after the American Egyptologist, Edwin Smith (1822-1906), who acquired it at Thebes (1862) and even attempted its decipherment at a time when knowledge of hieratic was limited; his daughter, Leonora Smith, presented the document to the New York Historical Society. Our present knowledge of this unique papyrus is due exclusively to James Henry Breasted: his preliminary interpretations (1922) have culminated in the publication of the Edwin Smith Surgical Papyrus (1930), containing historical introduction, translation and commentary (vol. i), with facsimiles in color (vol. ii). Breasted is the foremost of American Egyptologists, and his many books on the subject are standard. His great edition of the Edwin Smith Papyrus places all scholars in his debt.

III—MEDICINE IN ANCIENT GREECE

Aesculapius—There are three references to Aesculapius in the Iliad (ii, 731; iv, 194; xi, 518); it must be remembered that in the Homeric poems Aesculapius had not yet become the god of medicine.—Ovid: Metamorphosis (in Frank Justus Miller's version for the Loeb Classical Library, the references to Ovid's treatment of the Aesculapius myth will be found in vol. ii, p. 434).—Further references in Leonhard Schmitz (William Smith's Dictionary of Greek and Roman Biography and Mythology, 1844, i, 44-6).—Edward Theodore Withington: Medical History from the Earliest Times (1894), the best work of its kind (appendix ii, 370-9); also his Asclepiadae and Priests of Asclepius (Charles Singer's Studies in the History and Method of Science, 1921, ii, 192-205).

Homer—The reader will naturally keep to his favorite version. Our quotations from both the Iliad and Odyssey are from the Loeb Classical Library (A. T. Murray, 4 vols.).—Charles Daremberg: La médecine dans Homère (1865; on the drugs, anatomy, physiology, surgery and medicine in the Homeric poems).—Hermann Frölich (Die Militärmedizin Homers, 1879) argues that Homer was a physician!—See the great bibliography by George Sarton: Introduction to the History of Science (From Homer to Omar Khayyam, 1927, i, 53-6).

Hippocrates—The oldest Hippocratic manuscripts (Vindobenensis med iv; Parisinus 2253; Marcianus Venetus 269; Laurentianus 74, 7; Vaticanus graecus 276) are from the tenth-twelfth century, and not earlier than the ninth. For references to the printed editions, see Index-Catalogue of the Surgeon-General's Office (1885, 246-55; 1902, 148-66). The standard Hippocratic texts of the nineteenth century are those of Carolus Gottlob Kühn (1825-7) and Emile Littré (1839-61); other editions contain special features, as J. E. Petrequin: Chirurgie d'Hippocrate (1877-8). The early English translations of Hippocrates are now of historic interest only. In the absence of a complete edition of Hippocrates in English, we are fortunate in Francis Adams: Genuine Works of Hippocrates, prepared for the Sydenham Society (1849); and in W. H. S. Jones: bilingual Hippocrates, prepared for the Loeb Classical Library (1923-31, 4 vols.); the surgical volume is by Withington (1927).

Greek Biology—A satisfactory history of general biology has been lacking, and even Singer's work on this subject (1931) proved disappointing.—A masterly survey of Greek biology, with many illustrations, by Charles Singer: Greek Biology and its Relation to the Rise of Modern Biology (in his Studies, 1921, ii, 1-101); Greek Biology and Greek Medicine (Chapters in the History of Science, 1922).

Aristotle—Recent editions of Aristotle have been undertaken chiefly by the Oxford University Press; the most valuable volume for our purpose is the translation, with notes, of the History of Animals, by D'Arcy Wentworth Thompson (1910). Bibliography in Sarton's Introduction (i, 127-36); by the same author, Aristotle and Phyllis (Isis, 1930, 8-19, 5 illustrations).

Theophrastus—Enquiry into Plants, first English translation, by Arthur Fenton Hort (Loeb Classical Library).

Thucydides—The description of the plague of Athens is the first masterpiece in the history of infection (ii, 47-54; in Charles Foster Smith's version for Loeb Classical Library, vol. i, pp. 341-57).

Surgical Instruments—William Alexander Greenhill: Chirurgia (William Smith's Dictionary of Greek and Roman Antiquities, 1842, 219-23).—John Stewart Milne: Surgical Instruments in Greek and Roman Times (1907, 187 pages of text, 54 plates).

IV—GREEK MEDICINE IN ALEXANDRIA

Alexander the Great—In the Loeb Classical Library, from which our quotations are taken, Bernadotte Perrin's edition of Plutarch (1914-26) occupies eleven volumes (the Alexander is in vii, 223-439).

General Survey—Charles Daremberg: Histoire des sciences médicales (1870), contains a useful chronological table of the Alexandrian physicians (i, 159-69).—Heinrich Haeser: Geschichte der Medicin (1875, i, 229-53, with bibliography).—Johann Hermann Baas: History of Medicine (tr. by H. E. Handerson, 1889, 118-30).—Max Neuburger: History of Medicine (tr. by Ernest Playfair, 1910, i, 172-94).

The Empirics—References above, and Daniel Le Clerc: Histoire de la Médecine (1723^3, 341-80).—Greenhill: Empirici (Smith's Dictionary, 1842, 379-81).—Withington's History (1894, 66-70), brief and valuable.—A chief original source is the preface of Celsus (infra).

Herophilus—Revival of interest in Herophilus dates from the scholarly synthesis of Karl Friedrich Heinrich Marx (Herophilus, Ein Beitrag zur Geschichte der Medicin, 1838, 1842).—J. F. Dobson (Proceedings Royal Society of Medicine, 1925, 19-32).

Erasistratus—Galen: On the Natural Faculties (Arthur John Brock, 1916, 95, 105, 135-7, 153-77); Aulus Gellius: Attic Nights (John C. Rolfe, 1928, xvi, 3; xvii, 11); Plutarch: in life of Demetrius (1920, ix, 93-7); all of the above in Loeb Classical Library.—J. F. Dobson (Proceedings of Royal Society of Medicine, 1927, 21-8).

Alexandrian Papyri—Karl Sudhoff: Arztliches aus griechischen Papyrus-Urkunden (Puschmann Foundation Studies, 1909, 1-296, 17 reproductions).

V—GREEK MEDICINE IN ROME

General Survey—Thomas Clifford Allbutt: Greek Medicine in Rome (1921).

Gods of Health—Jayne: The Healing Gods of Ancient Civilizations (1925, 371-499, bibliography, 536-8).

Psychopathology—Much psychopathology can be dug out of the Lives of the Caesars by Suetonius, who was certainly a gossip, in fact, a pioneer muckracker, but the essential truth of his accusations has been substantiated beyond denial (2 vols., tr. by J. C. Rolfe, Loeb Classical Library).—Tacitus, in Bohn's Classical Library, and recently in Loeb.—Martial and Juvenal!

Celsus—Following the Editio princeps (Florence, 1478), there have been over 100 editions of Celsus; modern texts are based on Daremberg's Celsus (1859); the latest English translation by Walter George Spencer (1935-38) summarizes the arguments for regarding Celsus as a medical practitioner.

Pliny—As an index of changing tastes, the most popular author of the Middle Ages has not yet been completed in the Loeb Classical Library (scheduled for ten volumes); for Pliny's extraordinary popularity in the past, see the review of 222 editions by E. W. Gudger (Isis, 1924, 269-81; "it seems as if nearly every town in northern Italy had set up a press especially to issue an edition of Pliny").—The English version by Philemon Holland (2 folio vols., 1601) is still vigorous and readable; our quotations are from the edition of John Bostock and Henry Thomas Riley (Bohn's Classical Library, 6 vols., 1855-7).

Aretaeus—First 19th century edition by Kühn (1828), who was evidently fated to produce indispensable editions which arouse scholarly indignation.—Discussion of previous texts in the Sydenham Society bilingual edition of Francis Adams: Extant works of Aretaeus the Cappadocian (1856), from which our quotations are taken.

Galen—Extensive bibliography in Sarton's Introduction (i, 301-7) and in Bibliotheca Osleriana (1929, items 350-427).—Galen students now go to Kühn (1821-33, 20 vols.), though doubting at times his Greek transcription and complaining of his Latin; the truth is that the modern student must be in love with his theme to be able to read much of Galen (the technical treatises) in any language.—Charles Singer wrote a letter (Annals of Medical History, 1917, 433-4) about the formation of a Galen Society and a project to translate into English the entire works of Galen, but nothing has come of it.—J. S. Prendergast: Background of Galen's life and activities, and its influence on his achievements (Proceedings of Royal Society of Medicine, 1930, 53-70).—By Joseph Walsh: Galen's discovery and promulgation of the function of the recurrent laryngeal nerve (Transactions of College of Physicians of Philadelphia (1925, 677-92); Galen's studies at the Alexandrian School (Annals of Medical History, 1927, 132-43); Galen clashes with the medical sects at Rome (Medical Life, 1928, 408-43); Galen's second sojourn in Italy and his treatment of the family of Marcus Aurelius (ibid., 1930, 473-506); first English translation of Galen's Exhortation to the study of the arts, especially medicine (ibid., 1930, 507-30).

VI—ARABIAN MEDICINE IN THE MIDDLE AGES

General Survey—Many of the Arabian writers were put into medieval Latin, but others await the translating zeal of Oriental scholars; the most quoted European sources for Arabian medicine are Ferdinand Wüstenfeld's Geschichte der arabischen Aerzte und Naturforscher (1840), Lucien Leclerc's Histoire de la médecine arabe (1876), Carl Brockelmann's Geschichte der arabischen Litteratur (1898), and the monumental labors of the archivist Moritz Steinschneider.—John Freind: History of Physick (1785^5, vol. ii, "containing all the Arabian writers").—Francis Adams: Seven Books of Paulus Aegineta, translated from the Greek with a commentary embracing a complete view of the knowledge possessed by the Greeks, Romans, and Arabians (Sydenham Society, 1844-7; appendix, On the substances introduced into the Materia Medica by the Arabians, vol. iii, 424-80).—Budge: The Syriac Book of Medicines (1913; vol. i, introduction and Syriac text; vol. ii, English translation and index).—Sarton's Introduction (1927) is particularly rich in Oriental references; see also the chapter East and West (pp. 73-124) in his History of Science and the New Humanism (Colver lectures, 1931).—Withington: Medical History (1894, 138-75).—Neuburger: History of Medicine (1910, i, 343-94). —Edward Granville Browne: Arabian Medicine. (Fitzpatrick lectures, 1921; pp. 81-91 devoted to Arabian psychotherapy.)

Hunain ibn Ishaq—Researches of Gotthelf Bergsträsser (1913-25). —Max Meyerhof: The book of the ten treatises on the eye ascribed to Hunain (Government Press, Cairo, 1928); New Light on Hunain and his Period (Isis, 1926, viii, 685-724); several valuable studies by Meyerhof have appeared in Isis, this one being especially serviceable.

Moslem Hospitals—The first issue of Janus (1846) reproduces the Arabic text of al-Macrizi's description of Moslem hospitals, with Wüstenfeld's German translation (pp. 28-39), from which our account of the Mansurian Hospital of Cairo is taken.

Rhazes—Treatise on Smallpox and Measles, tr. from the Arabic by Greenhill (Sydenham Society, 1848; with introduction and notes; Rhazes on quacks, 80-2).—George Spiers Alexander Ranking: Life and Works of Rhazes, from original sources (International Congress of Medicine, London, 1913, section xxiii, 237-68).

Avicenna—Islam's most influential philosopher and scientist, the dominating medical figure of Asia and Europe until well after the Renaissance, is still a potent physician in the East, since his tomb at Hamaden is visited for its curative power by numerous pilgrims; in the West, however, Avicenna has long receded to the academic realm of the incunabula and the Latin translations of Gherardo of Cremona. For Avicenna's surgery, see Ernst Julius Gurlt: Geschichte der Chirurgie (3 Bände, Berlin, 1898, i, 650-9).

Maimonides—L. J. Bragman translated Maimonides' tracts on Physical Hygiene (Annals of Medical History, 1925, 140-3) and Poisons (Medical Journal and Record, 1926, 103-7, 169-71), but we have no English translations of his medical works from the original Arabic.—His Guide for the Perplexed was thus translated by Michael Friedländer (1904^2).—Heinrich Graetz: (History of the Jews, 1894, iii, 445-93; "his medical aphorisms . . . are nothing further than extracts from and classifications of older theories. In spite of his almost absolute lack of originality in the province of medicine, Maimuni nevertheless enjoyed a wide reputation as a medical author," p. 473). This judgment, which is correct enough, is censured in the uncritical Life of Maimonides by David Yellin and Israel Abrahams (1903; useful notes, 219-33).—Isaac Broydé and J. Z. Lauterbach: Moses ben Maimon: (Jewish Encyclopedia, 1905, ix, 73-86 passim).—Julius Pagel: Maimuni (1908).—James J. Walsh: Old-Time Makers of Medicine (1911, ch. iv, 90-108; contains 21 health rules of Maimonides).—Reuben Levy: The Tractatus de Causis et Indiciis Morborum, attributed to Maimonides (Singer's Studies, 1917, i, 225-34; shows that it is not by Maimonides).—Maimonides' Prayer for Physicians was written by Marcus Herz (1747-1803), physician to the Jewish Hospital in Berlin; it was first published under his name in the Hebrew periodical Meassef (1790, vi, 242-4); for the legend of the Prayer, see

Bibliotheca Osleriana (item 5114); for the Prayer itself, W. W. Golden (Transactions West Virginia Medical Society, 1900).

VII—EUROPEAN MEDICINE IN THE MIDDLE AGES

General Survey—George Sarton's Introduction to the History of Science, to appear in several volumes, is the most comprehensive survey yet attempted; vol. I (1927), which we have frequently cited, covers the IXth B.C.-XIth A.D. centuries. "Vol. 2 of my introduction, From Rabbi ben Ezra to Roger Bacon, XIIth & XIIIth centuries, is now printing. It will be far more thorough and important than vol. 1." (Personal communication, March 29, 1931). Sarton's Introduction (1927-1931) went out of print, and was practically unobtainable by 1943; even modern books may become bibliographical rarities.—Lynn Thorndike: History of Magic and Experimental Science during the first Thirteen Centuries of our Era (1923, 2 vols., based on original printed sources and unpublished medieval manuscripts; challenges various accepted opinions; stimulating contribution which has become indispensable to all workers in this field); also his: Study of Western Science of the Fourteenth and Fifteenth Centuries (Medical Life, 1925, 117-27); Magic and Medicine (ibid., 1929, 148-55); Science and Thought in the Fifteenth Century (1929).

Anglo-Saxon Medicine—Extant Anglo-Saxon medical MSS. were collected and translated into English by Oswald Cockayne: Leechdoms, Wortcunning and Starcraft (1864-6, 3 vols., containing Leech Book of Bald, *c.* 900-50 A.D.)—Joseph Frank Payne: English Medicine in the Anglo-Saxon Times (Fitzpatrick lectures, 1904).—Charles Singer: Early English Magic and Medicine (1920, 34 p.).

Frederick II and Michael Scot—The writer of the article on Michael Scot in the Dictionary of National Biography (1897, li, 59-62) utilized the proofs, and followed the conclusions, of James Wood Brown: An Enquiry into the Life and Legend of Michael Scot (1897), which has also been followed by Comrie (Edinburgh Medical Journal, July 1920, reprint of 11 pp. with plates).—Brown's biography is still the main source of our knowledge of Scot, but his statements must be checked up with the critical researches of Haskins: Michael Scot and Frederick II (Isis, 1922, iv, 250-75); and Thorndike (1923, ii, 307-37). Haskins' various studies of the period have been collected in his important History of Medieval Science (1924; 1927^2,

242-326; ch. xiv gives an analysis of Frederick's zoölogical treatise).

Roger Bacon—E. T. Withington: Roger Bacon and Medicine (in Andrew George Little's VIIth centenary Bacon essays, 1914, 337-72), and his translation of Bacon's De erroribus medicorum (Essays presented to Karl Sudhoff, 1924, 139-57).—John Henry Bridges: Essays and Addresses (1907, 159-88) and Life and Work of Roger Bacon (1914; passing of rays, 100-1).—Robert Steele: Roger Bacon and the state of Science in the thirteenth century (Singer's Studies, 1921, ii, 121-50).—Thorndike: History of Magic (1923, ii, 616-91; important critical study of the legends and over-estimation of Bacon).— Tenney L. Davis: Roger Bacon and his Sound Views on Medicine (Medical Life, 1924, 473-8).

Papal Bulls—Decretal in 1300, of Boniface VIII, forbidding cooking the bones of the dead (in Latin, Medical Library and Historical Journal, 1904, ii, 13-14; in English, ibid., 1906, iv, 265-6).—Decretal, at Avignon about 1317, of John XXII, forbidding alchemies (in Latin, ibid., 1905, iii, 252-3; in English, 250-2). For both the Latin transcriptions and English translations of these papal bulls we are indebted to James J. Walsh. Also in his: The Popes and Science (1908).

Medieval Anatomy—Robert von Töply: Studien zur Geschichte der Anatomie im Mittelalter (1898).—George W. Corner: Anatomical Texts of the Earlier Middle Ages (1927).—Charles Singer: Evolution of Anatomy (1925, 62-86).—Mortimer Frank: Manuscript Anatomic Illustration of the Pre-Vesalian Period (Ludwig Choulant's History and Bibliography of Anatomic Illustration, ed. and tr. by Mortimer Frank, 1910, 49-87; based on Sudhoff).—Lynn Thorndike: Medicine versus Law in Late Medieval and Medicean Florence (Romanic Review, 1926, 8-31, Salutati's reasons for preferring jurisprudence).

Traditional Anatomy—Sudhoff is here the master. From the manuscripts he dug up the texts and pictures for his Puschmann-Foundation studies (Tradition und Naturbeobachtung, 1907; Anatomie im Mittelalter, 1908). By his comparative studies of anatomical drawings throughout several centuries, Sudhoff demonstrated the stationary character of pre-Vesalian illustrations.

Fasciculus Medicinae of Johannes de Ketham—A collection of medical tracts circulating in MS.; when printed, memorable as the first incunabulum illustrated with anatomical woodcuts. The first edition, Latin, printed by Giovanni and Gregorio de Gregorii (Venice, 1491);

two years later the brothers printed Sebastiano Manilio's Italian version of the collection (1493), containing more illustrations and Mondino's Anatomy. Both the 1491 and 1493 Fasciculus have recently been reproduced in perfect facsimile (by R. Lier & Co., Florence, 1924-5). In a supplementary volume, Charles Singer furnished an English translation of Mondino's Anatomy, with highly valuable discussions and explanations, and an atlas of 90 illustrative figures from MS. and printed sources. The facsimiles are vols. 1 and 2 of Monumenta Medica.

Medieval Universities—Hastings Rashdall: The Universities of Europe in the Middle Ages (1895, 3 vols.)—Charles Homer Haskins: The Rise of Universities (Colver lectures, 1923); Renaissance of the Twelfth Century (1928, 368-97).

School of Salerno—Unpublished documents and tracts edited by Salvatore de Renzi: Collectio salernitana (1852-9, 5 vols.).—Salernitan bibliography is so extensive that in the first series of the Index-Catalogue it occupies 7 columns (1891, xii, 469-72) and since then, among many others, we have had the investigations of Sudhoff and his pupils, particularly Friedrich Hartmann (1919).—John Ordronaux: Regimen Sanitatis Salernitanum (1871^2, introduction, 11-43, and bilingual translation, 46-167).—Henry Ebenezer Handerson: School of Salernum, An historical sketch of medieval medicine (1883). —Charles and Dorothea Waley Singer: Origin of the Medical School of Salerno, the first university, an attempted reconstruction (Essays presented to Sudhoff, 1924, 121-38).—Karl Sudhoff: Salerno, A medieval health resort and medical school on the Tyrrhenian sea (Essays in History of Medicine, 1926, 229-47).—John Conrad Hemmeter and Arthur Oehm: Wandering and Musing about Salerno and Monte Casino (Medical Life, 1927, 198-217).—Leopold Vaccaro: School of Salerno (ibid., 1929, 271-84).—Kate Campbell Hurd-Mead: Trotula (Isis, 1930, 349-67, in defense of her historicity).

Social Conditions—George F. Fort: History of Medical Economy during the Middle Ages (1883; on prostitution, 336-47).—E. Belfort Bax: German Society at the Close of the Middle Ages (1894; first signs of social revolt).

Separation of Medicine and Surgery—Allbutt: Historical Relations of Medicine and Surgery (1905, xvi-125 p.).

Petrarch—Our section on Francesco Petrarca is based, in part, on Eugen Holländer: Karikatur und Satire in der Medizin (1921^2,

73-8), and Pagel-Sudhoff: Geschichte der Medizin (1922[3]); English trans. in Medical Life (1931, 187).

VIII—MEDICINE IN THE RENAISSANCE

Incunabula—William Osler: Incunabula Medica, Study of Earliest Printed Books, 1467-80 (Bibliographical Society, 1923, 152 p., 16 plates).

Leonardo da Vinci—Quaderni d'Anatomia (ed. by C. L. Vangensten, A. Fonahn, H. Hopstock, facsimile of drawings and notes, German and English translation, 1911-16, 6 folio vols.).—Halfdan Hopstock: Leonardo as Anatomist (trans. from Norwegian by E. A. Fleming, Singer's Studies, 1921, ii, 151-91, 25 figs., valuable essay).— Sarton's preface, xv-xx, to James Playfair McMurrich: Leonardo da Vinci, the Anatomist (1930).—Sigmund Freud's psychoanalysis of Leonardo (Eine Kindheitserinnerung des Leonardo da Vinci) has been translated by A. A. Brill (Leonardo da Vinci, A psychosexual study of an infantile reminiscence, 1916), and criticized by J. C. Hemmeter (Master Minds in Medicine, 1927, 484-503).

Paracelsus—The young Sudhoff won his first laurels in medical history by his studies of the Paracelsus manuscripts; after an elapse of half a century, new leaves were entwined with the early wreath, for our venerable master climaxed his career by issuing, with notes and commentary, the definitive edition of Paracelsus in fifteen volumes; an important feature of this enterprise is that for the first time it assembles all the unprinted manuscripts.—John Ferguson: Bibliographia Paracelsica (1877-90).—The Life of Paracelsus, by Anna M. Stoddard (1911), which is frequently cited, is uncritical.—Impartial monograph by John Maxson Stillman (1920), further valuable because of its literal translations from the original.

Canano—Facsimile edition of his Dissectio, annotated by Harvey Cushing and Edward Clark Streeter, with epilogue on extant copies by Arnold Carl Klebs and Virgilio Ducceschi (R. Lier & Co., Florence, 1925, vol. 4 of Monumenta Medica).

Vesalius—No amount of reading about Vesalius can take the place of an inspection of the original edition of the Fabrica (1543) itself.— The chief biography is by Moritz Roth: Andreas Vesalius Bruxellensis (Berlin, 1892).—In English we have the noteworthy works of James Moores Ball: Andreas Vesalius, Reformer of Anatomy (1910), and Marion Harry Spielmann: Iconography of Andreas Vesalius

(1925).—Charles Singer: Evolution of Anatomy (1925, 110-35), a summary of his actual achievements, followed by a Vesalian Atlas, 187-205; in Ball's folio, mentioned above, the illustrations are larger. —Brief sketches, dwelling dramatically upon his nocturnal body-snatching exploits, are numerous, since a composition along this line is apt to be the first offering of the beginner in medical history.

Servetus—Bibliography in Hemmeter: Master Minds in Medicine (1927, 392-8).

Renaissance Surgery—The chief surgical treatises of the Renaissance are John de Vigo's Practica in arte chirurgica copiosa (1514), Hans von Gersdorff's Feldtbuch der Wundartzney (1517), Berengario da Carpi's Tractatus de fractura calvariae seu cranei (1518), Paracelsus' Chirurgia magna (1536), Walther Hermann Ryff's Gross Chirurgei (1545), Pierre Franco's Traite des hernies (1561), Felix Würtz's Practica der Wundartzney (1563), Thomas Gale's Treatise of wounds made by gonneshot (1563), Ambroise Paré's Oeuvres (1575), William Clowes' Proved practise for all young chirurgians (1591), Fabricius Hildanus' De gangraeno et sphacelo (1593), Peter Lowe's Whole course of chirurgerie (1597), and Tagliacozzi's De curtorum chirurgia per insitionem (1597). Vigo was Englished by Bartholomew Traheron (1543) and Paré by Thomas Johnson (1634); the standard edition of Paré is by Malgaigne (1840), supplemented by the family papers and documents found in the national archives by Claude Stéphane Le Paulmier (1884-7).

Venereal Disease—Ernest Roucayrol: Considérations historiques sur la blennorragie (Paris thesis, 1907, 244 pp., with 38 figs., from original documents).—Earliest Printed Literature on Syphilis, being ten tractates of 1495-8 (in complete facsimile, with introduction and other accessory material, by Karl Sudhoff, adapted by Charles Singer, published by R. Lier & Co., of Florence, 1925, vol. 3 of Monumenta Medica).

Fracastorius—Nahum Tate ("England's worst poet laureate," who mangled other men's plays, and did not hesitate to change shakespeare) deserves credit for his version (1686) of Fracastoro's Syphilis. —An anonymous prose translation from the Latin appeared in St. Louis (1910).—Important study by Charles and Dorothea Waley Singer: The Scientific Position of Girolamo Fracastoro (Annals of Medical History, 1917, 1-34).—Bilingual edition of Contagion, with translation and notes by Wilmer Cave Wright (History of Medicine Series, issued under auspices of Library of New York Academy of Medicine, 1930).

William Gilbert—In 1900, on the tercentenary of the publication of "De magnete," the members of the Gilbert Club translated this work from the Latin into English, reproducing the folio's format, and adding valuable notes about the First Electrician; 250 copies printed.

IX—MEDICINE IN THE SEVENTEENTH CENTURY

Harvey—Robert Willis: The Works of William Harvey, translated from the Latin, with a life of the author (Sydenham Society, 1847, xcvi-624).—John Aubrey: Brief Lives, chiefly of contemporaries, set down between the years 1669-96 (ed. from the MSS. by Andrew Clark, 1898, i, 295-305).—K. J. Franklin: Valves in Veins (Proceedings of Royal Society of Medicine, 1927, 1-33), comprehensive and well-illustrated survey, tracing the subject from the sixteenth century onwards, of importance because of its relationship to Harvey's discovery.—Bibliotheca Osleriana (Harvey and his forerunners, 1929, items 692-918).—The Harveian Orations are many, but relatively few are worth consulting.—The tercentenary of the publication of De motu cordis (1628-1928) produced considerable Harveiana, including Geoffrey Keynes: Bibliography of William Harvey (a sumptuous work), and the new and sprightly translation (with valuable notes) by Chauncey D. Leake. Harvey's (p. 17) "Sed me hercule porositates nullae sunt, neque demonstraripossunt," is translated in the first English text (1653), "But by my troth there are no such pores, nor can they be demonstrated"; by Willis (p. 17), "But, in faith, no such pores can be demonstrated, neither in fact do any such exist"; and by Leake (p. 21), "But, damn it, no such pores exist, nor can they be demonstrated."—Lytton Strachey: Elizabeth and Essex (1928, p. 51, passim).

Malpighi—Michael Foster: Malpighi and the Physiology of Glands and Tissues (History of Physiology, 1901, 84-120).—William George MacCallum: Marcello Malpighi (Johns Hopkins Hospital Bulletin, 1905, 275-84).—His first published work (two letters written in 1661 to Borelli, announcing his discovery of the capillaries) translated from the Latin by James Young: Malpighi's "De Pulmonibus" (Proceedings of the Royal Society of Medicine, 1929, 1-11).—Arturo Castiglioni: Antonio Maria Valsalva (Medical Life, 1923, 466-89).

Individuals—Beginning with this period, so many important workers emerge, that individual names must be consulted in the standard bibliographies already cited.—See also, Fielding H. Garrison: Available Sources and Future Prospects of Medical Biography (Bulletin of New York Academy of Medicine, 1928, 586-607).

The Royal Touch—Richard Wiseman: Several Chirurgicall Treatises (1676, p. 87, passim).—T. Longmore: Biographical Study of Richard Wiseman (1891, 137-42).—Illustrated monograph by Raymond Crawfurd: The King's Evil (1911, 187 pp.).

Witchcraft—Malleus Maleficarum, by the inquisitors Jacob Sprenger and Henricus Institoris, was first issued about 1486, and went through many editions until the close of the 17th century; Osler had the edition of 1669, which was one of the most complete; see the numerous items indexed under Witchcraft in Bibliotheca Osleriana.— Sir Thomas Browne: Religio Medici, 1642; in the edition of C. H. Herford for Everyman's Library, Browne's remarks on witchcraft are on p. 34; A. H. Bullen's article on Browne (Dictionary of National Biography, 1886, vii, 64-72).—Henry Charles Lea: History of the Inquisition of the Middle Ages (1887, vol. iii, 492-549, important chapter on the early persecutions for witchcraft).—The librarian of Bamberg, F. Leitschuch, published the letter of Johann Junius (Beiträge zur Geschichte des Hexenwesens in Franken, 1883).—E. T. Withington: John Weyer and the Witch Mania (Singer's Studies, 1917, i, 189-224; we are much indebted to this valuable essay; the Johann Junius episode and letter on 208-12).—Numerous papers by George Lincoln Burr listed in the bibliography of Preserved Smith: A History of Modern Culture (1930, i, 641-4; Smith's chapter on Superstition, 425-58).

X—MEDICINE IN THE EIGHTEENTH CENTURY

Foremost Contributors—In his latter years, Sir William Osler (1849-1919) compiled a list of the greatest names in medicine from Hippocrates to Röntgen. Of these outstanding 67, the following 17, in the order indicated, were admitted into his Bibliotheca Prima as contributors of first rank to the medicine of the eighteenth century: George Berkeley, Irish bishop and metaphysician; Stephen Hales, English clergyman, physiologist, inventor; Hermann Boerhaave, Dutch physician; Linnaeus, Swedish botanist; Joseph Black, Scottish chemist and physicist; Albrecht von Haller, Swiss physiologist; Giovanni Battista Morgagni, Italian pathological anatomist; Joseph Priestley, English liberal clergyman and man of science; Antoine Laurent Lavoisier, French chemist; John Howard, English prison reformer; Lazzaro Spallanzani, Italian physiologist; Henry Cavendish, English chemist and physicist; John Hunter, Scottish physiologist and surgeon; Luigi Galvani, Italian physiologist and electrician; John Dalton, English Quaker, chemist and mathematician; Edward Jenner, English physician; Thomas Robert Malthus, English clergyman and political economist (Bibliotheca Osleriana, items 1066-1300). Of several of the names in this list, there can be no dispute, but others are open to question, and the inclusion of Berkeley (conspicuous in medicine as the apostle of the tar-water panacea, and in science as the enemy of algebra) is inexcusable. In reference to his "primarians," Osler's editors say, very justly (p. xi): "No two competent judges would perhaps agree to endorse the whole list; a few of the names must surprise them." It was Osler's contention that catalogues of old medical books make interesting reading, and Bibliotheca Osleriana is undoubtedly the most inspiring catalogue ever published.

Weikard—Autobiography of Melchior Adam Weikard, A Picture of 18th Century Medicine in Germany, edited and translated by William Ferdinand Petersen (Medical Life, 1927, 52-82).

Théophile de Bordeu—Max Neuburger: Essays in the History of Medicine (1930, 105-15, a discussion of Bordeu as the precursor of the doctrine of internal secretions).—Arthur Weil: History of the Internal Secretions (Medical Life, 1925, 73-97).

Wolstein—Robert Rosenthal: A Controversy on Venesection in Vienna at the Close of the 18th Century (Janus; tr. in Medical Life, 1922, 585-90).

Thomas Fuller—Ludvig Hektoen: Thomas Fuller, Country Physician and Pioneer Exponent of Specificness in Infection and Immunity (Bulletin of Society of Medical History of Chicago, 1922, 321-333).

Quackery—John Cordy Jeaffreson: A Book about Doctors (1860, formulae of Joanna Stephens' medicines, 185-7).—Alfred Binet and Charles Féré: Animal Magnetism (1888, report of the Commission appointed to investigate mesmerism, 16-25).—A. C. Wootton: Chronicles of Pharmacy (1910, 2 vols.).

Social Conditions—Ernest Roucayrol (1907, l.c.).—Jacob Rosenbloom: Statements of Medical Interest from the Life of Jacques Casanova (Medical Life, 1923, passim).—Diderot's letter and de Branciforto incident in Léon Bizard: Souvenirs d'un Médecin des Prisons de Paris (1925[12], 177-9), an important social document by a physician whose official experience included 400,000 prostitutes; recently Englished (MS.).

Hygiene—Works and biographies of Stephen Hales, John Pringle, James Lind, John Howard, John Coakley Lettsom.—The indispensable volumes of Charles Creighton: History of Epidemics in Britain (1891, for typhus or jail-fever in 18th century, ii, 54-159).

XI—MODERNIZATION OF MEDICINE

Dissection of the Dead—Samuel Warren (Passages from the Diary of a Late Physician, 1830): "You expect us to cure you of disease, and yet deny us the only means of learning *how?* You would have us bring you the ore of skill and experience, yet forbid us to break the soil, or sink a shaft! Is this fair, *fair* reader? Is this reasonable?"— Other novels in which resurrectionists appear, by David Macbeth Moir (Life of Mansie Wauch, Tailor in Dalkeith), Bulwer-Lytton (Children of Night), Charles Dickens (A Tale of Two Cities), Robert Louis Stevenson (The Body-Snatcher, in Tales and Fantasies). The humorous verses of Thomas Hood (Mary's Ghost, A Pathetic Ballad), always quoted in this connection, are in extremely bad taste, and should be buried.—Bransby Blake Cooper: Life of Sir Astley Cooper (1843, i, 339-448).—Henry Lonsdale: Life of Robert Knox (1870, 54-116). —Sir Dominic John Corrigan: Reminiscences of a Medical Student Prior to the Passing of the Anatomy Act (British Medical Journal, 1879, p. 59).—George MacGregor: History of Burke and Hare and of the Resurrection Times (1884).—James Blake Bailey, editor of: The Diary of a Resurrectionist (1896).—S. S. Sprigge: Life and Times of Thomas Wakley (1897, several references to Henry Warburton).— Alexander Macalister: Memoir of James Macartney (1900).—Frank Baker: A History of Bodysnatching (Washington Medical Annals, 1916, 247-53).—William Roughead: Burke and Hare (1921, illustrated, full report of trial, 95-258).—James Moores Ball: Sack-'em-up Men (1928, 216 pp., considerable irrelevant material, but covers the subject, illustrated).

General Statement—As a rule, medical historians prefer to conclude their labors with the year 1800; fortunately, an exception is found in Fielding H. Garrison, half of whose standard volume is devoted to the modern period. References to most of the important medical investigators of the nineteenth and twentieth centuries are readily available in his History of Medicine (1929[4], 996 pp.).—The following essays on modern scientists are included in Victor Robinson: Pathfinders in Medicine (1929[2], 283-787): Berzelius, Samuel Guthrie, Laennec, Purkyně, Schleiden-Schwann, Henle, Darwin, Simpson, Duchenne of Boulogne, Claude Bernard, Hebra, Semmelweis, Elizabeth Blackwell, Pasteur, Koch, Metchnikoff, Pavloff.

Aviation Medicine—Paul Bert: La Pression Barométrique (Paris, 1878, 1168 pp.); the classic research in aviation physiology; flight surgeons (a term devised March, 1918) now regard Paul Bert as the father of aviation medicine.—Henry Graeme Anderson: The Medical and Surgical Aspects of Aviation (London, 1919); the first British textbook on aviation medicine.—Louis Hopewell Bauer: Aviation Medicine (Baltimore, 1926); first American textbook on the subject.

XII—MEDICINE IN AMERICA

Sources—The original source of publication of important contributions is given in Fielding H. Garrison: Texts Illustrating the History of Medicine (Index-Catalogue Library of Surgeon-General's Office, 1912, xvii, 89-178) which is practically complete for American references.

Revolutionary Period—James Thacher: A Military Journal during the American Revolutionary War (1827[2]).—Joseph Meredith Toner: Contributions to the Annals of Medical Progress and Medical Education in the United States before and during the War of Independence (1874); Medical Men of the Revolution (1876).—John E. Lane: Jean-François Coste, Chief Physician of the French Expeditionary Forces in the American Revolution (Americana, 1928, i, 30 pp.).

Journalism—Victor Robinson: The Early Medical Journals of America, founded during the Quarter-Century 1797-1822 (Medical Life, 1929, 553-85, with portraits of the pioneer editors and facsimile of McDowell's original article on ovariotomy).

Anesthesia—Osler collected over 150 documents on anesthesia, some of great rarity (Bibliotheca Osleriana, items 1352-1506).

Centennial Year—Edward H. Clarke, Henry J. Bigelow, Samuel D. Gross, T. Gaillard Thomas, John S. Billings: A Century of American Medicine (1876).—S. D. Gross: History of American Medical Literature from 1776 to the Present Time (1876). The history of American surgery has had no more prolific contributor than Gross (1851-61-76); his writings retain a certain value, but their florid enthusiasm must frequently be checked by sharp incisions from the pen of Billings.

Medical History in America—The simple-mannered man who hitched his horse to a fence and walked to the White House was the only American president interested in science. Thomas Jefferson (1743-1826), the correspondent of Jenner, was our first comparative philologist, pioneer vertebrate paleontologist, and the founder of the University of Virginia. Jefferson, as Rector of the University, imported from the mother country an Englishman to teach anatomy, surgery, medical theory, physiology, materia medica, pharmacy and the history of medicine. So the youthful savant, Robley Dunglison, amid his multifarious duties, delivered lectures on the history of medicine, which were later published in a volume.

One would suppose that medical history in America, beginning under such auspicious circumstances, would develop logically and systematically. But a country passing through the throes of pioneer days, looks toward the future and not the past. Most of our medical students were then trained by preceptors, and a doctor who carries his office in his saddle-bags is not equipped to discuss the ancients. After the preceptor system was supplanted by college training, we did not find leisure to add instruction in medical history to the curriculum. Now and then some member of the faculty would come across a copy of Le Clerc or Freind, and excited by his discovery, would arrange to cover the subject within a few hours. The course was optional, illattended, there were neither source-books nor incunabula, not even an empty cigar-box was put aside as a foundation for a museum or an institute, and by the following semester the lecturer's enthusiasm was apt to be at an end. Over many of these courses it is simply an act of charity to throw the mantle of silence. Students who heard them must have conceived an unconquerable aversion for medical history.

Although specialism in America developed alarmingly, the idea prevailed that medical history, if mentioned at all, could be taught by any lecturer without special training. Of the existence and methods of medical historiography, our schools knew nothing. Even if the lecturer devoted himself to the subject and was well-informed, he failed to gain academic recognition for medical history. For example, Eugene Fauntleroy Cordell (1843-1913) was only honorary professor of history of medicine at the University of Maryland, and when he passed away no attempt was made at the time to secure a successor. As an instance of the neglect of medico-historical instruction in the United States, Cordell was once asked by a well-known Johns Hopkins professor, "Who is Aretaeus?" (Personal communication).

It cannot be denied that the situation became a reproach. What was permissible in 1800, was inexcusable in 1900. While Pagel at Berlin, Sudhoff at Leipzig, and Neuburger in Vienna, were showing their students the tools of medico-historical research, America remained under the impression that medical history meant a collection of interesting anecdotes about famous physicians. Without the schools, however, we began to learn, and a genuine extra-curricular interest grew and developed, fostered by the example of such leading men as Abraham Jacobi, Silas Weir Mitchell, John Shaw Billings, William Osler, and William Henry Welch. Until well within the twentieth century, the American devotees of medical history were few; as Jacobi stated in the introduction to the first edition of Pathfinders in Medicine (1912, p. 7): "In America the history of medicine is almost never taught, and as long as our universities do not teach it, the pupils feel encouraged to neglect it. We have no journal devoted to the history of medicine, and our books on the subject are few." The following year the situation was changed by the appearance of Garrison's important History of Medicine (1913). Jacobi (1830-1919) lived to see the founding of the Annals of Medical History (New York, 1917). A few years later, Medical Life was established (New York, 1920) as the first monthly journal in the English language devoted to the history of medicine.

In spite of increasing interest in various directions, the academic taboo seemed unbreakable, yet it arrived with a dramatic suddenness which made it front page news. Our newspapers informed us (November 7, 1926) that the Johns Hopkins University of Baltimore had set aside an appropriation for a complete department of medical history under the professorship of Welch. At the dedication of the William H. Welch Medical Library (Fielding H. Garrison, then Librarian), Harvey Cushing delivered the main address; the following day (October 18, 1929), after introductory remarks by Welch, the Department of History of Medicine of Johns Hopkins University was inaugurated by Karl Sudhoff, who at the age of seventy-six came on his initial voyage to America for that purpose. Always a beautiful sight to see Sudhoff and Welch together, never was it more so than on the memorable occasion when medical history in America ceased to be an academic stepchild. Other universities have since instituted courses, and some have established chairs.—Victor Robinson: The Teaching of Medical History in America, remarks at the University of Amsterdam, July 22, 1927 (Sixième Congrès International d'Histoire de la Médecine, Leyde-Amsterdam, 1929, pp. 274-5).

XIII—SOCIOLOGY IN AMERICA

Since John Stuart Mill knew considerable Greek at the age of three, studied linguistics and Euclid at eight, and mastered numerous disciplines in his youth, it is not surprising that at thirty he cast about for a new science to conquer. He experimented (1836) with such phrases as the natural history of society, speculative politics, social economy, social philosophy, and social science, but in the following year Auguste Comte introduced the word sociology (1837), whereupon Mill, with characteristic generosity, adopted and popularized that now familiar term.

The story of medicine is incomplete if it fails to recognize its sociological background. A Curriculum Guide for Schools of Nursing (National League of Nursing Education) allots 30 hours to sociology and the same amount of time to social problems in nursing service. The Quarterly Cumulative Index Medicus (American Medical Association) classifies current articles under Social Conditions, Social Hygiene, Social Insurance, Social Medicine, Social Security, Social Service.

References—How the Other Half Lives (1890), by the Danish-born journalist, Jacob August Riis.—Lillian D. Wald: The House on Henry Street (1915); Windows on Henry Street (1934), the title suggested by Ernest Poole; Miss Wald, who founded the first nurses' settlement (1893), in that year introduced the winged phrase, "public health nurses."—Encyclopaedia of the Social Sciences (1930-34), 15 vols. edited by Edwin Robert Anderson Seligman and Alvin Johnson. —Dictionary of American Biography (1928-36), 20 vols. edited by Allen Johnson and Dumas Malone.—Dictionary of American History (1940), 6 vols. edited by James Truslow Adams.—Russell H. Kurtz (ed.): Social Work Year Book (Russell Sage Foundation, 1943).

INDEX

INDEX

Aaron of Alexandria [7th century], 158
Abdallatif of Bagdad [1161-1231], 191-2
Aben, Ezra, *See* Abraham ibn Ezra
Abernethy, John [1764-1831], 385
Abnormal hunger (*boulimia*), first description of, 71
Abracadabra, 193-4
Abraham ibn Ezra [1092-1167], 202
Adam of Cremona [*fl.* 1227], 204
Adam's missing rib, 256
Adams, Robert [1791-1875], 392
Addison, Joseph [1672-1719], 342
Addison, Thomas [1793-1860], 392, 433
Adelard of Bath [12th century], 202
Aegidius of Corbeil (Gilles de Corbeil) [*fl.* 1170], 220
Aeschylus [525-456 B. C.], 40
Aesculapius, 33-37, 41, 46, 48, 51, 83, 91, 119, 314, 329, 465
Aëtius of Amida [6th century], 110
Agnodice, 69-70
Ahmad ibn Yusuf [*fl.* 900], 202
Akhnaton (Amenophis IV) [*reigned* 1375-1358 B. C.], 22-25
Albertus Magnus (Albert Bollstädt) [*c.* 1206-80], 183, 216, 280, 320
Albinus, Bernhard Siegfried [1697-1770], 328
Albucasis (Abulqasim Zahrawi, Abulcasis, Alsaharavius) [1013-1106], 164-7, 191, 202, 230, 243
Alcmaeon of Crotona [6th century B. C.], 38, 56, 68
Alderotti, Taddeo [1223-1303], 220-1

Alexander the Great [356-323 B. C.], 55-56, 61-64, 208
Alexander of Hales [*d.* 1245], 183
Alexander the Paphlagonian [2nd century], 119-20, 134
Alexander VI (Rodrigo Borgia) [1431-1503], 238-9
Alfraganus (al-Farghani) [*fl.* 850], 202
Alhazen (Ibn al-Haitham) [*c.* 965-1039], 202, 206
Ali ibn Abbas. *See* Haly Abbas
Ali ibn Isa (Jesu Haly) of Bagdad [11th century], 191
Ali ibn Ridwan of Cairo [*c.* 998-*c.* 1061], 202
Ali al-Tabari (Abul Hasan Ali ibn Sahl ibn Rabban al-Tabari), [*fl.* 850], 151-2, 158, 160
Alkaloids, 393
Alkindus (al-Kindi) [9th century], 202, 206
Alpharabius (al-Farabi) [*d.* 950], 160, 179
Alpino, Prospero [1553-1617], 246, 328
Althaus, Julius (electrolysis), 393
Amatus Lusitanus [1511-62], 252
American medical journalism, origin of, 455-64
Ammianus Marcellinus [*c.* 325-*c.* 391], 67
Ammonius Lithotomus (Ammonius the Lithotomist) of Alexandria [*c.* 1st century B. C.], 77
Amulets. *See* Magic
Amyntas II, father of Philip of Macedon, 77

INDEX

Ana, Countess of Chinchon [17th century], 313
Anaritius (al-Nairīzī) [-922], 202
Anatoli (Anatolio, Abtalion) Jacob [fl. 1194-1256], 204
Anaxagoras [c. 500 B. C.], 40, 133
Anaxarchus [c. 340 B. C.], 62
Anaximander [c. 611-547 B. C.], 38
Anaximenes of Miletus [6th century B. C.], 38
Andral, Gabriel [1797-1876], 392
Andrew the Jew, 203
Anel, Dominique [1628-1725], 340
Anesthesia, 226, 420, 471-6
Animal-hospitals of Asoka, 141
Antisepsis, 226, 420-23, 476-9
Antonius Musa [fl. 23 B. C.], 96-7
Antyllus [2nd century], 111-12, 167
Apelles, 48, 62, 103, 129
Aphorisms, 52, 228-9
Apollo, 33-37, 83, 119-20, 475
Apollonius of Alexandria [2nd century], 66, 79
Appendicitis
American contributions, 484
Among Egyptians, 16
Celsus on, 98-9
First reference to, 50
Appia 1 of Alexandria [2nd century], 73
Aquinas, Thomas (Thomas of Aquino) [c. 1227-74], 183, 320
Archagathus [fl. 219 B. C.], 90
Archigenes of Apamea [2nd century], 109
Archimedes [c. 287-212 B. C.], 81-82, 196
Arctinus of Miletus [c. 744 B. C.], 33
Arderne, John of [fl. 1370], 209, 213, 318
Aretaeus [2nd century?], 110, 114-19, 158, 328, 418, 452
Aristarchus of Samos [3rd century B. C.], 196
Aristobulus of Paneas [3rd or 4th century B. C.], 180
Aristophanes [c. 448-385 B. C.], 40-1, 56
Aristotle [384-322 B. C.], 38, 55-64, 66, 103, 133, 136, 145, 149, 160-61, 171, 179-81, 183, 192, 196, 201, 203, 205-6, 221, 240, 243, 245-6, 280, 284, 289, 296
Artemis, goddess of childbirth, 43
Arterial surgery, creation of, 112
Artificial feeding of children, first case, 34
Arzachel (al-Zarqali) [c. 1029-c. 1087], 202
Asclepiades of Bithynia [1st century B. C.], 91-93
Aselli, Gasparo [1581-1626], 294
Asklepions (healing shrines of Greece), 34-37
Asoka [reigned 264-227 B. C.], 141
Astruc, Jean [1684-1766], 350
Atanus of Amid, 184
Athenaeus of Cilicia [c. 1st century], 110
Athletes, Galen's protest against, 129-30
Atom in antiquity, 92
Atra bilis of ancient pathology, 71, 91, 159
Attalus Philometor [d. 133 B. C.], 77
Aubrey, John [1626-97], 282, 284-7, 292
Auenbrugger, Leopold [1722-1809], 330-1, 372
Auerbach, Leopold [1828-97], 403
Augustine, Saint [354-430], 195, 213, 320
Aulus Gellius. See Gellius.
Automata at Alexandria, 80-1
Avendeut, John (John of Seville?) [fl. 1135-53], 202
Avenzoar (Ebn Zohr) of Cordova [1113-62], 164, 167-71, 191
Averroes of Cordova [1126-98], 164, 170-2, 191, 203, 268, 414
Avicenna (Ibn Sina) [980-1037], 160-4, 167, 179, 190-1, 199, 202-3, 206, 221-2, 230, 240-3, 245-6, 268-70, 280, 284

Bacon, Francis (Baron Verulam) [1561-1626], 283, 319, 454
Bacon, Roger [c. 1214-c. 1294], 184, 203, 205-8
Bacteriology, Eighteenth Century, 357-8; Greek, 117-18; Modern, 401-29;

Primitive, 10; Renaissance, 276-7; Roman, 96; Seventeenth Century, 309-10
Baer, Karl Ernst von [1792-1876], 386
Baglivi, Giorgio [1668-1706], 301
Bagnall, Anthony [17th century], 444
Bard, John [1716-99], 457
Bar Hebraeus (Abul-Faraj Gregorius) [1226-86], 184, 191
Bartels, Ernst Daniel August [1778-1838], 386
Bartholinus, Thomas [1616-80], 302
Bartlett, Elisha [1804-55], 454
Barton, Benjamin Smith [1766-1815], 435
Basedow, Carl Adolph [1799-1854], 436
Bassi, Laura Maria Caterina [1711-78], 338
Bayley, Richard [1745-1801], 457
Beaumont, William [1785-1853], 465-9
Bees, Aristotle on, 57
Behring, Emil von [1854-1917], 419
Bell, Benjamin [1749-1806], 423
Bell, Sir Charles [1774-1842], 385, 391
Bellini, Lorenzo [1643-1704], 295, 328
Bellonius (Pierre Belon) [1517-64], 246
Benjamin of Tudela [12th century], 186
Berkeley, George [1685-1753], 345
Bernard, Claude [1813-78], 429-31, 433, 450, 469
Berzelius, Jöns Jakob [1779-1848], 388, 393
Bethencourt, Jacques de (on venereal disease), 274-5
Bezoar Stone, 167-8
Bibago, Abraham (Bibas-Vivas) [fl. 1446-89], 180
Bichat, Marie-François-Xavier [1771-1802], 373-4
Bigelow, Henry Jacob [1818-90], 473-4
Billings, John Shaw [1838-1913], 454
Bismarck, Otto Eduard Leopold von, Prince [1815-98], 399
Black Death, 231-2
Black, Joseph [1728-99], 345
Bleeder's disease (*hemophilia*), First modern description, 457; First reference to, 166-7

Blondus, Michael Angelus (Biondo) [1497-1565], 245
Boccaccio, Giovanni [1313-75], 232-3
Body-snatching. *See* Resurrectionists
Boeck, Carl Wilhelm (leprosy), 418
Boerhaave, Hermann [1668-1738], 327-9, 336, 376, 408
Bohun, Lawrence [-1622], 444
Bonet, Théophile [1620-89], 337
Bonnet, Charles [1720-93] of Geneva, 333
Boniface VIII (Benedetto Gaetano) [*Pope*, 1294-1303], 222
Bontius, Jacobus [1592-1631], 311
Bordeu, Théophile de [1722-76], 339-40
Borelli, Giovanni Alfonso [1608-79], 295-8
Bosquillon, Édouard-François-Marie [1744-1814], 423
Bossuet, Jacques Bénigne [1627-1704], 303
Bouchard, Charles-Jacques [1837-1915], 393
Bourignon, Antoinette [1616-80], 304
Boyle, Robert [1627-91], 296, 307
Brasavolus, Antonius Musa [1500-55], 244, 275
Bretonneau, Pierre [1778-1862], 392
Briggs, Henry [1561-1630], 319
Bright, Richard [1789-1858], 391
Brissot, Pierre [1478-1522], 241
Brodie, Sir Benjamin Collins [1783-1862], 385, 462
Bronze Age, origin of, 11
Brookes, Joshua [1761-1833], 375
Brosses, Charles de [1709-77], 353
Broussais, François-Joseph-Victor [1772-1838], 372-3
Brown, Charles Brockden [1771-1810], 461
Brown, John [1735-88], 334
Brown-Séquard, Charles Edouard [1817-94], 430, 432-4
Browne, Launcelot [*d.* 1605], 282
Browne, Sir Thomas [1605-82], 318, 323
Brunfels, Otho [1464-1534], 246-7
Brunner, John Conrad [1653-1727], 319
Bruno, Giordano [*c.* 1548-1600], 278

Bruno of Longoburgo [*c.* 1252], 226-7, 230
Bucer, Martin [1491-1551], 260
Buddha (Gotama) [*c.* 560-*c.* 480], 37, 139-44
Buddhism in medicine, 141-3
Buffon, George Louis Leclerc, Comte de [1707-88], 353
Bull of Boniface VIII, 222-4
Burke, William [1792-1829], 378-85
Burns, Robert [1759-96], 357, 380

Cadwalader, Thomas [1708-79], 449
Caelius Aurelianus [*c.* 400], 68, 94, 112
Cæsar, Gaius Julius [102-44 B. C.], 87, 96, 435
Cæsarian section, Apollo delivers Æsculapius by, 34; First case of, in America, 469-70
Caius, John [1510-73], 244, 281
Calcar, Jan Stephen van [1499-1546], 254
Caldwell, Charles [1772-1853], 354, 450, 458
Callimachus [*fl.* 250 B. C.], 66, 79
Calvin, John [1509-64], 261, 263, 265
Canano, Giambattista [1515-79], 251-2
Cancer, 110, 169-70
Canvane, Peter (oleum ricini), 355
Capillary circulation, 73, 296-7
Capillary phenomena, first experiments in, 248
Casanova de Seingalt, Giovanni Jacopo [1725-98], 345, 352
Case-histories, the first, 50-51, 54
Casserio, Giulio [1561-1616], 282, 319
Cassiodorus [*c.* 490-*c.* 580], 199
Catherine the Great [1729-96], 333, 335, 353
Cato the Censor (Marcus Porcius Cato) [234-149 B. C.], 84-85, 97, 234, 236
Catullus, Gaius Valerius [? 84-54 B. C.], 87
Cautery, 167, 227, 272-3
Cave-chronology, Aurignacian (Aurignac cave), 6; Azilian (cave Mas d'Azil), 5, 7; Madelenian (Magdalenian), from the cave La Madeleine

Gabriel de Mortillet, 5, 7; Mousterian (Le Moustier cave, Gabriel de Mortillet), 6; Solultrean (Solutré cave, Gabriel de Mortillet), 6
Caventou, Joseph Bienaimé [1795-1877], 393
Cell-theory, anticipation of, 75
Celsus, Aurelius Cornelius [25 B. C.-50 A. D.], 67, 94, 97-100, 134, 169, 240-1, 435
Celsus [*fl.* 178], author of *True Word*, 134-5
Cervantes Saavedra, Miguel de [1547-1616], 258, 319
Cesalpine, Andrea [1524-1603], 291
Champier, Symphorien [1472-1539], 261
Charaka, the Hindu Hippocrates, 139-42
Charcot, Jean-Martin [1825-93], 393, 434, 436
Chassaignac, Charles-Marie-Édouard [1805-79], 411
Cheselden, William [1688-1752], 343
Cheyne-Stokes respiration (described by Hippocrates), 392
Chiron the Centaur, 33-34
Chopart, François [1743-95], 340
Chosroes the Blessed (Nushirwan the Just) [531-79], 139, 143-4
Christodorus of Thebes [*fl.* 491-518], 57
Chrysippus of Cnidus [*c.* 365 B. C.], 67
Cicero (Marcus Tullius) [106-43 B. C.], 87, 93, 98, 121, 236, 261, 284
Circulation of blood, 249, 264-5, 288-92, 296-7, 359
Circumcision, 14, 164, 182
Claparède, Jean-Louis-René-Antoine-Édouard [1832-70], 388
Clayton, John [1693-1773], 355
Clement VI (Pierre Roger) [*Pope*, 1342-52], 231, 234, 236
Clift, William [1775-1849], 462
Clinical medicine, foundation of, 54
Clusius, Charles de l'Escluse [1526-1609], 313
Cobbett, William [1762-1835], 451
Cohn, Ferdinand Julius [1828-98], 402-4, 425
Cohnheim, Julius [1839-84], 403-4

INDEX 549

Coindet, Jean-François (iodine in goiter), 436
Coiter, Volcher [c. 1534-76], 280
Coitus as a therapeutic measure, 90, 93, 182
Colle, Giovanni [1558-1631], 311
Colles, Abraham [1773-1843], 392
Colombo (Matthaeus Realdus Columbus) [1494?-1559?], 274, 280, 291
Concussion of the brain, first work on, 227
Condorcet, Marie-Jean-Antoine-Nicolas-Caritat, Marquis de [1743-94], 366
Confucius (Kung tsze [550-478 B. C.], 37
Constantinus Africanus [c. 1020-87], 200-1, 206, 242
Contagion. See Infection
Contraria contrarius curantur, 94
Cooper, Sir Astley Paston [1768-1841], 375-8, 385, 420, 462
Copernicus, Nicolaus [1473-1543], 239, 256, 278, 390, 440
Copho of Salerno (*Anatomia porci*), 291
Cordus, Euricius [1486-1535], 246-7
Cordus, Valerius [1515-1544], 246-8
Corrigan, Sir Dominic John [1802-80], 375, 392
Corvisart, Jean-Nicolas [1755-1821], 371-2
Coschwitz, George Daniel [1679-1729], 332
Cosmas and Damian (patron saints of medicine and pharmacy), 216
Cotbian House, 187-8
Cowley, Abraham [1618-67], 306
Crateuas (Cratevas) [*fl.* 70 B. C.], 79
Crawford, Jane Todd (McDowell's patient), 463-4
Crawford, John [1746-1813], 452
Credé, Carl Siegmund Franz [1819-92], 425-6
Crookes, Sir William [1832-1919], 394
Cross-sections in anatomy, origin of, 250
Ctesias of Cnidus [5th century B. C.], 103, 195
Cullen, William [1710-90], 345, 354

Culpepper (Culpeper) Nicholas [1616-54], 447
Curie, Marie [1867-], 441
Curie, Pierre [1859-1906], 441
Curling, Thomas Blizard [1811-88], 436
Currie, James [1756-1805], 357
Curtois, Bernard (iodine), 436

Daniel of Morley (Merlai, Merlac, Marlach) [*fl.* 1170-90], 203, 210
Danielssen, Daniel Cornelius (leprosy), 418
Dante Alighieri [1265-1321], 280
Darius twists his foot, 39
Darwin, Charles (Robert) [1809-82], 376-7, 389-91, 399, 440
Darwin, Erasmus [1731-1802], 461
David, Jean-Pierre [1737-84], 340
Daviel, Jacques [1696-1762], 340
Davy, Sir Humphry [1778-1829], 393, 462, 472
Decompression operation, 10
Dee, John [1527-1608], 277-8
Democedes of Crotona [6th century B. C.], 38-40
Democritus [460?-350? B. C.], 40, 49, 92
Demonology. See Magic
De Quincey, Thomas [1785-1859], 380
Desault, Pierre-Joseph [1744-95], 373
Descartes, René [1596-1650], 319, 342
D'Eslon, Charles (mesmerism), 348-50
Despars, Jacques (Jacobus de Partibus), 241
Dhanvantari (Hindu medicine), 141
Diaz, Francisco [*fl.* 1575], 271
Diderot, Denis [1713-84], 353
Digby, Sir Kenelm [1603-65], 446
Dio Chrysostom [40-115], 65
Diocles of Carystus [*fl.* 350 B. C.], 68
Diodorus Cronus [4th century B. C.], 70-1
Diodorus the Sicilian (Diodorus Siculus) [*fl.* 21 B. C.], 16, 25
Diogenes of Apollonia (Diogenes Apolloniates) [c. 460 B. C.], 68
Diogenes Laërtius [*fl.* 222-35?], 60
Dionysius of Halicarnassus, 117

Dioscorides, Pedacius [40-90], 94, 101, 126-7, 145, 149, 184, 243, 245, 247, 355-6, 420, 474
Diphtheria, 115, 418-19
Disease-demons, 3-4, 12, 197-8
Dissection, 7, 57, 59, 67-8, 90, 122, 146, 192, 219-25, 249-60, 280-9, 294, 319, 373-85, 387
Dolet, Etienne [1509-46], 261
Domingo Gundisalvo (Dominicus Gondisalvi), 202
Donato, Marcello (pathology), 266
Dorsey, John Syng [1783-1813], 462-3
Dover, Thomas [1660-1742], 316
Drake, Daniel [1785-1852], 469
Drake, Joseph Rodman [1795-1820], 459
Drugs, Arabian, 145-7, 156; Eighteenth Century, 354-7; Egyptian, 22; Graeco-Roman, 101, 116, 124-6; Medieval, 226, 230-1; Modern, 393, 476; Pontine, 77-9; Renaissance, 246-8, 263; Seventeenth Century, 311-17
Dryden, John [1631-1700], 279, 306, 342
Du Bois-Reymond, Emil [1818-96], 388
Duchenne, Guillaume-Benjamin-Amant [1806-75], 393
Duclaux, Émile [1840-1904], 410
Duns Scotus (Doctor Subtilis) [1265?-1308?], 183
Duttha Gamani [d. 161 B. C.], 138

Edessa, Nestorian medical school at, 137-8, 145
Ehrlich, Paul [1854-1915], 426-7, 429
Electricity, 38, 277-9, 345-50, 393-4, 449
Electrotherapy, origin of, 100-1
Elsholz, Johann Sigmund [1623-88], 308
Empedocles [c. 490-430 B. C.], 40, 109
Empiric Tripod (Glaucias), 76
Empirics of Alexandria, 73-7
Endocrinology, 118, 339-40, 429-38
Ent, Sir George [1604-89], 287-8
Ephraem Syrus (Ephraim the Syrian) [4th century], 137

Epicurus [342-270 B. C.], 92, 135
Epilepsy, 3, 9, 14, 51, 117
Erasistratus [4th century B. C.], 67-75, 82
Erasmus, Desiderius [1466-1536], 244, 268-70
Eratosthenes of Cyrene [c. 276-c. 194 B. C.], 196
Estienne (Etienne) Charles [1505?-1564], 269
Eternity of Matter, 38, 181
Euclid [3rd century B. C.], 80-1, 133, 149, 160, 201, 206, 277
Eudemus of Rhodes (editor of Aristotle), 59
Euphronius (vase-painting), 40
Eupolis [c. 446-411 B. C.], 40
Euripides [480-406 B. C.], 40, 70
Eye-glasses, first medical reference to, 213
Evelyn, John [1620-1706], 318, 323
Evolution, Anaximander, first evolutionist, 38; Aristotle, a forerunner of, 58; Nineteenth Century, 389-91

Fabricius, Hieronymus (Fabrizio, Geronimo) [1537-1619], 281-2, 284, 296
Fabricius Hildanus. See Fabry, Wilhelm
Fabry, Wilhelm (Fabricius Hildanus) [1560-1624], 271, 350, 417
Facies Hippocratica, 49
Falcucci, Niccolo [d. 1412], 280
Fallopius, Gabriel [1523-62], 252, 258-9, 273, 280
Faraday, Michael [1791-1867], 393
Faraj ben Salim (Moses Farachi of Girgent) [13th century], 201
Favorinus (See under Gellius), 72
Feeding experiments, the first, 59
Feigned diseases, 125
Felix, Charles-François (Louis XIV's surgeon), 318
Fergusson, Sir William [1808-77], 382
Fernel, Jean [1497-1558], 242, 266
Finsen, Niels Ryberg [1860-1904], 441
Fistula-in-ano, 210, 213, 318-19
Fitzer, Wilhelm (Harvey's printer), 288

INDEX

Fitz-Roy, Robert [1805-65], 389
Flajani, Giuseppe [1741-1808], 436
Flamsteed, John [1646-1719], 319
Floyer, Sir John [1649-1734], 311
Fodere, François-Emmanuel [1764-1835], 435
Foesius, Anutius [1528-95], 243
Foligno, Gentile da [14th century], 280, 417
Foramen ovale, persistent, 250
Foreest, Pieter van (Petrus Forestus) [1522-97], 241
"Four Masters" of Salerno, 226
Fournier, Alfred [1832-1914], 393
Fracastorius (Girolamo Fracastoro) [1484-1553], 275-6, 280, 289, 310
Fractures, prehistoric, 8
Franco, Pierré [fl. 1560], 271
Franklin, Benjamin [1706-90], 345, 349, 447-9, 451
Frederick II [1194-1250], 203-5, 211-12, 218-19, 222
French, John [1616?-1657], 447
Freud, Sigmund [1856-], 440-1
Fries, Lorenz (Avicenna's defender), 243
Frobenius (Joannes Froben) [c. 1460-1527], 243, 268-9
Fryer, Thomas [d. 1623], 443
Fuchsius (Leonhard Fuchs) [1501-66], 244, 246-7, 356
Fuller, Samuel [1580-1633], 444
Fuller, Thomas [1654-1734], 357

Gaddesden, John of [1280?-1361], 210, 212, 230
Galen [130-200], 29, 68, 73, 74-5, 77, 79, 94, 97, 109-10, 120-22, 124, 127-28, 130-34, 136, 145, 150-51, 154, 158, 163, 169-70, 181, 184, 192-93, 196, 199, 201-2, 206, 221-22, 229-30, 237, 241-42, 244-6, 249, 251-4, 256, 261-2, 268-70, 272, 284, 290, 295, 311, 327, 329, 435, 452, 461
Galileo Galilei [1564-1642], 280, 295, 319, 390, 426
Galvani, Luigi [1737-98], 350
Gardane, Joseph-Jacques de (ethics in venereal disease), 351-2
Geber [Jabir ibn Haiyan], 191

Gedaliah ibn Yahyah, the Chronicler, 180
Geissler's vacuum tube, 394
Gellius, Aulus [c. 130-180], 59, 68, 72, 86, 96, 103, 195
Genetics, 438-40
Geologist, the first, 60
Gerard of Cremona [c. 1114-87], 202
Gerson, Johann [fl. 1467], 243
Gesner, Conrad, 244, 248
Geynes, John [d. 1563], 311
Gilbertus Anglicus (Gilbert the Englishman) [fl. 1250], 209-11
Gilbert, William [1544-1603], 277-9
Gilino, Corradino (tract on syphilis, 1497), 274
Giovanni of Monte Cassino, the illuminator, 201
Girdles of chastity, 214-15
Girolamo da Carpi (Canano's illustrator), 252
Glauber, Johann Rudolf [1604-68], 312
Glaucias [? 3rd or 2nd century B. C.], 76
Glisson, Francis [1597-1677], 304, 311-12, 332
Gmelin, Leopold [1788-1853], 388
Godwin, William [1756-1836], 366
Goethe, Johann Wolfgang von [1749-1832], 371, 385
Goiter, 87, 270, 434-8
Gold-headed cane, origin of, 9
Goliards, rhymes of the, 217
Gordon, Bernard de [1285-1318], 212-13
Graaf, Regner de [1641-73], 319
Graham, James [1745-94], 345-7
Grancher, Jacques-Joseph [1843-1907], 413-14
Graves, Robert James [1796-1853], 392
Gray, Stephen [-1736], 350
Gregory of Tours [538-94], 197
Gregory X (Tebaldo Visconti) [Pope, 1073-85], 215
Gregory X (Tebaldo Visconti) [Pope, 1271-6], 211-12
Grew, Nehemiah [1641-1712], 300, 312
Gross, Samuel David [1805-84], 433, 459
Grünpeck, Joseph (tract on syphilis, 1496), 274

Guarinonius, Christophorus [*fl. c.* 1600], 311
Guericke, Otto von [1602-86], 319, 350
Guérin, Jules [1801-86], 411
Guido de Vigevano (anatomical text, 1345), 224
Guillemeau, Jacques [1550-1612], 294
Guinterius (Guinterus, Guintherius, Guintherus, Joannes Andernacus, John Winter of Andernach) [1487-1574], 253, 262
Gull, Sir William Withey [1816-90], 436
Gutenberg, Johann [*c.* 1398-1468], 241
Guthrie, Samuel [1782-1848], 470-1
Guy de Chauliac [1300-68], 229-31, 246
Gwinne, Matthew [1558?-1627], 443

Haeckel, Ernst [1834-1919], 391
Haen, Anton de [1704-76], 327, 330-1, 347
Hahnemann, Samuel Christian Friedrich [1755-1843], 335
Haller, Albrecht von [1708-77], 331-3, 341, 345, 386, 391, 435
Halley, Edmond [1656-1742], 309, 319
Haly Abbas (Ali Abbas, Ali ibn Abbas) [*d.* 994], 158-60, 191, 200-1, 206, 221, 230
Hansen, Armauer [1841-1912], 418
Hare, William [*fl.* 1829], 378-85
Harris, Walter [1647-1732], 311
Harun al-Rashid [*c.* 766-809], 149, 186
Harvey, William [1578-1657], 281-93, 295, 302, 326, 328, 344, 359, 443
Hasdai ibn Shaprut (Abu Yusuf ben Isaac ben Ezra) [*c.* 915-*c.* 90], 191
Hauksbee, Francis, the elder [*d.* 1713?], 350
Havers, Clopton [-1702], 319
Hawkins, Sir Cæsar [1711-86], 343-4
Haymen, Georges (hematology), 393
Hayward, George [1791-1863], 479
"Healing by first intention," 226
"Healing by second intention," 226
Heberden, William [1710-1801], 354, 462
Heister, Lorenz [1683-1758], 341
Heliodorus the Surgeon, 110-11
Heliotherapy, origin of, 25

Helmholtz, Hermann Ludwig Ferdinand von [1821-94], 387
Helmont, Johannes Baptista van [1577-1644], 386, 409
Henle (Friedrich Gustav) Jakob [1809-85], 388, 395-6, 398-401
Henry, Joseph [1797-1878], 393
Henslow, John Stevens [1796-1861], 377
Heraclides of Tarentum [*c.* 240 B. C.], 82
Herder, Johann Gottfried von [1744-1803], 371
Hermann the German, 201
Hermes Trismegistus ("the thrice great Hermes"; Thoth, "scribe of the gods"), 26
Hernandez, Jean-François (inoculation of gonorrhea), 423
Herodicus of Thrace [5th century B. C.], physician-gymnast, 41-42, 50
Herodotus [*c.* 484-425 B. C.], 11, 15, 38-9, 40, 46-8, 57, 103
Herondas (Herodas) [3rd century B. C.], 79
Hero (Heron) of Alexandria [? 1st century B. C.], 80-1
Herophilus [4th century B. C.], 67-75, 77, 82
Hertz, Heinrich (Rudolf) [1857-94], 394
Hery, Thierry de [-1599], 275
Hesiod [? 8th century B. C.], 38, 196
Hewson, Thomas Tickell [1773-1848], 463
Hildebrand. *See* Gregory VII
Hildegard, Saint [1098-1179], 218
Hindu medicine, 139-43
Hipparchus [*fl.* 146-126 B. C.], 80
Hippocrates [460-370 B. C.], 40, 48-55, 66, 68, 75-6, 91, 94, 99-101, 117, 122, 126-8, 133, 145, 149, 158, 169, 181, 184, 196, 206, 218, 220-1, 234, 241-2, 243, 245, 261, 271-3, 280, 295, 315, 317, 344, 373, 392, 394, 418, 454-5
Hippocratic Oath, 54-5, 100
Hobbes, Thomas [1588-1679], 288
Hodgkin, Thomas [1798-1866], 391-2
Hodgson, Joseph [1788-1869], 391
Holmes, Oliver Wendell [1809-94], 424, 453, 458, 474-9

INDEX

Homer [*c.* 1000 B. C.], 29-33, 41, 64, 66, 79, 196, 233-4, 236, 240
Hooke, Robert [1635-1703], 296, 308-9
Hooker, Sir Joseph Dalton [1817-1911], 390
Horace (Quintus Horatius Flaccus) [65-8 B. C.], 87, 97, 245
Horror vacui, 73, 75
Horsley, Sir Victor [1857-1916], 436-7
Hosack, David [1769-1835], 460, 465
Hospitals, 138, 141, 146, 158, 185-9
Howard, John [1726-90], 362-3
Hubaish ibn al-Hasan of Bagdad [9th century], 150
Hugh of Lucca [*fl.* 1250], 226, 228, 230
Hugo, Victor [1802-85], 431
Humboldt, Alexander von [1769-1859], 385, 397-9, 474
Humoral pathology, 71, 159
Hunain ibn Ishaq (Joannitius) [809-77], 146-51, 184, 191, 202
Hunter, John [1728-93], 363-6, 374, 385, 408, 423
Hunter, William [1718-83], 341
Huxley, Thomas Henry [1825-95], 391
Huygens, Christian [1629-95], 319
Hydrostatics, founder of, 81
Hygiene in eighteenth century, 359-63
Hyginus, Gaius Julius [-?10], 70
Hypatia [*c.* 370-415], 136
Hypodermic syringe, origin of, 81

Ibn el-Chatib (on contagion), 191
Ibn Ezra. *See* Abraham ibn Ezra
Ibn Khallikan (Abul Abbas Ahmad ibn Khallikan) [1211-82], 152
Ibn Tibbon, Samuel [1150-1230], 177
Iliad, medicine in, 29-33
Imhotep [*fl.* 2900 B. C.], 33
Immunity, 78, 171, 370
Incunabula (cradle books), 242-3
Infection, 48, 95-6, 117-18, 210, 229, 276-7, 357-8, 401
Innocent VIII (Giovanni Battista Cibo) [*Pope,* 1484-92], 320
Intravenous medication, origin of, 307-8

Intraventricular moderator band, discovery of, 250
Ion of Chios [5th century B. C.], 40
Isidore of Seville (Isidorus Hispalensis) [*c.* 560-636], 215
Isocrates [436-338 B. C.], 117
Isaac Israeli the Elder (Isaac Judaeus, Ishaq al-Israili) [832-932], 191, 200, 206, 211
Island of Æsculapius, 83
Itch mite (Acarus scabiei), early description of, 168

Jabir ibn Haijan. *See* Geber
Jackson, Charles Thomas [1805-80], 473-5
Jackson, James [1777-1867], 465
Jail fever (typhus), 360-3
James, Robert [1705-76], 344
Jehuda ben Solomon Cohen (Spanish encyclopedist), 204
Jenner, Edward [1749-1823], 369-70, 412, 462
Jerome, Saint (Eusebius Sophronius Hieronymus) [*c.* 340-420], 197
Joannitius. *See* Hunain ibn Ishaq
Jobert de Lamballe, Antoine-Joseph [1799-1867], 479, 482
John the Grammarian, 149
John XXI (Petrus Hispanus) [*Pope,* 1276-7], 211, 217
John the Saracen (Joannes Saracenus), [*c.* 1040-*c.* 1103], 201
Johnson, Samuel [1709-84], 344
Joly, Nicolas [1812-85], 410
Jonathan of Lunel [12th-13th centuries], 182
Jones, Margaret [-1648], 445
Jonson, Ben [1573-1637], 286
Josephus, Flavius [*c.* 37-*c.* 95], 180
Juba, King of Mauritania ("the African Varro"), 97, 102
Judah ibn Shoshan, 173
Jundisapur, 138-9, 144-7, passim
Junius, John. *See* under Witchcraft
Jupille, Jean Baptiste (Pasteur's patient), 414-15
Juvenal (Decimus Junius Juvenalis) [*c.* 60-140], 87, 94, 110, 113, 435

Kämpf, Johann [18th century], 334
Kelly (Kelley) Edward [1555-95], 277
Kepler, Johann [1571-1630], 319, 390, 426
al-Khwarizmi [-c. 850], 145, 202
King's Evil, 317-18, 445
Kircher, Athanasius [1602-80], 310
Kirkland, Thomas [1722-98], 477
Kitasato, Baron Shibasaburo [1852-1931], 405, 407
Klebs, Edwin [1834-1913], 419
Knox, Robert [1791-1862], 378-85
Koch, Robert [1843-1910], 401-7, 425-7
Kocher, Theodor [1841-1917], 436
Kölliker, Albert von [1817-1905], 388
Kuhn, Adam [1741-1817], 355

Laennec, René-Théophile-Hyacinthe [1781-1826], 372-3, 386
Lancisi, Giovanni Maria [1655-1720], 301
Lanfranchi of Milan [-1315], 227-8
Lange, Johannes [1485-1565], 241
Larrey, Felix-Hippolyte, Baron [1808-95], 415, 482
Lavoisier, Antoine-Laurent [1743-94], 349
Lead poisoning (*plumbism*), 116
Leeuwenhoek, Anthony van [1632-1723], 305, 310
Leibnitz, Gottfried Wilhelm [1646-1716], 319
Leo Africanus (Johannes Leo, Giovanni Leone) [c. 1494-1552], 172
Leo X (Giovanni de' Medici) [*Pope, 1513-21*], 239, 251
Leonard of Pisa (Leonardus Pisanus) [13th century], 204
Leonardo da Vinci [1452-1519], 248-51
Leoniceno, Niccolò [1428-1524], 241-246, 273-274
Leprosy, 99, 100, 210, 212-13, 215, 270, 418
Lettsom, John Coakley [1744-1815], 362
Licensure, origin of, 185-6, 218-19
Lichtheim, Ludwig [1845-1928], 403
Liebig, Justus von [1803-73], 408-9
Ligature, Alexandrian knowledge of, 73; Graeco-Roman knowledge of, 99, 111-12; Reintroduced by Paré, 272
Linacre, Thomas [1460?-1524], 244, 281
Linnæus (Carl von Linné) [1707-78], 332, 354, 391
Lister, Joseph, Baron [1827-1912], 421-3, 474, 478
Liston, Robert [1794-1847], 374, 420, 474
Livy (Titus Livius) [59 B. C.-17 A. D.], 109, 117
Locke, John [1632-1704], 306, 319
Loculus, the first puzzle, 81
Löffler, Friedrich August Johannes [1852-1915], 419
Long, Crawford Williamson [1815-78], 471-2, 475
Lonsdale, Henry [1816-76], 382
Lopez, Roderigo [-1594], 283-4
Louis, Pierre - Charles - Alexandre [1787-1872], 392
Lover's pulse, 74
Lovesickness, treatment of, 159
Lowe, Peter [c. 1550-c. 1612], 243
Lower, Richard [1631-91], 296, 307
Lucan (Marcus Annæus Lucanus) [39-65], 63, 87, 164
Lucian of Samosata [120-180], 73, 119-20, 134-5
Lucilius Junior (correspondent of Seneca), 182
Lucretius (Titus Lucretius Carus) [c. 98-55 B. C.], 92-3, 117, 276
Ludwig, Carl (Friedrich Wilhelm) [1816-95], 388
Lull, Raymond [c. 1235-1315], 218
Luther, Martin [1483-1546], 239, 269
Lycophron [*fl.* 285-247 B. C.], 79
Lyell, Sir Charles [1797-1875], 390-1

Macartney, James [1770-1843], 385
Macaulay, Thomas Babington, Baron [1800-59], 385
Machaon, son of Æsculapius, 33
Magendie, François [1783-1855], 393, 408, 430
Magic, Arabian, 145, 167-8; Egyptian, 12-13, 19, 21, 25-7; Greek, 35-7; Medieval, 193-6, 203, 207, 209-10,

INDEX

216, 233; Primitive, 3-5, 9-10; Renaissance, 239, 270-1; Roman, 85, 102-9
Maimon (Maimun) Ben Joseph [12th century], 172-3
Maimonides (Moses ben Maimon) [1135-1204], 164, 172-5, 177-183, 191, 201, 204, 243
Malmesbury, Oliver of [*fl.* 1066], 216
Malpighi, Marcello [1628-94], 294-6, 298, 302, 305
Malthus, Thomas Robert [1766-1834], 366-7, 369, 390
Manardi, Giovanni [1462-1536], 241
Man's origin, 92
Mansur Gilafan (Mansurian Hospital), 187-8
Manutius, Aldus [1450-1515], 243-4
Maqrīzi (al-Macrizi, Makrīzi, Taqi ud-Din Ahmad ibn Ali) [1364-1442], 187-9
Marcellus Empiricus of Bordeau [*fl.* 385], 194
Marcus Aurelius Antoninus [121-180], 124-5, passim
Martial (Marcus Valerius Martialis) [38 ?-102 ? A. D.], 87, 95, 113, 164
Masarjawaih (smallpox), 158
Mather, Cotton [1663-1728], 323, 444
Mather, Increase [1639-1723], 323
Matthew Paris [-1259], 204
Maurus, Rabanus (Opus universum, 1467), 243
Maxwell, James Clerk [1831-79], 394
Mayerne, Theodore Turquet de [1573-1655], 311-12
Mayow, John [1643-79], 296
McDowell, Ephraim [1771-1830], 463-4
Mead, Richard [1673-1754], 344
Meckel, Johann Friedrich [1781-1833], 387
Medical slaves, 85-6
Medicine Man, 3-10
Meibomius, Henricus [1638-1700], 319
Meigs, Charles Delucena [1792-1869], 449-450, 477
Meister, Joseph (Pasteur's patient), 413, 415
Melanchthon, Philip [1497-1560], 260

Mendelssohn-Bartholdy, Jakob Ludwig Felix [1809-47], 399
Mendel, Gregor Johann [1822-84], 439-40
Menecrates of Zeophleta [*fl.* 34], 97
Meningitis, early reference to, 98
Menon [4th century B. C.], 59
Menstruation, 105-7
Mercurialis, Hieronymus [1530-1606], 243, 246
Mesmer, Franz Anton [1733-1815], 347-50
Messahala (Mashallah) [-c. 820], 202
Mesuë (Mesua), Johannes. *See* Yuhanna ibn Masawaih
Metabolism, first experiment in, 71
Metchnikoff, Eli [1845-1916], 427-9
Methodics, School of, 112
Mettauer, John Peter [1787-1875], 479
Microscope, 280, 296-301, 308-10, 386
Miller, Edward [1760-1812], 456, 460
Milon the wrestler, 40
Milton, John [1608-74], 306, 319
Mineralogist, the first, 60
Minoan civilization [*c.* 4000 B. C.], 28-9
Mitchell, John [1680?-1768], 355, 451
Mitchell, Silas Weir [1829-1914], 459
Mitchill, Samuel Latham [1764-1831], 456-62
Mithridates Eupator (Mithradates), [-63 B. C.], 77-9, 93
Mohammed (Mahomet, Muhammad), Chapter VI, passim
Mohammed ibn Tumart, 171-2
Molière (Jean Baptiste Poquelin) [1622-73], 294, 314, 319
Molyneux, Sir Thomas [1661-1733], 309
Monardes, Nicholas [1493-1588], 246
Monastic Medicine, 199
Mondeville, Henri de [-c. 1315], 228-9, 301
Monro, Alexander, primus [1697-1767], 345, 376
Monro, Alexander, secundus [1733-1817], 376
Monro, Alexander, tertius [1773-1859], 376, 384
Montanus (Giovanni Battista della Monte) [1497-1557], 273

Montesauro, Natale (tract on syphilis, 1498), 274
Morgagni, Giovanni Battista [1682-1772], 336-7
Morgan, John [1735-89], 449, 465
Morton, William Thomas Green [1819-68], 473-5
Moses, 19, 28, 181, 198, 320
Mott, Valentine [1785-1865], 465, 481
Müller, Johannes [1801-58], 387, 395, 397, 399
Mummification, 15-18
Mundinus (Mondino de' Luzzi) [c. 1276-1326], 221-4, 240
Murray, George Redmayne (thyroid feeding), 436
Musitanus, Carolus [1635-1714], 311
Musset, Alfred de [1810-57], 431
Mynsicht, Adrian [fl. 1631], 312
Myron [5th century B. C.], 40

Nägeli, Karl Wilhelm von [1817-91], 439
Napier, John [1550-1617], 319
Neckam, Alexander [1157-1217], 208, 220
Nefertiti, Queen [fl. 1350 B. C.], 23-4
Neisser, Albert [1855-1916], 425
Nélaton, Auguste [1807-73], 482
"Nerve-muscle preparation," 328
Nestorians, 136, 160 (Chapter VI)
Nestorius of Constantinople [-c. 451], 136-7
Newton, Sir Isaac [1642-1727], 309, 319, 344, 358, 360
Nicetas [11th century], 111
Nicholas V (Tomaso da Sarzana, Tomaso Parentucelli) [Pope, 1447-55], 240, bis
Nicholas the Fish, 205
Nicolaus Salernitanus (Antidotarium), 220, 226
Nightingale, Florence [1820-1910], 421
Nizami of Ganja, 191
Nizami of Samarcand, 191
Nodier, Charles [1780-1844], 431
Noeggerath, Emil [1827-95], 424-5
Norman, Robert [fl. 1590], 279
Nureddin (Arabian hospitals), 186-7

Octopus, Aristotle on, 57
Odyssey, medicine in, 32-33
Oglethorpe, James Edward [1696-1785], 360-1
Oldenburg, Henry [1615?-1677], 305
Omar Khayyam [-1123], 162
Oporinus, Joannes [1507-68], 255
Optics, 80, 280, 309
Ord, William Miller (myxedema), 436
Organotherapy, origin of, 14-15
Oribasius [325-403], 68, 111, 149, 158, 193
Origen [c. 185-c. 254], 135-6
Osler, Sir William [1849-1919], 454
Otto, Adolf Wilhelm [1786-1845], 386-7
Otto, John Conrad [1774-1844], 457, 463
Ovariotomy, the first, 463-4
Ovid (Publius Ovidius Naso) [43 B. C.-17 A. D.], 87, 117, 276
Oviedo y Valdes [1478-1547], 246, 273

Pancoast, Joseph [1805-82], 480
Papyri: Papyrus of Mother and Child, 19; Surgical Papyrus of Thebes (Edwin Smith), 19-21; Therapeutic Papyrus of Thebes (Papyrus Ebers), 21-22; Veterinary and Gynecologic Papyri from Kahun, 18-19
Paracelsus (Philippus Aureolus Theophrastus Paracelsus Bombastus von Hohenheim) [1493-1541], 266-70, 451
Parchment (pergamena), origin of, 120-1
Paré, Ambroise [1510-90], 271-3, 294, 317, 319, 419, 451, 479
Paris Faculty, 293-4, 311-12, 318
Parkinson, James [-1824], 391
Parkinson, John [1567-1650], 356
Parotid duct, discovery of, 302
Parry, Caleb Hillier [1755-1822], 435
Pasicrates [2nd or 1st century B. C.], 82
Pasteur, Louis [1822-95], 407-16, 423, 478
Patin, Guy [1601-72], 318
Patrick, Saint [c. 389-], 194

Paulus Ægineta [625-90], 111, 149, 158, 165, 193, 435
Pavloff, Ivan Petrovich [1849-   ], 469
Pecquet, Jean [1622-74], 294
Pelletier, Joseph [1788-1842], 393
Peony root, 34
Pepys, Samuel [1633-1703], 306-7, 318
Percussion, 116, 330-1, 371-2
Periclean age, 273, passim
Perkins, Elisha [1741-99], 456
Persius (Aulus Persius Flaccus) [34-62], 87
Peruvian bark (*Cortex Cinchonae*), 313-15, 393
Peter, Charles-Felix-Michel [1824-93], 416
Petit, Jean-Louis [1674-1750], 340, 417
Petrarch (Francesco Petrarca) [1304-74], 220, 230-37, 24 , 280
Petronius (Petronius Arbiter), 87
Petrus Hispanus. *See* John XXI
Petrus Lombardus [*c.* 1100-*c.* 1160], 216-17
Petty, Sir William [1623-87], 319
Pfeufer, Carl [1806-69], 400
Phaenarete, midwife, mother of Socrates, 42
Phagocytosis, discovery of, 427-9
Philetas of Cos [4th century B. C.], 48
Philinus of Cos [280 B. C.], 76-7
Philip the Acarnanian [*c.* 340 B. C.], 62
Philip II, king of Macedonia [382-336 B. C.], 55, 61
Phryne, the Athenian hetaira, 129-30
Physical diagnosis, 116, 308, 330-1, 371-3
"Physicians' skin," 20
Physick, Philip Syng [1786-1837], 456, 462
Pier della Vigna (Petrus de Vineas) [*c.* 1190-1249], 204
Pietro d'Abano (Peter of Abano) [1250-1320], 280
Pietro da Eboli (healing waters), 204
Pilatus, Leontius (Leonzio Pilato) [-1366], 233
Pindar [*c.* 522-443 B. C.], 40
Pinel, Philippe [1745-1826], 452
Piorry, Pierre Adolphe [1794-1879], 411

Pitard, Jean [1228-1315], 227
Placental development of dog-fish, 58
Plague, 33, 123-4, 231-2, 317, 367
Plant illustrations, the first, 79
Plastic surgery, 99, 111, 271
Platearius, Matthaeus [*c.* 1150], 206, 220
Plato [427-347 B. C.], 40-6, 48, 56, 59, 133, 135-6, 149, 179, 221, 291, 474
Plautus, Titus Maccius [-184 B. C.], 236
Plenciz, Marcus Anton von [1705-86], 358
Pliny the Elder (Gaius Plinius Secundus) [*c.* 23-79], 63, 68-9, 86, 90, 93-8, 101-9, 195, 206, 234, 236, 245-6, 435
Pliny the Younger (Publius Caecilius Secundus, Gaius Plinius Caecilius Secundus) [*c.* 61-*c.* 113], 102, 104-5, 109
Plotinus [204-70], 197
Plutarch [*c.* 46-120], 48, 61-3, 68, 73, 77, 81, 96, 117
Pluto (Hades), 34, 83
Pneumatic theory (forerunner of Oxygen theory), 73
Podalirius, son of Æsculapius, 33
Poisoned fruits, 77
Polyclitus [5th century B. C.], 40
Polygnotus [5th century B. C.], 40
Porphyry [233-*c.* 304], 160, 197
Postulates of Bacteriology, Henle on, 401; Koch on, 405
Post, Wright [1766-1828], 457
Pot, John [*c.* 1625], 444
Pott, Percival [1713-88], 365
Pouchet, Félix-Archimède [1800-72], 410
Powder of Sympathy, 446
Praxagoras of Cos [*fl.* 330 B. C.], 67-8, 73
Praxiteles [4th century B. C.], 129
Preventive medicine, pioneer treatise on, 72
Priessnitz, Vincenz [1799-1851], 394-5
Priestley, Joseph [1733-1804], 350, 355
Primrose (or Primerose), James [-1659], 290
Pringle, Sir John [1707-82], 422
Proclus (Proculus) [410-85], 80

Prosser, Thomas (Derby neck, 1769), 435
Prostitution, 3, 11, 47, 87-90, 100, 110, 129-30, 198, 213-15, 238-9, 352-4
Protoplasm, 387, 389, 442
Psychoanalysis, 440-1
Psychotherapy, 189-91
Ptolemy (Claudius Ptolemaeus) [- 162], 149, 151, 160, 201-2, 206
Ptolemy Euergetes [reigned 246-221 B. C.], 65
Ptolemy of Lucca, 211
Ptolemy Philadelphus [309-246 B. C.], 65
Ptolemy Soter [4th century B. c.], 65
Pulse, 5, 53, 67-9, 71, 73-4, 110, 125, 311, 359
Purkinje, Johannes Evangelista (Jan Evangelista Purkyně) [1787-1869], 385-7
Pus, 5, 226, 231, 270, 272
Pyrrho of Elis [c. 360-270 B. C.], 70, 76
Pythagoras [6th century B. c.], 40

Quackery, 9, 94-5, 119-20, 156-7, 314-15, 342-52, 456
Quintilian (Marcus Fabius Quintilianus), [c. 35-95], 86, 164

Rabbula [5th century], 137-8
Rabelais, François [c. 1490-1553], 261
Radiology, anticipation of, 208-9; discovery of, 441
Radium, discovery of, 441
Ramazzini, Bernardino [1633-1714], 311
Rameses II [reigned 1292-1225 B. C.], 16
Rameses III [c. 1198-1167 B. C.], 16
Ramsay, David [1749-1815], 454
Ramus, Petrus (Pierre de la Ramée) [1515-72], 246
Raphael Sanzio [1483-1520], 251
Rauwolf, Leonhard [-1596], 246
Ravaton, Hugues (double-flap amputation), 340
Ray, John [1627-1705], 358
Rayer, Pierre-François-Olive [1793-1867], 393

Raymond, archbishop of Toledo, 201-2
"Read the Ancients," 335
Read, Sir William [-1715], 342
Réaumur, René Antoine Ferchault de [1683-1757], 339
Rectal feeding, origin of, 170
Red blood corpuscles, discovery of, 299
Redi, Francesco [1626-97], 310
Regeneration of removed parts, 339
Reichert, Karl Bogislaus [1811-83], 388
Rejuvenation, 21, 207, 434, 484
Remak, Robert [1815-65], 388, 393
Rembrandt (Rembrandt Harmens van Rijn) [1606-69], 319
Renan, Ernest [1823-92], 414, 442
Resurrection-bone, 256
Resurrectionists, 253, 255, 374-85
Reverdin, Jacques-Louis (thyroidectomy), 436
Rhazes (Abu Bakr Muhammad ibn Zakariya al-Razi) [850-923], 111, 152-8, 160-1, 186, 189-92, 199, 206, 221, 226, 230, 242-3, 268
Richard of Wallingford [1292?-1336], 215
Richmond, John Lambert [1785-1855], 469
Richter, August Gottlieb [1742-1812], 341
Ricord, Philippe [1799-1889], 423-4
Riggs, John Mankey [1811-85], 472
Roentgen, Wilhelm Konrad [1845-1922], 441
Roger II [1093-1154], 203-4, 218
Roger of Palermo (Ruggiero) [c. 1210], 226
Roland of Parma [c. 1250], 226
Roman deities of childbirth, 83-4
Rondelet, Guillaume [1507-66], 245
Rondelles, 9
Roux, Emile (experimental syphilis), 429
Royal Society of London, 300, 306-9, 358
Royal Touch. See King's Evil
Rubens, Peter Paul [1577-1640], 319
Rudolphi, Karl Asmund [1771-1832], 387
Ruini, Carlo (anatomy of the horse), 292

INDEX

Rusch, Adolf ("R" printer), 243
Rush, Benjamin [1745-1813], 449-56, 460, 465
Russell, Walter [fl. 1608], 443
Rutherford, Daniel [1749-1819], 355

Sahl al-Tabari [9th century], 151
Saint-Marc Girardin [1801-73], 431
Saint Martin, Alexis (Beaumont's patient), 466-9
Saladin [1138-93], 175-7, 181
Salerno, 219-20, 226, 338, passim
Salicet, William of (Guilelmo Salicetti, Guilelmus Placentinus) [1210-75], 227-8
Sallust (Gaius Sallustius Crispus) [86-34 B.C.], 353
Salutati, Coluccio (Law vs. Medicine, 1399), 224
Sanctorius (Santorio Santorio) [1561-1635], 280, 319
Sarpi, Paolo [1552-1623], 292
Scanaroli, Antonio (tract on syphilis, 1498), 274
Scarburgh, (Scarborough) Sir Charles [1616-94], 287
Schaudinn, Fritz [1871-1906], 426
Scheele, Karl Wilhelm [1742-86], 355
Schellig, Konrad (tract on syphilis, 1496), 274
Schelling, Friedrich Wilhelm Joseph von [1775-1854], 335
Schiff, Moritz [1823-96], 436-7
Schiller, Johann Christoph Friedrich von [1759-1805], 371
Schleiden, Matthias Jacob [1804-81], 399
Schwann, Theodor [1810-82], 399
Scot, Michael [1175-1234?], 203-6, 222
Scot, Reginald (Reynold Scott) [1538?-99], 322
Scribonius Largus [c. 45], 100-1
Seabury, Samuel [-1680], 447
Seignette, Pierre [1660-1719], 312
Sekhetenanch [c. 3533 B.C.], 26
Semmelweis, Ignaz Philipp [1818-65], 421, 478-9
Seneca, Lucius Annaeus [c. 3 B.C.-65 A.D.], 87, 94, 164, 182

Serenus Sammonicus (Samonicus), Quintus [3rd century], 193-4
Sergius of Resaina [-536], 148, 151, 184
Sertürner, Friedrich Wilhelm Adam [1783-1841], 393
Servetus, Michael [1509?-1553], 260-5, 291, 453
Sévigné, Marie de Rabutin-Chantal [1626-96], 314-15, 446
Sewall, Samuel [1652-1730], 323
Sextus Empiricus [fl. 193], 68, 70, 76
Sextus Placitus of Papyra [fl. 370], 194
Sexual impotence
 first description of, 49
 medieval treatment of, 209
Sexual perversion in Rome, 87-90
Shakespeare, William [1564-1616], 281, 292, 319
Sharp, Samuel [1700-78], 343
Shippen, William [1736-1808], 449
Silliman, Benjamin [1779-1864], 471
Simpson, Sir James Young [1811-70], 420-1, 471, 477
Sims, James Marion [1813-83], 479-83
Sincipital-T, 9
Sleeping sponge (*spongia somnifera*), 226
Sloane, Sir Hans [1660-1753], 344
Smallpox, 157-8, 171, 210, 316, 367-70, 447
Smith, Elihu Hubbard [1771-98], 456, 460-2
Smith, Captain John [1579-1631], 443-4
Smith, Nathan [1762-1829], 452, 465
Socrates [469-399 B.C.], 40, 42-6, 59, 70, 82, 218
Solidist pathology, 91-5
Sophocles [495-406 B.C.], 40, 68
Soranus of Ephesus [2nd century], 94, 112-13, 199, 425
Sostratus [c. 250 B.C.], 80
Spallanzani, Lazaro [1729-99], 338-9
Specific gravity, discovery of, 81
Spermatozoa, discovery of, 310
Spinoza, Baruch [1632-77], 305, 319, 328
Stahl, Georg Ernst [1660-1734], 234

Stafford, Ed. (instructions to Winthrop), 445
Stearns, John [1770-1848], 457
Steno (Stenon, Stenonis, Stensen), Nicolaus (Niels) [1638?-86], 302-3, 305
Stephen of Antioch, 201
Stephen of Pisa, 200
Stephens, Joanna [*fl.* 1739], 343-4
Stertinius [1st century], 95
Stethoscope, invention of, 373
Stevens, Eduardus (on digestion), 339
Stokes, William [1804-78], 392
Strato (quoted by Aristotle) [6th or 5th century B. C.], 73
Stukeley, William [1687-1765], 358
Suetonius Tranquillus, Gaius [*fl.* 90-140], 87-8, passim
Surgical anatomy, pioneer treatise, 227
Susruta [6th century B. C.], 37, 140-1
Swammerdam, Jan [1637-80], 304-5, 328
Sweating-sickness, first treatise on, 281
Swieten, Gerard van [1700-72], 327, 330-1, 347
Sydenham, Thomas [1624-89], 312, 315-17, 328
Syllogism of Diodorus Cronus, 70-1
Sylvius (Franciscus de le Boë) [1614-72], 312
Sylvius, Jacobus (Jacques du Bois) [1478-1555], 244, 256-7, 262

Tacitus, Cornelius [*c.* 55-120], 87, 89
Tagliacozzi, Gasparo (Gaspar Taliacotius) [1546-99], 271
Tait, (Robert) Lawson [1845-99], 425
Talbor (Tabor), Sir Robert [1642?-1681], 314-15
Thacher, Thomas [1620-78], 446-7
Thales of Miletus [640-546 B. C.], 37-8, 277
Themison of Laodicea [*c.* 50 B. C.], 93-4
Theocritus [3rd century B. C.], 79, 298
Theodora [-547], 213
Theodoric of Cervia [1205-98], 226-8
Theodorus Priscianus [4th century], 86
Theomnestus [*c.* 480] 149
Theophrastus of Eresos, Lesbos [*c.* 372-287 B. C.], 59-60, 64, 101, 247, 355
Thermometer, 280, 329-30
Thessalus of Tralles, [*fl.* 60], 94-5
Thomas of Cantimpré [1201-70], 218
Thucydides [5th century B. C.], 40, 47-8, 117, 125
Titian (Tiziano Vecellio) [*c.* 1477-1576], 254
Tomitan, Bernard [1506-76], 275
Torre, Marcantonio della [1473-1506], 251
Torrella, Caspare [*fl.* 1497], 274
Torricelli, Evangelista [1608-47], 319
Tragus, Hieronymus [1498-1560], 246-7
Translations, 147-51, 184, 199-205, 220, 240, 243-4
Traube, Moritz [1826-94], 403
Trepanation (trephination), 8-9
Tribunus [6th century], 139
Trotula [11th century], 219, 338
Trousseau, Armand [1801-67], 392
Truss, origin of, 230
Tuberculosis, 17, 50-1, 114, 125-6, 277, 392, 405
Twilight, treatise on (Alhazen), 202

Universal antidote of antiquity, 78-9, 124
Urinary calculi, earliest observations on, 49
Useibia, [1203-69], 191
Uterine inertia, 8

Valsalva, Antonio Maria [1666-1723], 337
Van Dyck, Sir Anthony [1599-1641], 286, 319
Varro, Marcus Terentius [116-27 B. C.], 95-6, 103, 117
Vauquelin, Louis-Nicolas [1763-1829], 393
Velasquez, Diego Rodriquez de Silva y [1599-1660], 319
Velpeau, Alfred-Armand-Louis-Marie [1795-1867], 474, 481-2
Venables, James M. (Long's patient), 471-2

INDEX

Venereal disease, 17, 155-6, 162-3, 213, 228, 230-1, 273-6, 286, 311, 350-2, 364-5, 393, 423-9
Venereal prophylaxis, origin of, 228
Venesection (bloodletting), 8, 50, 67, 116, 341-2, passim
Venus of Laussel, 6
Venus of Willendorf [22,000 B. C.], 6
Vesalius, Andreas (André Vésale) [1514-64], 253-9, 262, 272, 280-2, 302, 319, 328, 336, 374, 435
Vesico-vaginal fistula, 479-83
Vierordt, Karl [1818-84], 388
Vigo, Giovanni de [c. 1460-1519], 266, 271-2, 274
Villemin, Jean-Antoine [1827-92], 392
Vincent of Beauvais [-c. 1264], 183
Virchow, Rudolf (Ludwig Karl) [1821-1902], 330, 388, 408
Virgil (Publius Vergilius Maro) [70-19 B. C.], 97, 117, 241
Vis medicatrix naturae (healing power of nature), 50, 54, 271, 454
Vitruvius (Marcus Vitruvius Pollio), 81
Voit, Carl von [1831-1908], 441
Volta, Alessandro [1745-1827], 350
Voltaire, François Marie Arouet de [1694-1778], 334, 353, 424
Votive offerings, 34-36, passim
Vulpian, Edme-Félix-Alfred [1826-87], 434

Wakley, Thomas [1795-1862], 385
Walafrid Strabo [807-48], 199
Wallace, Alfred Russel [1822-1913], 390
Wallis, John [1616-1703], 319
Warburton, Henry [1784?-1858], 385
Warren, John Collins [1778-1856], 472-4
Wassermann, August von [1866-1925], 427
Water-closet at Knossos, 29
Webster, Noah [1758-1843], 456
Weigert, Carl [1845-1904], 403
Weikard, Melchior Adam [1742-1845], 335-6
Wells, Horace [1815-48], 472-5

Wells, Sir Thomas Spencer [1818-97], 425
Wesley, John [1703-91], 344
Weyer, Johann (Wierus) [1515-88], 322
Wharton, Thomas [1614-73], 303, 317, 435
White, Charles [1728-1813], 477
Whytt, Robert [1714-66], 345
Wieland, Christopher Martin [1733-1813], 371
William of Auvergne, 183, 218
Willis, Thomas [1621-75], 311
Winter, John. *See* Guinterius
Winthrop, John [1588-1649], 444-6
Winthrop, John [1606-76], 446
Wiseman, Richard [1625-86], 317
Witchcraft, 3, 239, 320-6, 330, 445-6
Withering, William [1741-99], 356-7
Wöhler, Friedrich [1800-82], 388-9
Wolff, Caspar Friedrich [1733-94], 333-4
Wollaston, William Hyde [1766-1828], 393
Wolstein, Johann Gottlieb [1738-1820], 341-2, 452
Wood, Anthony à [1632-95], 285-6
Wooton, Thomas [c. 1607], 443
Wotton, Edward [1492-1555], 281
Wren, Sir Christopher [1632-1723], 307-8, 319
Würtz, Felix [1518-75], 246

Xenophanes of Colophon [6th century B. C.], 38

Yellow fever, 449-62, 485
Young, Edward [1683-1765], 345
Yuhanna ibn Masawaih (Musuë, Mesuë Major, Masuya), [777-857], 146-7, 151, 191, 242, 268

Zeno of Elea [6th-5th centuries B. C.], 40
Zenodotus [*fl.* 280 B. C.], 66
Ziemssen, Hugo von [1829-1902], 393
Zoroaster [c. 500 B. C.], 37, 139, 158
Zoser, King [c. 2980-2900 B. C.], 13

INDEX TO SOCIOLOGY CHAPTER

Abbott, Samuel Warren [1837-1904], pioneer hygienist, 519
Accidents as national wastage, 516-18
Addams, Jane [1860-1935], 501-2, 508
Adler, Felix [1851-1933], 489
Ambulance, first municipal, 496-7; ambulance surgeons, first examination for, 497
American fever, 487
American Public Health Association, founding of, 513
Andrews, John Bertram [1880-   ], (battle against phossy jaw), 515
Animals, protection of, 498-99
Antin, Mary (The Promised Land, 1912), 491-2
Ash-heap blossoms into a garden, 503
Audubon, John James [1785-1851], 508
Automobile, 517-18

Bacteriology, American pioneers of, 513-14
Barnett, Samuel Augustus [1844-1913], first warden of Toynbee Hall, 500
Bartram, John [1699-1777], America's first botanist, 486-7
Bath-room, 492-4
Bathtub, 492
Beers, Clifford Whittingham (mental hygiene movement), 515
Bergh, Henry [1811-88], 498-99
Biggs, Hermann Michael [1859-1923], 514
Billings, John Shaw [1838-1913], 518
Brace, Charles Loring [1826-90], 498
Brazil, visitor from, 494
Bridgman, Laura [1829-89], 508-9
Burbank, Luther [1849-1926], 508

Cabot, Richard Clarke [1868-1939], 510-12
Cannon, Ida Maud (hospital social service), 511
Child care, 497-500
Children, protection of, 498-99
Cholera, 514

Code of Hammurabi, 488
Coit, Henry Leber [1854-1917], originator of certified milk, 514-15
Coit, Stanton (founder of first Settlement in America), 501
Colonial bathtubs, 492; homes, 486-7
Comfort-stations, 493

Dalton, Edward Barry [1834-72], 496-7
Dirt, 494-5
Drainage, defective, 493

Eliot, Jared [1685-1763], colonial clergyman-physician, 486

Flagg, Ernest (house planning), 490
Forbes, Gerrit (pioneer report on slums, 1834), 488
Frankel, Lee Kaufer [1867-1931], 507
Franklin, Benjamin [1706-90], 487, 492

Gautier, Theophile [1811-72], 493
Gerry, Elbridge Thomas [1837-1927], 498-500
Gihon, Albert Leary [1833-1901], 515
Girard, Stephen [1750-1831], 492
Gorgas, William Crawford [1854-1920], 495
Griscom, John Haskins [1809-74], report on housing horrors, 488

Hamilton, Alice (industrial toxicology), 515
Health survey, 503
Heart disease, 517
Hospital social service, 510-12
House planning, pioneer of, 490
Howe, Samuel Gridley [1801-76], 497, 508-9
Hygiene, 489, 504, 512-16

Industrial poisons, 515

INDEX

Jacobi, Abraham [1830-1919], 498, 514

Keller, Helen [1880-], 508-9

Letterman, Jonathan [1824-72], 496
Life-table, earliest in America, 518
Long, Crawford Williamson [1815-78], 508
Lowell, Josephine Shaw [1843-1905], 489

Maplewood fever (typhoid), 493
Mary Ellen, case of, 498-99
Medical social service, 510-12
Mental hygiene, 515
Military hygiene, 515
Milk: bacteriology of, 514; certified milk, 515; milk bottle, the first, 515
Moses, Israel [c. 1827-70], military surgeon, 496
Munson, Edward Lyman [1868-], military hygiene, 515

Naval hygiene, 515
Newsboys, first lodging house for, 498
Nurses: Cannon, Ida Maud, 511; Pelton, Garnet Isabel, 511; Richards, Linda, 505; Wald, Lillian D., 489

Pearl, Raymond [1879-1940], 519
Pelton, Garnet Isabel (first nurse in Hospital Social Service), 511
Playgrounds, origin and development of American, 503, 505-6
Plumber, first American, 492
Plumbing, 493
Preventive medicine, 512, 516
Privy, outdoor, 492-3
Prudden, Theophil Mitchell [1849-1924], 513
Psychiatry in social case work, 510
Psychology: displaced by psychiatry in social case work, 510
Public health, 494, 513
Pump-handle era of milk, 514

Reed, Walter [1851-1902], 496, 508
Richards, Linda [1841-1930], America's first trained nurse, 505
Richmond, Mary Ellen [1861-1928], (social case work), 509-510
Rosenau, Milton Joseph [1869-], preventive medicine, 516

Sade, Louis-Donatien-François-Alphonse de [1740-1814], 498
Salmon, Daniel Elmer [1850-1914], 513
Sand pile into playground, 505-6
Scarlet fever, 508
Sedgwick, William Thompson [1855-1921], 513-14
Settlements, social, 500-505
Shattuck, Lemuel [1793-1859], America's first sanitary statesman, 513, 516
Ship fever, 488
Sickness and old age insurance, 500
Silicosis, 515, 517
Slums, 487-92
Smith, Stephen [1823-1922], 489, 513
Smith, Theobald [1859-1934], 513
Social case work, 508-10
Social ethics, 511
Social forces, 520
Social hygiene, 516
Social work, 506-8
Socialization of medicine, 512, 520
Sternberg, George Miller [1838-1915], 513
Stover, Charles Bunstein [1861-1929], champion of parks and playgrounds, 501
Straus, Nathan [1848-1931], apostle of pure milk for the masses, 514
Street-cleaning, 494-5
Strong, William Lafayette [1827-1900], 495
Sullivan, Anne Mansfield [1866-1936], 508-9

Taylor, Graham [1851-1938], 502
Tenement-House, 487-91
Tenement House Law, the first, 489
Thatcher, Hervey D. (the first milk bottle), 515

Toynbee, Arnold [1852-83], 500-1
Typhoid epidemics, 513-14

Vaughan, Victor Clarence [1851-1929], 495
Veiller, Lawrence (housing reform), 490-91
Venereal diseases, 514
Vital statistics, 518-19
Vitamins, bibliography of, 515

Wald, Lillian D. [1867-1940], founder of first Settlement for nurses, 489
Waring, George Edwin [1833-98], sanitary engineer, 495-6
Water, polluted, 513-14
Water-closet, 493, 502

Welch, William Henry [1850-1934], 513
Wheeler, Etta Angell (case of Mary Ellen), 498-99
White, Alfred Tredway [1846-1921], first seaside home for poor children, 489
White Wings, 496
Wigglesworth, Edward [1732-94], father of vital statistics in America, 518
Woods, Robert Archey [1865-1925], social worker, 504
Wounded, transportation of, 496

Yellow fever, 495-6

Zakrzewska, Marie Elisabeth (Doc Zak) [1829-1902], 505-6